Inviting the Spirit of Play to Transform Trauma

Healing for All Ages

Monica C. Blum

Routledge
Taylor & Francis Group

NEW YORK AND LONDON

I0127811

Designed cover image: Getty Images

First published 2026
by Routledge
605 Third Avenue, New York, NY 10158

and by Routledge
4 Park Square, Milton Park, Abingdon, Oxon, OX14 4RN

Routledge is an imprint of the Taylor & Francis Group, an informa business

© 2026 Monica C. Blum

All rights reserved. No part of this book may be reprinted or reproduced or utilised in any form or by any electronic, mechanical, or other means, now known or hereafter invented, including photocopying and recording, or in any information storage or retrieval system, without permission in writing from the publishers.

Trademark notice: Product or corporate names may be trademarks or registered trademarks, and are used only for identification and explanation without intent to infringe.

ISBN: 978-1-032-82933-3 (hbk)
ISBN: 978-1-032-82932-6 (pbk)
ISBN: 978-1-003-50949-3 (ebk)

DOI: 10.4324/9781003509493

Typeset in Times New Roman
by codeMantra

"A wonderful, practical, and creative synthesis of cutting-edge foundations in treating traumatized individuals, this highly readable and practical book offers us a new, important aspect for our work: the use of humor and play in the treatment journey across the lifespan. Using illustrative examples and clear invitations on how to open our clinical presence to enable a more engaging, inspiring, and empowering relational experience for both client and therapist alike, Monica Blum provides us with a treasure trove of compassionate insights, readily applicable tools, and a deep understanding of the interpersonal neurobiology of trauma and its treatment. Bravo for this Bluming buzzing garden of therapeutic delights!"

Daniel J. Siegel, MD, *founder and director of education, Mindsight Institute, and New York Times bestselling author of* Personality and Wholeness in Therapy, IntraConnected, *and* Aware

"Monica Blum has crafted a remarkable integration of modern trauma treatment, weaving together contemporary neuroscience, attachment theory, polyvagal insights, and transformational approaches like AEDP and IFS to illuminate how, in a deeply relational context, play can catalyze deep healing. The book artfully balances cutting-edge science with therapeutic wisdom, offering vivid clinical examples that demonstrate how the transformative power of play, combined with attuned presence, can bypass defenses, activate innate healing capacities, and access and heal trauma's deepest layers. Whether working with children, adults, or the wounded child within, clinicians will find this book to be an invaluable guide to incorporating therapeutic playfulness in trauma-informed practice. Monica Blum's work validates what many therapists have known intuitively— that genuine play can coexist with and amplify profound therapeutic transformation. A must-read for clinicians working with clients of any age."

Diana Fosha, PhD, *AEDP founder and author/editor of* Undoing Aloneness and the Transformation of Suffering into Flourishing: AEDP 2.0

"Monica Blum offers fledgling and experienced trauma (and all) therapists a neuroscientifically grounded and clinically profound, practical, and landmark book on how to playfully transform entrenched human suffering. Thank you, Monica, for gifting the healing community with this inspirational and educational gem."

Stuart Brown, MD, *founder of the National Institute of Play and New York Times bestselling author of* Play: How It Shapes the Brain, Opens the Imagination, and Invigorates the Soul

"Monica Blum's book is a must read for all trauma therapists! Chapters are packed with important research plus clinical examples and suggestions that promote a fun and refreshing approach to deep healing and growth. A playful spirit is essential in therapists and clients alike."

Terry Marks-Tarlow, PhD, *author/editor of* Play and Creativity in Psychotherapy, Clinical Intuition in Psychotherapy, *and* Awakening Clinical Intuition

"With a radically integrative perspective, Monica Blum reveals how engaging playfully can not only transform trauma with clients of all ages into well-being but also open the intuitive therapeutic relationship to exciting, new creative processes for stimulating growth and development through right-hemisphere dynamics."

Sharon Stanley, PhD, *author of* Relational and Body-Centered Practices for Healing Trauma: Lifting the Burdens of the Past

"Read this book! Monica Blum has written a very important and very serious book about the vital place of playfulness in healing traumatized clients. With creative imagination, wisdom, spiritual sensitivity, and skill, she weaves state-of-the-art theory and research with wonderful examples of playfulness (from stomach rumblings in therapy to conversations about duck poop) and strategies for using play to transform therapy and clients' lives."

Kenneth I. Pargament, PhD, *professor emeritus, Bowling Green State University, and author of* Working with Spiritual Strategies in Psychotherapy: From Research to Practice

Inviting the Spirit of Play to Transform Trauma

This unique and accessible book unites leading-edge trauma approaches with the power of playful practice to treat traumatized clients of all ages.

Abundant case examples and exercises show new and established therapists how to relationally engage a playful mindset—not play therapy—to accelerate trauma healing and transformation. This book grows up the wisdom embedded in child-based playfulness and grows down complex, adult-focused trauma theory. Readers will discover how to playfully integrate scientifically supported healing principles of Polyvagal Theory, Interpersonal Neurobiology, Coherence Therapy, Accelerated Experiential Dynamic Psychotherapy, Sensorimotor Psychotherapy, and Internal Family Systems, along with broaden-and-build theory, affective neuroscience, structural dissociation, mindfulness, spirituality, and more.

Most importantly, this book will empower therapists working at the heart of trauma treatment to compassionately hold space for the depth of trauma's painful, isolating effects while embodying play's life-affirming, joyful, and transformational qualities to make trauma healing more fun, creative, engaging, and effective.

Monica C. Blum, PhD, is a clinical psychologist treating trauma in clients of all ages. She provides consultation/supervision and training on how to integrate somatics and playfulness into trauma treatment.

To everyone who has inspired me with their courage and strength to survive, heal, thrive, and play. You make the world a better place and you have made me a better person.

And to Jeff, Jeremy, and Matthew—you are my world.

Contents

Figures

Acknowledgments

This book has been my third child. Fittingly, my husband Jeff was at its conception. After multiple attempts at stuffing my ideas into a short article for a peer-reviewed journal failed, he urged me, "This is not an article, it's a book. Write the book!" And so, the active gestation of this book project began. Thank you, Jeff, for your patience and unfailing support in encouraging me to "write the book" even though it meant I abandoned you for thousands of hours. I am so appreciative of the ways you flexed and wore many hats to help me at every level of this project—conceptual/theoretical, editorial, practical, emotional, and marketing. This baby has brought us closer together even though it kept us apart. Thank you.

Thank you to my sons, Jeremy and Matthew, who lost their otherwise patient and available mother to their new book sibling. Matthew sarcastically captured his jealousy toward his new sibling poignantly, "I'm a book too, you know"—pay attention to me. Meanwhile, Jeremy repeated, "Trauma, trauma, trauma," just to get my attention. Despite you both feeling displaced, I so deeply appreciate your love, encouragement, and pride in my authoring this career-long exploration.

Thank you to my dear and steady-making accountability partners: Lisa Kohn, Sima Bernstein Kern, and Louisa Kathryn Aspden. Throughout my undertaking, you've been my sounding boards, practical publishing advisors, and my dear friends who found ways to help me believe in the importance of what I had to say.

Thank you to Marsha Heiman—my colleague, supervisor, friend, and deeply wise mentor for over 30 years. I realize the full gestational period of this book baby has been through our entire relationship! You have supported my development to embody my best therapist self. You've enriched me with your knowledge. You've supported and encouraged me to express my organic, playful, style and gain comfort in drawing outside of prescribed theoretical lines. I appreciate all the ways you have nurtured this book baby's development. Thank you.

Thank you to Ken Pargament, my graduate program mentor/advisor, who has left an indelible impression on me about the importance of infusing spirituality into therapy and taught me what a mensch truly is. Thank you to Diana Fosha a fellow Barnard alumna, who has created Accelerated Experiential Dynamic Psychotherapy, a deeply relational healing treatment that has enriched my work, and that of countless others. Diana's brilliant deconstruction of what makes change and transformation possible has enlivened my practice and gifted my clients with ways to metabolize hope. Thank you to Dan Siegel, the father of Interpersonal Neurobiology, whose international impact on therapists and parents has taught me how to be a mindful, whole-brain therapist and being. Thank you to Terry Marks-Tarlow whose contributions to play, creativity, and intuition have fueled my pursuit to buttress these messages. Thank you to Sharon Stanley, a fellow transtheoretical trauma therapist, whose integrative work with mind, body, emotions, and spirituality motivated my own. Finally, thank you to Stuart Brown, the father of play science and the founder of the National Institute for Play for your 60+ years documenting and demonstrating the benefits of and need for free and creative play and its ability to spread joy and deep engagement. Your messages have supported and inspired my truth!

Thank you to my dear friends and colleagues Harriet Achtentuch Hessdorf, Jessey Bernstein, Rosa Bianco, Patrick Connelly, Wendy Eisenberg, Ava Hanson, Maureen Hudak, Elena Kazakina, Deirdre Kramer, "Alli" List Hutner, Sandy Shamoon Watson, Toni Teixiera, and my mother-in-law Beverly Savlov who have consistently shared their love, empathy, encouragement, perspective, and faith in me and the worth of this project as I experienced premature labor and extended gestational periods along the way.

Thank you to Alicia Patterson who has consistently and securely held me with deep care, grounded me, and reflected her deep belief in me and my work.

Thank you to Skye Kerr Levy, my developmental editor who held, taught, and guided me with love, devotion, compassion, grace, and profound insight and talent to bring this book baby to full term. I am profoundly grateful for our teamwork in nurturing and developing this book baby into what it is today. Your skills and your presence in my life are invaluable. Thank you.

Thank you to Heather Marie Evans who joined me in the final stages of gestation with your concise-making edits and easing my book project to delivery.

Thank you to Routledge and Anna Moore for supporting this endeavor and seeing the promise held in its many pages.

Thank you to my parents David and Lottie Blum who are watching and supporting me from above. They showed me how it is possible to survive a genocide and love, learn, grow, dance, sing, laugh, and play again.

Finally, thank you to all my clients over the years. Through this book, I hope I have captured your vulnerability and resilience; honored your voices, spirits, and truths; and conveyed your teachings, courageousness, and receptivity to being playful together in the work of healing. I feel blessed to do this work because each of you, in your own way, has been a blessing and inspiration to me. Thank you. And remember to thank yourselves.

Prologue

Embracing Playfulness in Treating Trauma

I wanted to share a little about myself to give you a sense of how this book came to be.

Back in the late 1980s and early 1990s, I was trained in a clinical-community psychology PhD program at Bowling Green State University. I specialized in child/family systems psychotherapy and trauma. My training was eclectic, featuring a smorgasbord of classes and supervision experiences spanning psychodynamic/psychoanalytic-developmental, family and community systems, play, neuropsychological, and behavioral and cognitive approaches. What a mouthful! Thanks to my mentor and committee chair Kenneth Pargament, I learned to integrate spirituality with psychotherapy—an uncommon offering at many graduate programs. I was schooled in designing and implementing prevention, intervention, and postvention programs, too.

Through externships, internships, and my job after graduation in a community mental health center and school-based program, I became steeped in the world of child trauma. I worked with the systems in which my child and adolescent clients were involved, such as families, schools, child protective services, the juvenile justice system, community programs, religious institutions, and the courts. I learned to support my clients as they tried to prosecute, confront, and reconcile with their offenders. Working with the young and innocent victims, who were often further victimized by ineffective and overwhelmed systems, left me vicariously traumatized. I felt like Sisyphus, pushing upward and forward toward healing and repair against oppressive, broken systems destined to recreate ruptures and downward spirals. Treating traumatized clients was heart-wrenching and painful.

It sucked, yet it motivated me. Like other new trauma therapists, my overwhelm with the complexity and difficulty of the work drove my hunger to learn and devour all I could get my hands on and afford. I was all in.

I pursued my own psychotherapy, supervision, and additional trauma training to satisfy my broad style. I learned about: Play Therapy, Psychodrama,

Process-Oriented Psychotherapy, Accelerated Experiential Dynamic Psycho-therapy (AEDP), Sensorimotor Psychotherapy, Eye Movement Desensitization and Reprocessing (EMDR), Internal Family Systems (IFS), Sound-Healing, Somatic, and Spirituality-Based Therapies, IMAGO, Rogerian, and dynamic and different relational approaches. I continued to explore different religious/spiritual practices and weave them into my work. I became certified by the New Jersey Governor's Task Force in the assessment and treatment of child sexual abuse. I attended countless workshops and purchased more books than my shelves could hold about the neurobiology of play and trauma, mindfulness, spirituality, psychotherapy, body-mind therapy, relationality, and attachment.

Once I had my own children, working with victimized little ones grew too emotionally difficult. I developed needed boundaries and shifted into a private practice seeing mainly adolescents and adults—in early, middle, and late adult-hood. But my reputation as a trauma therapist followed me. Colleagues referred the most difficult cases to me: adult survivors of complex, chronic trauma—clients they didn't know how to or want to treat. All the while I worked with these adults, my roots in and passion as a child therapist tugged at me. Being a mother of two young children kept me connected with my playful spirit, which trickled into my professional practice. So, despite having paused my profes-sional work with very young people, I found myself moving back to nonverbal and play modalities with older clients, particularly when treatment seemed to loop or get stuck. These types of interventions helped me connect with the very young, traumatized parts of these grown-up clients.

As necessity is the mother of invention, I created ways to integrate somatic and playful modalities with adult trauma therapies to shift "stuckness" in severely traumatized clients. I developed embodied mirroring (Blum, 2015), an experiential, relational, body-based technique to help very dissociative, vul-nerable, and primitive-presenting adolescent and adult clients move through treatment and relational impasses. An outgrowth of my play orientation with young clients, this technique combined right brain–reliant approaches (including aspects of EMDR, Sensorimotor Psychotherapy, Psychodrama, IFS, and AEDP) with creativity, playfulness, and spontaneity in the therapist-client relationship, transforming the client's traumatized state.

After teaching embodied mirroring in workshops, webinars, and supervision groups, attendees contacted me after using it with their clients. I was deeply moved to hear how embodied mirroring was helping therapists connect with their clients with more meaning, empathy, and compassion. Most importantly, overwhelmed and burnt-out therapists reported feeling reinspired and rejuve-nated in their work with formerly exhausting and hopelessness-inducing clients. This reenergized my conviction to explore and define other ways to bring play-fulness to my work with clients of all ages while staying true to trauma theory.

While the embodied mirroring technique powerfully facilitates movement, it didn't always meet the clinical need at hand. The technique requires time to move into and through a clinical stuck point. Its efficacy rests on the ability to slow down and metaprocess the many rich, relational, intrapersonal, and somatic realizations. So, I flexibly kept exploring different directions and opportunities to help my clients using deep attunement. I remained open to spontaneously, and often unconsciously, injecting playfulness when and with whom it seemed right enough. Also, because my sons were growing into prickly, loud, yet lovable teenagers, I felt comfortable welcoming little children back into my private practice. I found myself bringing more of my play therapist mindset to clients of all ages with varied and extensive trauma histories.

I permitted myself to use dolls, balls, stuffed animals, action figures, dress-up materials, pencils, paper, pillows, blankets, pipe cleaners, or whatever I could find to objectively act out and personify insights or conflicts. My supervisor of over 30 years, Marsha Heiman, herself a child and adult trauma therapist, was fully encouraging. I leaned into my acting and Psychodrama experience to use different voices or literally act out ways clients' internal parts spoke or argued with each other. When I felt confused—lacking words or ways to ground myself or my clients—I leaned into the body's wisdom and movement. I sometimes called upon whatever spiritual or higher power my client believed in—even if it was their beloved pet. For example, we'd appeal to the loving attunement of their God or pet and translate what they might be saying or guiding them and me to do. Other times I'd asked clients for permission to join or watch me take a moment to follow what my body was trying to let me know. Then I'd ask them what their body was saying and use it to guide our movement together.

Experientially and with curiosity, we'd dance, draw, squeeze and mold Play-Doh, play music, sing, scream, and assume yoga asanas, often with my client leading the way with my encouragement. Other times, we'd pull tarot cards, silently follow their imagination, rhythmically move in sync, or even pray together. Just like being with my preverbal clients and my own children, I playfully used sensation and movement in attuned ways, to calm or energize the state we co-experienced. I jumped up with excitement, waved my hands in the air, or did a happy dance to celebrate a client's click of recognition or a moment of change. I mindfully and intentionally suggested clients look into my eyes and breathe with me, slowly, in soothing ways. I injected humor—corny comments, juvenile puns, wit, sarcasm—into sessions with clients of all ages. In nearly every session, my clients and I laughed and shared many smiles filled with recognition and connection. If lucky, we shared a deep belly laugh or cry together with laughter.

Infusing a playful attitude with the intense trauma work I do has been refreshing, invigorating, and fun for me and my clients. Incorporating playfulness in trauma treatment with grown-ups and kids has felt like an antidote to burnout, as well. Most importantly, inviting the spirit of play in trauma work has promoted movement and growth in profound ways I could never have imagined.

Blending a playful mindset with my broad-ranging practice and study of trauma has profoundly affected my work and my personhood. It has intensified my respect for the human spirit of survival. It has highlighted the brilliant, creative, and spontaneous ways we adapt under threat. It has deepened both my humility and respect for my clients' bravery to share their aloneness, hopelessness, and excruciating pain; their willingness to take risks to connect with laughter, joy, and lightness; and their desire to change for the better (Fosha, 2000). As a result, my eagerness and motivation to integrate all I have learned continue to mushroom, as has my passion to be a trauma therapist, trainer, and supervisor/consultant. Inviting the spirit of play to aid the unburdening of my clients' trauma has led me to become a more skilled and compassionate therapist. It has guided me to be a wiser client in my own therapy, unburdening the intergenerational trauma I carry as a daughter of two Holocaust survivors. Finally, it has inspired me to be a better, more self-reflective mother, spouse, friend, and person.

The Promise of This Book and My Wishes for You

This book is unique, the first of its kind to scientifically show you *why* it is important to bring the powers of playfulness to trauma healing <u>and</u> *how* to do so with clients of all ages. While academically rigorous, I have written this book with simpler language than is typical. This is because I want you to understand and feel supported by trauma theory and the powers of playfulness to more readily integrate them into your practice. As you read, you will grow appreciation for how trauma disconnects us from our full sense of Self, truth, and essence, while embodying and engaging the universally shared language and spirit of play reconnects us.

This book is replete with clinical examples and vignettes that illustrate how to practically apply trauma theory in real clinical situations. While I have protected the identity and confidentiality of the incredible people I've worked with, I have done my best to convey a felt sense of their deeply touching voices and profound teachings. You may even want to share relevant portions of this book with your clients if you feel it relates.

This book is respectful of and complementary to all theories and orientations for working with all clients and their parts of mind. By practicing what you learn across the chapters, you will successfully integrate the spirit of play without needing to learn a new therapy or approach that is costly and time-consuming. By promoting a more fun and inviting attuned healing process, you will increase treatment engagement, motivation, and commitment—perhaps for both you and your clients! Playfully practicing what you learn in the following chapters will build your personal and relational creativity, intuition, and trust. As a result, your confidence to experiment with and blend your and your clients' organic, playful styles will grow. You may find yourself integrating your evolving playful spirit with protocolized and manualized treatments and yield better results. Integrating playful practice with theory will support your trauma healing work to become more *real* and *relational*—which I believe makes change and transformation possible, richer, and more meaningful.

Because of the times we live in, deep, experiential, playful connection is humanizing and needed more than ever before. Therapists and clients must cope in tandem with global traumas—the COVID-19 pandemic, wars, food and water insecurity, climate change, economic hardship, and racial, political, religious, and socioeconomic instability and divisiveness. What's more, our coping is further challenged by so many systemic factors including, but not limited to, cellular, neurobiological, intrapsychic, interpersonal, community, institutional, religious, spiritual, or universal levels. It makes sense that an unprecedented number of therapists are feeling vicarious and simultaneous traumatization by and with their clients. Therefore, infusing the positivity of play into trauma treatment offers an antidote to therapists and clients alike, connecting us to our shared humanity and wish to have fun and feel alive.

You may have selected this book because you were intrigued. Or because you wanted to learn about play's important role in healthy development, repairing ruptures, and transforming trauma for people of all ages. Or maybe this book is required reading for the trauma course you are taking. Whatever brought you here, I request you bring curiosity to the pages that follow as we enter together into a deep consideration of trauma and play. I hope you find something that speaks to you, makes you smile, and is transformative in your work. I hope the material in this book touches your heart, satisfies your intellect, inspires your inquisitiveness, and encourages you to try something new and intriguing.

Monica C. Blum

References

Blum, M. C. (2015). Embodied mirroring: A relational, body-to-body technique promoting movement in therapy. *Journal of Psychotherapy Integration, 25*(2), 115–127.
Fosha, D. (2000). *The transforming power of affect: A model for accelerated change.* New York: Basic Books.

A Playful Introduction to Trauma Treatment

Invitations to Embrace a Playful Spirit in Trauma Treatment

Lizzy, Larry, and Quackers

I will always remember the day when two of my clients, 8-year-old Lizzy and her 5-year-old biological brother Larry, came to meet me for a session with their foster mother Chelsea and their big, lumbering pet—a duck named Quackers. Lizzy was a sweet, devoted, and protective older sister. By age 4, she was often left alone for long periods of time to care for 1-year-old Larry when their mom disappeared to drink and get high. Their father had only been in their lives at conception. Lizzy would soothe hungry baby Larry with Coca-Cola and whatever food she could find that he wouldn't choke on. She figured out how to change his soiled diapers. Larry, by contrast, was a true victim of neglect, acting out of self-preservation rather than loyalty or connection. He often was self-absorbed or dissociative, scanning for the next abandonment. Child protective services found Lizzy and Larry neglected and placed them in foster care. They moved multiple times before being placed in the home of two stable foster parents— Bob and Chelsea—where they lived with Quackers, some chickens, a dog, and two cats.

Quackers was one of the biggest ducks I had ever seen. He stood nearly 3½ feet tall and 2 feet wide. He was the first duck I ever welcomed into therapy and was certainly the first to enter the clinic. At the time, I worked in a division of a large community-based mental health center treating sexually abused children from the inner city who were involved with multiple legal and social service agencies. Quackers' presence left the other clients and staff perplexed and intrigued.

After the family checked in with the receptionist, I led them in a procession through a labyrinth of long hallways to my office. I was followed by Chelsea, then Quackers, and finally by Lizzy and Larry. I asked them to supervise Quackers to make sure he stayed on course. Along the way, we got many strange and curious looks from my colleagues, the administrators, and a couple of the chronically

DOI: 10.4324/9781003509493-1

mentally ill clients. Most everyone smiled or smirked. This felt strangely thrilling and defiant to me; I enjoyed pushing the envelope of conventional therapy.

As we continued to wind our way back to my office, the siblings started giggling. Awkwardly, they announced, "Quackers is taking a crap!" Sure enough, Quackers was dropping many little poops down the processional route. The foster mom, Chelsea, was caught off guard and proceeded to mobilize us all to become Quackers' clean-up crew. Quackers was, of course, oblivious to the mess he'd left in his wake. Needless to say, Quackers was not invited back to the community mental health center once the director caught sight (and wind) of Quackers' deposits.

On that day, Quackers provided many symbols and metaphors about the crap these children had gone through, the messes they had to clean up, the loved ones who "crapped" on them through abandonment, and the need to keep waddling through life's unpredictable ups and downs.

The way I, Chelsea-Mom, and Rosena, the janitor who had a soft spot for all the abused child clients that ran through the center's hallways, responded to the Quackers Incident was unexpected to Lizzy and Larry, and very therapeutic. Together we cleaned up the mess, noticing its color, texture, and smell, holding our noses, rolling our eyes, and making jokes. The children's history had taught them that they would get punished physically, sexually, or emotionally if something bad happened—whether they did anything wrong or not. They had consistently been shamed, blamed, and left alone. However, during the Quackers' episode, Lizzy and Larry's confusion changed to relief. As the adults continued to reassure Lizzy and Larry that all was fine, they joined in with belly-laughs. We bonded in many ways around the Quackers event. In fact, I made a point to soothe Quackers, reminding him, "Of course you didn't know you couldn't poop here. There are no signs that say, 'Ducks, please do not plop your poops in the hallway.'" The kids giggled at this. I continued, "And you're just a young duck, you can't read! All of us are here to help you. And even if you *could* read and decided to plop your poops all over, we would still be here to help you." To deal with rejection I said, "As for the clinic director, I know he won't let you visit here again. I feel sad about that. I will miss you. He doesn't know what fun he missed with you today. But I know Lizzy and Larry will keep playing with you and Chelsea-Mom will feed you when you get back home."

Through this playful reframe, Lizzy and Larry were reminded that they weren't alone and even big, unpredictable messes caused by others they cared about could be handled with loving support and laughter. They also learned if they made mistakes, it was safe to tell, and things could be cleaned up as best as possible.

The Quackers' Incident was not the last crappy experience Lizzy and Larry had, nor was it the last time those whom they loved would unfairly and painfully dump on them and run. This was not intentional play therapy, per se. What was therapeutic was how Chelsea, Rosena, and I showed up with spontaneous playfulness in the face of an unpredictable, crappy event. While facing an unexpected event with them, I kept in mind Lizzy and Larry's trauma scripts so I could metaphorically offer new healing themes and meet the invitation to get playful with repairing trauma scripts with them.

Len and Eeyore

Then there was Len, a 52-year-old client who'd suffered a traumatic brain injury at age 38 that nearly killed him. He had lost his ability to work in his coveted, high-ranking, corporate job. Len struggled to maintain his balance when walking or moving, which prevented him from playing freely with his 10-, 7-, and 4-year-old children, or adequately attending to the medical needs of his infant son. He now relied on his wife as the sole breadwinner. He wrestled with feelings of deep inadequacy, an eviscerated former identity, and profound grief. His anger and irritability usually kept profound depression and shame from surfacing. However, when they did, they crushed his energy and spirit.

One day as we sat together in session, I felt drawn to Len's energy drain, lethargy, downward-cast gaze, drooped shoulders, and statements of despair and worthlessness. I asked Len if he would welcome all that he was getting in touch with and just sit with it, with me by his side. He was pensive and curious. After a long minute in silence, he asked, "Do you know Eeyore from *Winnie the Pooh*?"

I replied, "Sure I do."

Len said, "Well, that's me. I feel like Eeyore."

I suggested, "Oh, you are connecting with your Eeyore side. Let him know we both are welcoming him to join us."

With a strange glance at me, he refuted, "You might be welcoming him, but I'm not!"

"Well, he's here whether you welcome him or not," I replied, "so as you've told me: Keep your friends close and your enemies closer."

Len smirked in resistant agreement.

We continued to play with his Eeyore part, intentionally embodying his breathing patterns, movements, and speaking like him, saying things like, "It's all for naught." "The only cloud in the sky is raining, right on me. Somehow, I'm not surprised." When I asked him to see how Eeyore was trying to help him, Len said how strange and right that sounded. He realized that Eeyore was the side of him that held his deeply depressed feelings of loss and grief. He started to grow appreciative of this part.

Then I shared, "What a true buddy Eeyore has been to you; he's protected you from the overwhelm of it all." Len smiled and nodded. He conveyed that he sensed his Eeyore part was saying, "Thanks for noticing me"—another Eeyore catchphrase.

Len told his Eeyore part, "How lucky I am to have my Eeyore." He then turned to me and said, "Who knew that reading *Winnie the Pooh* stories to my kids could be so helpful to *me*?" Len's mood eased and burdened posture lifted. Playing with his Eeyore side had shifted his mood. Len shows us how engaging playfully with the effects of trauma in adults is as fruitful and productive as it is with children.

Receiving Treatment Guidance from All My Clients

These case examples offer great wisdom. The Quackers' Incident illustrates how the most vulnerable, multiply-traumatized children can teach all healing professionals how to embrace a deep, relational, playful spirit to transform aloneness, overwhelm, helplessness, shame, abandonment, and ruptures intrapsychically and with others. Lizzy and Larry's resiliency blossomed more fully not just by providing them safety and stability, seeing and soothing them, and grieving their pain, but through celebrating and luxuriating in the joy and laughter that accompanies states of change, growth, and thriving. Meanwhile, embracing playful creativity with Len and his Eeyore side demonstrated how unique and creative adaptations to trauma emerge at any point in life.

Lizzie, Larry, Quackers, Len, and Eeyore—along with the other children, teens, and adults I've treated for 35 years—inspired me to synthesize how to infuse the spirit of play and a playful mindset to heal and transform trauma with clients of all ages. This book is that synthesis. It reflects how practicing with clients young and old taught me how to become a whole-brain, integrative trauma therapist. To fit clients across the lifespan, especially adults traumatized as children, I looked to "grow up" youth-inspired playfulness—not develop a play therapy technique or treatment—and "grow down" knowledge of adult trauma treatment and theory. I leaned into and embraced the creativity, emotions, and spontaneity of my right brain and my left brain's rich ability to clarify, conceptualize, and organize theory.

This is how I found myself on a decades-long quest to integrate a vast academic literature with playfully spirited practice and experimentation. The literature revealed two consistent themes: right brain–based approaches previously used mainly with children, like creative arts and movement therapies, are being increasingly integrated into formerly left brain–based (e.g., pure talk or cognitive) therapies with adults. And, science–based theories, like neurodevelopment and affective neuroscience, are getting increasingly integrated with right-brain, play-based approaches for children. A paradigm shift was in process. Everything seemed relevant and interrelated, but something was not connecting.

Bridging Child and Adult Trauma Treatment through the Spirit of Play

As I continued to learn and practice, I realized how engaging playfulness, or a playful spirit, was a connector, a bridge, between child and adult practice and between right brain– and left brain–based trauma treatment theories. Playfulness, not play therapy specifically, serves as a unifier and integrator of the trauma field which, until recently, has had relatively separate and distinct paths. My experience also showed me that while playful approaches with children and trauma-informed adult practices were each impactful, synthesizing and integrating the two made trauma treatment so much better and more fun.

I learned how my playfully spirited approach with adults facilitated access to their younger ego states or child parts of mind. This was especially important when working with adult clients traumatized preverbally or in childhood. Playfulness also appealed to the kid in each client, softening their defenses, fostering their spontaneity, creativity, problem-solving, and resiliency. It was so amazing!

Meanwhile, my playful adaptations to adult-focused trauma theories and techniques revealed new avenues for healing my young clients—preverbal ones through teenagers. Making developmentally relevant changes helped them benefit from integrating Polyvagal Theory, Eye Movement Desensitization and Reprocessing, Sensorimotor Psychotherapy, Internal Family Systems, Structural Dissociation of the Personality, Interpersonal Neurobiology, affective neuroscience, and Accelerated Experiential Dynamic Psychotherapy, among other approaches.

Interestingly, the deep change that emerged from engaging a playful attitude often allowed my clients to connect more easily with their spirit, life force, and personal truth. The playfully spirited relational practice was compatible with my clients' (and my own) spirituality; we could even be playful when engaging their beliefs in and support of their higher powers.

Best of all, bridging child play therapy practices with adult trauma treatment approaches, helped me infuse a lighter, more hopeful energy into the often-crippling work of healing trauma. Infusing a playful mindset in my work mitigated the painful effects of vicarious traumatization. Instead of feeling burnt out, I became more motivated in the playful relational work as many clients shifted faster through stuck points.

By integrating child and adult trauma treatment and theories with practice, I realized play and trauma were *perfectly suited* to promote healing and change. They had more in common than I initially appreciated. What emerged was synergistic and became the meat, potatoes, and gravy of this book.

What This Book Offers You, the Trauma Therapist

This book was born from my career-long journey and supports the emerging zeitgeist in trauma treatment. It breaks new ground, innovatively delving into why and how engaging a playful spirit with clients of all ages can be a robust facilitator, even game-changer, to heal and transform trauma. This book will enrich and benefit novice and veteran therapists, aligning with and complementing all theoretical orientations and trauma treatment therapies.

Although filled with rich academic material and evidence-based theory, this book is designed to be playful and accessible. I want you to enjoy learning the substance behind the fun and have fun with the substance. You may want to share sections of this book with clients for psychoeducation to empower their learning about trauma in ways that are light yet relevant, important, and meaningful.

While this book will teach you how play is a universal, wired-in language shared by all people, you will appreciate that its expression and spirit are unique. Playfulness is an expression of personal creativity. I encourage you to learn about your own playful style and find wise ways to experiment and blend it into your practice.

Infusing attuned playfulness in trauma work promotes a refreshing and fun healing process that fosters greater treatment engagement, motivation, and commitment for both you and your clients. Engaging a playful spirit may even accelerate change and deepen relational healing work, allowing transformation. Just like Lizzy and Larry showed us, playfulness will help the "poop" of trauma feel less crappy and will nurture greater intimacy with our clients. Meanwhile, Len reminds us that engaging our playful spirit yields positivity which eases aloneness and despair and connects us to our creativity, curiosity, laughter, joy, deepest humanity, and resiliency.

Ultimately, by reading this book, you will discover and awaken your playful spirit and learn how to engage it in deeply attuned ways with your traumatized clients. Engaging your playful spirit will enable you to:

1. Lean into and capitalize on the right-brain powerhouse of healing trauma;
2. "Grow up" playfulness to effectively and respectfully treat adults;
3. "Grow down" adult trauma treatment knowledge to wisely treat young clients;
4. Complement and enrich your personal theoretical orientation and method of practice;
5. Integrate compatible, resonant, and appropriate spiritual practices; and
6. Infuse light, hope, fun, and laughter when treating trauma with clients of all ages.

How This Book Is Organized

To help you get the most out of this book, I have organized it into five parts. You can read each chapter separately as each can stand alone and offers valuable theoretical and practical clinical material. However, I have written the book in a stepwise and sequential fashion: each part, with its included chapters, forms a building block for the next, all meant to unify trauma treatment and theory with playfully spirited practice.

Part I: Trauma includes two chapters that integrate theory to help therapists understand trauma, its characteristics, and its effects. Chapters dive into the specific definitions and features of trauma, as well as explain how trauma causes dysregulation, disintegration, and disconnection. Cognitive protections, Polyvagal Theory, Affective Neuroscience, Interpersonal Neurobiology, Attachment Theory, Internal Family Systems, and Structural Dissociation of the Personality are discussed. Case examples practically illustrate theory and deepen the reader's appreciation of the survival-driven functions of trauma adaptations.

Part II: Play has two chapters that center around play. They help all therapists whether or not they are trained in child treatment or creative arts/play therapy, familiarize themselves with, and gain comfort integrating a playful mindset and spirit into their practice. The chapters explore different types of play, play's developmentally related, growth-promoting functions, and the continuum of play. Therapists gain knowledge in selecting the type of playfulness best suited to each client and themselves and opportunities for expanding growth through playfulness. Play's therapeutic powers are discussed in the presence of safe, healing relationships.

Part III—How Play Meets Trauma and Trauma Welcomes Play has two chapters that present the theoretical bedrock of why clinicians need to bring playfulness to trauma treatment and healing. It also shows how trauma symptoms present opportunities for playful engagement. The chapters detail how the right hemisphere-based superpowers of play hold relevance to treating traumatized clients across the lifespan by facilitating healing and transformation. Readers are offered a playful framework to work with trauma symptoms and given practical clinical examples.

Part IV—Infusing a Playful Spirit into Trauma Treatment has two chapters that detail practical ways therapists can bring the spirit of play into creating and utilizing the therapy setting and therapy relationship while promoting safety and connection. The chapters present many in-person and online therapy examples and cases. They demonstrate how to playfully engage the five senses and movement and magnify attunement in unique-to-therapy ways that are developmentally sensitive to all parts of the client's mind. The positivity of the therapist's playful spirit in setting and relationship is shown to be a healing catalyst.

Part V—Synthesis and Integration: Playing with the Elements Needed to Promote Change in Trauma Treatment presents five chapters in which the rubber meets the road and playful, clinical practice comes to life with the greatest detail and depth. Each chapter focuses on a different trauma theory and ways of practicing playfully with clients of all ages. Chapters explore how to use: Accelerated Experiential Dynamic Psychotherapy's metaprocessing and engage spiritual practices playfully to deepen, expand, and elevate positive change and promote transformation; Polyvagal Theory and Interpersonal Neurobiology to metaphorically frame and guide affect regulation practices; Coherence Therapy to support trauma memory reconsolidation around challenging multiplicities and dialectics; Sensorimotor Psychotherapy and different somatic approaches to develop healthy boundaries and attachments; and verbal and nonverbal modalities to safely facilitate creating and telling a coherent trauma narrative that promotes resolution.

The concluding chapter offers therapists a realistic sense of when the client's trauma is treated and transformed enough for the time being. It presents clinical examples highlighting how even in cases of ongoing, excruciating trauma, therapists relationally attuned with a playful spirit, impart hope, and promote meaningful and lasting change for our clients and for ourselves.

With the history and vision behind this book and an outlined sense of what awaits, you can now start this playful journey and enjoy the first chapter—an essential exploration into what trauma is and isn't.

Part I

Trauma

Chapter 1

What Is Trauma?

Before we can show up with a playful spirit to treat and transform trauma, we need to know what trauma is. In this chapter, we will define trauma's subjective nature, broadly describe its objective features, and identify its universal impact. We'll gain appreciation for how trauma victims, witnesses, and healers protect themselves from trauma's full impact through the continuum of awareness and mental acrobatics. Finally, we'll consider the ways therapists can learn from and help clients define when something is traumatic and wisely intervene.

What Makes Trauma Traumatic? It's Personal

Trauma is not *what* happens. Trauma is *how* we uniquely and subjectively feel about and appraise what happens.

The coronavirus is a perfect example that illustrates how the same collective experience caused disparate reactions in individuals of all ages. Online learning benefitted some children and harmed others. Some of my clients with learning disabilities or social anxieties blossomed academically for the first time and became more confident and in charge. Others were unable to learn, felt depressed, became socially phobic, and focused on how unwanted and unending the pandemic was. Getting poor grades due to online learning triggered despair and suicidality in one competitive teenager; another teen became motivated and chose to study more and "kick ass." Working remotely enabled some adults to thrive while others became traumatized. Some clients felt more relaxed and savored greater control over their schedule, not getting dressed up for work, or socializing with annoying co-workers. By contrast, others became depleted and consumed by the impossibility of separating work and home life. For many, parenting homebound young children, homeschooling others, and caregiving elderly parents was an impossible balancing act. Some adults recovering from near-death experiences felt blessed and grateful, finding new meaning and purpose in their lives; others became emotionally paralyzed by physical and cognitive losses and risk-averse which limited their exploration and growth.

DOI: 10.4324/9781003509493-3

The pandemic affected relationships and bonding, too. Some infants thrived in their attachments with their primary caregivers who were present round-the-clock. By contrast, some teenagers and young adults who were thwarted from socializing and individuating felt suffocated and helpless to change their situation. Some elderly parents who moved in with their adult children and grandchildren felt more connected and grew a sense of purpose, while others felt guilty, disconnected, and burdensome to their loved ones. These examples highlight that what makes an event or situation traumatic is entirely subjective.

So, what makes trauma traumatic to us? It is the combination of our internal body awareness or *felt sense* (Gendlin, 1981) of what happened (or might happen) and related feelings and personal appraisals. Together, they affect our ability to deal with the experience. Trauma, by definition, is "personally experienced" as "unbearable and intolerable" (van der Kolk, 2014), and a threat to life, integrity, or identity. We each have a unique tolerance for how much discomfort, pain, fear, shame, etc. we can bear. Feeling traumatized means we have left our personal window of affect tolerance (Siegel, 2020) which is influenced by developmental, emotional, and cognitive levels of functioning and life experience. In addition, something traumatic is appraised as "unwilled and unwanted" and evokes a "unitary sense of aloneness" (Fosha, 2009). Something is traumatic when we have a "lived experience" of suffering (Farrell et al., 2022) in which there is "fear without solution" (Duchinsky, 2018; Hesse & Main, 2006).

The Six UNs of Trauma

When we integrate these main points of what makes us *experience* something as traumatic (with ideas from Fosha, 2021; Nickerson, 2021; and Shapiro, 2018, p. 4), we get the six UNs:

1. UNsafe;
2. UNseen;
3. UNconnected (and alone);
4. UNbearable;
5. UNwilled (and unwanted); and
6. UNresolved.

The first three UNs refer to *what we feel*—the personally experienced aspects of the trauma—while the next three refer to *how we personally appraise, describe, and understand* the trauma. Our personal feelings and appraisals of a trauma interact. In addition, there can be psychic equivalency (Fonagy, 1995) in which we mistakenly equate our internal feelings or perceptions and external realities—what is objectively true and real. For example, we may feel trapped in a dark room, but the door is unlocked and we can leave anytime we're ready. Just because we feel UNsafe does not mean we are. Therapists need to acknowledge and unfold our traumatized clients' feelings and cognitions not determine their objective truth. (We will discuss our role in defining trauma with our clients later in this chapter.)

The six UNs are central to what makes an experience traumatic and, as a result, compromises functioning, adapting, relating, growing, flourishing, and resiliency. Each of the six UNs can be experienced and appraised along a range of intensity. Many factors can affect how disturbing something is experienced and appraised, including gender, culture, family history, age, race, and socioeconomic status. Let's now define each of the six UNs.

The Personal Experience of Trauma

The personal experience of trauma refers to how a person *feels* (including bodily and emotionally) UNsafe, UNseen, and UNconnected (and alone) in relation to the triggering event or situation.

UNsafe means we feel danger and/or threat to our life and/or identity. Our autonomic nervous system is in a state of fear ready to fight, flee, freeze, flop/faint (submit/shutdown), or fawn/friend (attach out of desperation). Feeling UNsafe can range in intensity from certain death to fear of some physical or emotional harm. Examples might be the following:

- Inevitable death: *I'm going to die* when my plane's engines fail and I hurtle toward Earth.
- Life threat: *I'm in danger* as the tornado is predicted to touch down in my neighborhood.
- Threat of identity/integrity: *I'm going to lose* my independence and mind as my dementia progresses.
- Fear of harm: *I'm going to break a leg* if I can't stop skiing in time to avoid hitting that tree.

UNseen means we feel invisible, irrelevant, invalidated, and unheard. We feel UNseen when our boundaries are dishonored when others get too close or intrusive—as in sexual abuse—or become too distant or disconnected—as in neglect. When victimization is random, as in a flood, we may feel UNseen by a higher power who failed to protect us. The intensity of feeling UNseen might range from partial to complete disregard of our personhood or basic needs. In ongoing relational trauma, misattunements leave people feeling minimized, unworthy, invalidated, ignored, and irrelevant to varying degrees, which can be devastating over time.

UNconnected (and alone) means we feel relationally alienated and intrapsychically self-alienated and fragmented (Fisher, 2017). With others, UNconnected feelings can range from feeling separate, left out or rejected, to paralyzing isolation, aloneness, and abandonment. Within ourselves, UNconnected feelings can show up as inner confusion and even dissociation, derealization, and depersonalization. Feeling UNconnected is neither willed nor wanted. Related experiences of shame, self-contempt, disgust, hopelessness, helplessness, despair, and despondency may emerge.

The Personal Appraisal of Trauma

The personal appraisal refers to how the triggering event is perceived as UNbearable, UNwilled (and unwanted), and UNresolved.

UNbearable appraisals mean the situation is believed to overwhelm our ability to manage and cope. It dysregulates us, autonomically affecting our mind, body, emotions, and spirit. We may experience a sense of defectiveness and an inability to cope with related pain, chaos, and confusion. The range of what seems unbearable and intolerable is highly person-specific and depends upon personal resiliency, life experience, and age. For example, a special forces soldier will likely have a greater threshold for tolerating torture, isolation, and deprivation compared with an infant.

UNwilled **(and unwanted)** appraisals of events mean we believe we have no control or agency over what happens to us and correspondingly lack choices, free will, and/or the power to change our situation. We do not consent. The range of intensity of perceiving a situation as UNwilled (and unwanted) can vary by context. For example, the sound of explosions is tolerated when we choose to go to see fireworks but not when our village is bombed.

UNresolved appraisals mean we believe we are unable to repair ruptures and cannot soothe or steady ourselves. Perhaps we become preoccupied with the need for closure, completion, or peace. The range of intensity of appraising a situation as UNresolved varies by individual, context, and life experience. For example, if an incestuous perpetrator suicides before trial, one victim may feel closure, while another may feel disturbed that justice was never served.

The six UNs remind us that "trauma isn't just what happens to you; it's actually more about what happens within you—in your mind, brain, and body" (Baldwin & Korn, 2021). The sine qua non of an event or situation being traumatic *always* rests in the victim's subjective experience and appraisal.

What Are the Features of Trauma? It's Objective

While trauma *is* a personally determined experience by the victim, what describes trauma is objectively perceptible.

Here, we will briefly review these characteristics of trauma. Remember: these features can describe any event, traumatic or not. It is the negative, fear-inducing, or life-threatening qualities that distinguish the events or dynamics as traumatic.

Objective Characteristics of Trauma

- *Frequency and duration.* Trauma can occur as a single or repeated incident or chronic situation. Chronic trauma can be complex, involving varied and multiple events or ongoing dynamics. Many cases in this book involve chronic, complex trauma. Traumatic events may be rare, like the 9/11 terrorist attack in New York City or more common, like poverty.
- *Time and timing.* Trauma can be something that has happened, is happening, or is anticipated to happen (e.g., *God won't let me into heaven when I die*) (Farrell et al., 2022). Trauma can occur at any age or developmental level of functioning. In part, unpredictable, untimely, or unexpected occurrences have the potential to be traumatic. When a 4-year-old and 90-year-old die of cancer, the unnatural timing of the early death makes it tragic and more traumatic, even if both suffered.
- *Context.* Trauma can be random and situational, like being in the wrong place at the wrong time, getting hit by a car, or struck by lightning. By contrast, trauma can be intentionally targeted, as in cyberbullying, cult mind control, or intimate partner abuse. Trauma can happen in relationship to oneself, others, the world, or one's spirituality. Respective examples are accidentally sawing off one's fingertip, getting beaten up by one's father, experiencing an earthquake that decimates one's town, and having one's prayers to save their child's life go unanswered.
- *Scope.* Traumas are often characterized as little "t" or big "T" events. Little "t" traumas may overwhelm our coping abilities and cause emotional distress and helplessness yet do not necessarily threaten our life or the integrity of our body or identity. A fender bender, getting sued, or breaking one's leg during the championship game are likely examples of little "t" traumas. Big "T" traumas are extraordinary, significant, and severely distressing events which, whether witnessed or personally experienced, are threatening to life, identity, and/or integrity. Their scope reaches further, and their negative effects go deeper than little "t" traumas. Examples might include a terrorist attack, being sex-trafficked or ritually abused. Both big "T" and little "t" traumas may induce helplessness, powerlessness, and lack of control.
- *Visibility.* Trauma may be visible, invisible, or somewhere in between. An armed robbery at the bank is a visibly obvious trauma. A less-visible or hard-to-see trauma might be sexual abuse where there is no visible physical damage. Another example is a boss making microaggressions—injurious discriminatory comments—about the employee's physical features, culture, race, ethnicity, or religious affiliation. Less-visible perpetrations are often subtle and therefore harder to detect. Also due to shame or fear of repercussions, the perpetrator can deny or gaslight, confusing the trauma victim about the reality of the trauma and questioning its felt-sense impact. Finally, invisible traumas can be the most difficult to detect and define because the

perpetrator and/or the victim may be unaware or in denial of its occurrence. For example, a town's residents may become medically harmed by drinking contaminated water due to old pipes leeching lead into the waterways, yet the township administrators are unaware.

One Universal Feature: Trauma Affects Us All

Trauma is an equal-opportunity experience, blind to age, ability, race, gender, religion, political affiliation, nationality, class, socioeconomics, or social status. No one is immune from trauma's effects as it directly impacts its victims, perpetrators, and indirectly affects its witnesses. Even if we have not personally experienced the trauma, we are impacted by its reverberations.

Large-scale brutality that affects countless layers of people demonstrates this point well. For example, the 9/11 attacks indiscriminately killed people of all socioeconomic means (e.g., janitors and CEOs), caused medical traumas (e.g., cancer) to those who lived and worked in the surrounding neighborhoods, and emotionally devastated the victims' families, friends, professional, and religious communities. People who watched the televised coverage across the world felt terrified, paralyzed, and helpless. Similarly, Russia's 2022 bombings in Ukraine that targeted and killed pregnant women and children in hospitals had global impact. Friends, relatives, and distant witnesses were forced to cope with barbaric deaths and grapple with unspeakable crimes against humanity seen on social media, while personally facing economic hardships like limited availability of wheat and fuel.

Other large-scale traumas, like the Holocaust, Great Depression, World Wars, slavery, colonization, or smaller scale relational traumas, like abuse and neglect, leave enduring legacies (Danieli, 1998) that affect subsequent generations. Research on the intergenerational transmission of trauma shows that trauma experienced by previous generations can lead to affect dysregulation and victimization scripts in offspring and relatives (Coburn et al., 2022; Hays-Grudo & Morris, 2020). Meanwhile, the field of epigenetics has uncovered how trauma's relational, behavioral, and environmental effects impact our resiliency, ability to bond with caregivers, and can change how our bodies read DNA sequences (Feldman et al., 2016).

In addition, all of us can also be traumatized simply by bearing witness to trauma as in vicarious traumatization: our schemas and beliefs, expectations and assumptions about self and others become disrupted with respect to dependency, safety, power, independence, esteem, and intimacy (McCann & Pearlman, 1990). When vicariously traumatized, we may feel overwhelmed and helpless to change things for the better and become frightened to explore our worlds or trust we will be safe anywhere. Early in my career when working exclusively with sexually abused children, I saw abuse everywhere. I felt and became suspicious of all caregivers—even the parents of my children's friends!

While the term "vicarious traumatization" originally (McCann & Pearlman, 1990) referred to ways therapists were affected by treating traumatized clients, we can appreciate that anyone exposed to painful and graphic traumatic material can have this experience. Clients and friends discuss how watching and hearing news about all things tragic harm their mood and outlook. Media coverage of poverty, oppression, sex trafficking, genocide, global warming effects, political divisiveness, structural racism, discrimination, or bigotry can have overwhelming effects on our minds, bodies, emotions, and spirit. Sometimes we can simultaneously experience vicarious and direct traumatization, as happened with first responders (e.g., police, firefighters, Emergency Medical Service workers, mental health and medical personnel) in the pandemic. They faced life and death with many for whom they cared and potential threat to their own health and safety.

Trauma's repercussions are broad-reaching and leave all of us vulnerable. Let's next examine how our awareness of trauma helps us manage its potentially destabilizing effects.

What Protects Us from Trauma's Full Impact?

Despite the inevitability of suffering, most of us would prefer to avoid experiencing and witnessing the disturbing, cruel, and sometimes unspeakable sides of life and human nature. All of us—helping professionals included—instinctively protect our minds, emotions, spirit, and nervous systems by pushing away harsh, threatening, or triggering realities. Frequent or chronic exposure to trauma may rattle us to our core. We may become hardened, numb, pessimistic, hopeless, and even paralyzed as we try to grapple with our spirituality and faith.

The horror of accepting traumatic realities often feels too unbearable and unthinkable, disabling us to act and sometimes even believe in the trauma itself. For example, I remember stories from my mother, a Holocaust survivor, who explained that when she came to America, she was visibly emaciated and shell-shocked. She told American co-workers and neighbors how from ages 12 to 16 she worked for the underground—the Nazi resistance. She said Americans accused her of lying because her stories of repeated escapes, heroism, devastation, family loss, and separation were too extreme and unbearable for them to tolerate or believe. Rather than get physical, financial, or emotional support, my mother described how people shook their heads in disbelief, called her a "liar," and walked away. While my mother felt abandoned and disappointed, people's inaction and distancing were understandable: it was all too horrific for them to process.

Even when we accept the reality that trauma is part of life, we must find ways to keep going, preserve hope, and foster healing through different types of distancing. As we briefly explore the range of ways all of us can distance ourselves from the deleterious effects of trauma, we'll gain compassion and patience for our own and clients' tendencies to make trauma a not-me experience.

The Continuum of Awareness: Full Awareness, Suppression, Denial, Repression, and Dissociation

The more we notice, the more we can sense, feel, think, and know. Practicing mindful awareness allows us to observe nonjudgmentally, with curiosity, while being embodied. However, when it comes to overwhelming trauma-related material, we often lack this type of balanced awareness. Instead, we move along a continuum of awareness that mentally distances and shields us from being overwhelmed by trauma-related behaviors, affects, sensations, and (static) knowledge or (dynamic) thoughts (see Braun, 1988). This continuum ranges from full awareness to suppression, denial, repression, and finally dissociation (Braun, 1988, p. 5). Each form of trauma awareness along this continuum can function adaptively and maladaptively. For example, while driving the school bus, Jardinia wisely suppresses her intolerable shame and avoids flashbacks of her spouse repeatedly kicking her and calling her "a worthless piece of shit." However, Jardinia gets hijacked by the same memories when tucking her son to sleep, causing him to stay awake and comfort her. We hope to ideally balance our awareness of trauma-related material to show up wisely whether as therapist, client, or person-in-the-world. Let's review the continuum of awareness of trauma that protects us from the full force of the pain, intolerability, and aloneness it can evoke.

Full awareness is full connection[1] with all trauma-related behaviors, affects, sensations, thoughts, and knowledge. Full awareness may correspond with mobilizing to rescue or heal trauma victims and undo its harmful effects. Examples might include social media campaigns to help people identify and advocate against racism, misogyny, or religious intolerance. On a smaller scale, stepping in to protect a victim of bullying or robbery reflects some positive effects of full awareness. By contrast, when full awareness isn't modulated, the opposite may occur, leading to burnout or vicarious traumatization and causing us to un/consciously move along the awareness continuum to suppression.

Suppression is the intentional, voluntary, conscious process of pushing away our awareness of unwanted, anxiety-provoking thoughts, memories, emotions, fantasies, desires, etc. Helpful suppression might include behaviors like not watching the news as frequently or removing social media apps that promote bullying, sexual exploitation, and anxiety. Similarly, more exercise, listening to music, spending time in nature, picking up a new hobby, playing more games and sports, or crafting can help distract from and suppress unwanted awareness about trauma. Extreme suppression might include withdrawing socially or using alcohol and substances to temporarily escape and distance from trauma's pain.

Denial, further along the continuum, is an intentional armoring of our awareness that distorts reality to the point that it seems as if a trauma didn't happen. In the 1960s sitcom *Hogan's Heroes,* Nazi Sergeant Schultz humorously

---

1 As Braun (1988) explains, "full" refers to as much awareness as our nervous system allows us to take in at a given moment.

epitomizes denial when learning the POWs whom he guards plan to steal a tank from the Germans. He says, "I see nothing. I was not here. I did not even get up this morning!" People who create false narratives or fake news deny their awareness by blocking out unwanted or feared information that may contradict their beliefs or values and destabilize their sense of security.

Repression and then dissociation are located further along the continuum and reflect the involuntary or unconscious ways we increasingly limit our awareness of trauma. Repression is involuntary suppression and is often associated with "repressed memories" of childhood trauma, whereby adults cannot access awareness of disturbing anxiety, shame, fear, and guilt-inducing memories. By contrast, dissociation induces separations between "mental and experiential contents that would normally be connected" (Howell, 2005, p. 18), causing a person to feel disconnected from their sense of who they are. (We will explore dissociation more fully as an adaptation to trauma in Chapter 2.)

Mental Acrobatics: Disbelieve, Downplay, Disown, and Blame

To help distance ourselves from trauma's impact, we can all engage what I call "mental acrobatics." Related to and co-occurring with the conscious and unconscious continuum of awareness, these mental twists and turns give us an illusory sense of safety, control over, and immunity from the experience of trauma. They help us maintain a positive perception of the world and humankind to continue living life. Ironically, because no one is immune from trauma, false perceptions of safety and control may leave us at more risk of victimization. Let's explore each of these mental acrobatics in turn: disbelieve, downplay, disown association with the trauma, and blame the victim.

Disbelieve

Because trauma can be so disturbingly shocking, we don't want to believe in its truth. Perhaps this is partly why we prefer to believe that privilege, power, wealth, or status (in the community or society) exempts a person from being a victim or victimizer, despite knowing it doesn't. Many express shock and disbelief when talented Hollywood stars, famous athletes, musicians, the ultra-wealthy, or esteemed religious figures harm people or are victimized. Similarly, we may resist believing a seemingly inspiring rags-to-riches story is one of fear, abuse, and exploitation.

In my work with abused children from privileged backgrounds, I have seen bias against bursting fairytale bubbles as well. People don't want to believe that an attractive, smart, and accomplished child living a seemingly positive life with their perfect pillars-of-the-community parents is in reality a victim of incest and physical abuse. In one case, family and friends tried to reconcile the deep and unbelievable incongruities, saying, "It's not possible. No father could do that to his son, especially him. He was married, straight, and an upstanding member of the community."

Downplay

When the shock and incredulity of the trauma wears off, victims, bystanders, and perpetrators may downplay or minimize trauma's impact so they can go on living as if everything is fine.

Particularly when victims downplay the harm and pain caused by trauma, they invalidate and gaslight themselves. It is a form of victim-blaming (discussed later) in which the victim holds themselves responsible for the trauma that befalls them. When doing this, the trauma survivor essentially internally mirrors and perpetrates what has been done to them. Here are examples of how victims downplay each of the six UNs of trauma:

- **UNsafe Downplay**: *The world can't be that unsafe or bad. I'm too sensitive or weak. I need a thicker skin.*
- **UNseen Downplay**: *If I'm the only one feeling/perceiving this, I must be wrong. It's all in my head; I must be going crazy.*
- **UNconnected (and alone) Downplay**: *I'm foolish and naïve to believe others will take care of me; I must be more self-sufficient and have my own back.*
- **UNbearable Downplay**: *It wasn't that bad. Others have it worse than me. Who am I to complain?*
- **UNwilled (and unwanted) Downplay**: *I probably had this coming to me. I deserved it. Who am I to want better?*
- **UNresolved Downplay**: *With time I'll just get over this one. Let bygones be bygones.*

Disown

When we disown our connection to the trauma, we convince ourselves it has nothing to do with us and doesn't need to affect us. Therefore, we don't need to do anything about it; it's a "you problem." This attitude may falsely lull trauma observers into believing they are safe and decrease their responsibility to help victims.

Disowning tendencies may reflect deeply baked-in biases such as racism, culturism, and nationalism. Attributing trauma to the victim's different socio-economics, educational background, type of employment, religious practices, race, or gender identification (among other qualities) is an attempt to distance. It strengthens beliefs like "We're not them (i.e., immigrants, BIPOCs, welfare recipients, Muslims, the uneducated or poor, etc.) or don't live like them so it can't happen to us." Disowning also reinforces a blame-the-victim mindset.

Blame

When we blame the victim, we hold the perpetrated partially or fully accountable for being harmed. As stated earlier, trauma victims can blame themselves too. When we imagine someone had some control over their victimization, we can believe the trauma was preventable. Therefore, if the perpetration was the victim's fault, we can feel less vulnerable in the world. In a trauma like getting pick-pocketed, we imply fault by asking, "Why didn't you keep your wallet in your front pocket where it's harder to access?" "Who would walk down *that* dimly-lit street?" The implication is that we know better how to protect ourselves, so it would not have happened to us.

For example, Joe's 82-year-old father had his identity stolen by sharing private information with a claimed phone company representative. Joe yelled at his father, blaming his age, slight cognitive decline, and hearing loss. He asserted, "Dad, how could you? I'd never be that naïve!" Joe deluded himself that he would never fall prey to the type of scam his father had, which left his father feeling more traumatized, vulnerable, and ineffective. However, four months later, Joe fell victim to identity theft when someone claiming to work for his computer's manufacturer called alerting him to a fatal error they detected in his computer. They requested private data, which Joe shared, causing his credit cards and bank accounts to be hacked. His financial life was turned upside down, which crippled him. Joe had duped himself into believing he was "too young and savvy" to be scammed like his elderly father. Joe apologized to his father and consolingly said, "They got me too, but they got me worse than you!"

Disbelief, downplaying, disowning, and blaming the victim can co-occur. Families and communities collude in disbelieving the truth that a beloved political or spiritual leader was an abuser. The stability of related systems can be deeply disturbed and threatened when someone of high repute and power masks a nightmare of deception, betrayal, and harm. Acceptance of the reality could uproot the group's moral, religious/spiritual, and ethical foundations, power, and cohesiveness. Downplaying the severity and ostracizing the accuser and their family can be the least destabilizing option.

We as healing professionals are responsible for examining our own mental acrobatics to best address those of our clients. We must get support and consultation to develop respectful and attuned approaches to help clients grapple with uncertainty, vulnerability, loss, and grief related to the trauma. Acceptance of trauma and its sequelae can be a challenging process for everyone, including the therapist. Let's explore this more deeply.

What Role Do Therapists Have in Defining the Client's Trauma Experience?

As therapists, our role in defining a client's trauma experience is to create a space where our client can define this truth for themselves. What a client defines as traumatic must be understood and not judged by supportive others, especially therapists. We must hold open curiosity as our clients share how they make meaning of their experiences.

In this section, we will dive into how therapists can connect with, support, and offer deep compassion to our clients as they define their own experiences, regardless of their presenting issues.

Honoring the Client's Developmental, Relational, and Contextual Influences

Trauma therapists benefit from taking a phenomenological approach—getting to see, know, and feel the client's world through their eyes and experience. More specifically, working phenomenologically helps healing professionals honor and consider the client's developmental, relational, and contextual (D-R-C) influences and related scripts/beliefs, affects, emotions, somatic (including sensorimotor), and spiritual components. Using a D-R-C lens with each client—whether trauma victim, perpetrator, or bystander—helps us get to know them and the unique tapestry of factors that inform their full narrative, identity, and trauma story.

The D-R-C lens recognizes that our clients' being, identity, emotions, and behavior are inextricably and reciprocally linked to multiple contexts and relationships in their life (Lerner, 1991), which may or may not be stable and secure. These may include how a person, particularly a growing child, is enveloped by emotional, mental, physical, economic, social, cultural, racial, religious, gender, spiritual, and global influences. When stable and supportive, these factors encourage growth and thriving. But especially for clients with complex and chronic trauma histories, this is not the case. It is very important for us to assess the levels of influence which can encourage or hinder development in additive, synergistic, or opposing ways. We also need to notice how the developmental stage during which traumatic experiences occur affects how a person encodes, remembers, and expresses trauma.

The D-R-C lens reveals how the client's past, present, and future interplay with their history, genetics, biology, environment, and all relationship experiences. For example, developmental influences can occur historically, prior to or around conception, in utero, perinatally, or at any other time in a person's life. Intrapsychic and interpersonal relationships are influenced by the systems and contexts through which people move between, including family, community, peers, educational, religious, medical, political, and other institutions. In turn, these influences interact with identity linked to gender, ethnicity, country, socioeconomics, generational mores, and cognitive, emotional, and physical abilities. Taking into account this non-exhaustive list of interactive D-R-C factors helps therapists more fully see, honor, and be sensitized to each client's unique trauma adaptations.

The D-R-C lens is transtheoretical and compassionate, supporting us to see our clients with fuller complexity and dimensionality. The D-R-C approach reveals the rich, diverse experiences that make each person vulnerable, unique in their survival adaptations, and focused to become their best self. The D-R-C lens offers therapists a wide, nonjudgmental view of how a person develops their full being and ways of relating to self, others, and the world, cognitive and spiritual belief systems, values, and how they sense, feel, emote, and move.

My use of a D-R-C lens has benefitted my work with child incest victims, their perpetrators, and bystander parents. It helped me appreciate how all family members were traumatized. By holding space, compassion, and understanding for the hurt of each person in the system, I could facilitate the family's healing. I learned, as the saying goes, that "hurt people, hurt people" intentionally or completely inadvertently. That's why, for example, one mother with unresolved childhood trauma could not protect her own daughter from abuse by her spouse. Using a D-R-C lens grows our ability to treat all clients with dignity and humanity.

Letting the Client Identify What Is Traumatic

As previously stated, a therapist does not determine what is traumatic: the client does through their subjective experience. Therapists must nonjudgmentally and compassionately support our clients to sit with and honor their personally experienced truth.

I learned this lesson early in my career when working with 10-year-old Michaela. Her older cousin, Hector, then 21, had been grooming her since she was 5 and molesting her since she was 8. Supposedly, he had perpetrated other children he babysat. After Michaela disclosed this to her school counselor, the county prosecutor became involved and heavily leaned on me to get Michaela to divulge the specifics of the sexually abusive behaviors—putting my role in dual conflict between therapist and evaluator. Once I clarified my role, I still held a bias and responsibility to keep Michaela and other children safe from Hector. However, Michaela loved Hector. He was the only adult in her family who paid attention to her. Hector helped her with homework, read her bedtime stories, played games with her, and even made the "best rice and beans ever!" Michaela also loved Hector's special name for her, "Mami Mimi."

Michaela did not experience anything about Hector's behaviors as abusive, violating, or traumatizing. Only when she learned that Hector had nicknamed her younger cousin Minadoras "Mami Mini" did she feel hurt; her specialness was minimized. She felt betrayed. However, Michaela never consciously experienced the inappropriate sexual touch as traumatic. In addition, her parents had grown up in the Dominican Republic where they explained that these touch behaviors were common within families and among close friends and were never prosecuted. They too were unwilling to file charges because, from their perspective, their nephew's behavior was not traumatic or a violation.

However, my questions to Michaela belied my viewing Hector as only a victimizer who exploited her boundaries rather than a loving caregiver. This jeopardized Michaela's trust in me as a supportive, neutral "feelings helper." Once cooperative and talkative, Michaela became reticent and made no eye contact. I left Michaela feeling not seen, heard, or validated. Clearly my values and biases were different than hers and her family's. Also, Michaela continued to function well at school and at home and had no significant emotional disturbance. It was her school counselor, Child Protective Services (CPS), the county prosecutor's office, and me who defined this as traumatic.

Protecting the Client's Safety

Above all else, therapists must act to protect our clients' safety and well-being, particularly when working with minors. In Michaela's case, all involved systems, her family, and I shared the common goal and intention of supporting Michaela's well-being. She remained at-risk of being groomed and perpetrated by others who would exploit her need for attention and love. In therapy, protecting Michaela's safety centered around providing psychoeducation to her and her family about appropriate touch and boundaries. I taught her somatic ways to self-empower. I helped her parents access childcare that would keep Michaela and her siblings safe.

However, when a client's safety—of life, integrity, or identity—is imminently threatened, the clinician, professional, caregiver, or witness is legally bound to protect them even if they deny abuse. In this case, what is deemed traumatic is not determined subjectively—by the jeopardized person's experience—but objectively by outside safety-ensuring people and organizations. When therapists blow the whistle on child abuse, sometimes children are placed in foster care, the police and courts may get involved, parents may be removed from the home or incarcerated, and families may be placed in shelters. When therapists report elder abuse, the elder's life may similarly become upended. Family members, community supports (e.g., religious), and friends may abandon the victims emotionally, physically, financially, etc. Disclosing abuse for the sake of protection may result in a cascade of additional traumas that can be even more unbearable, isolating, and traumatic than the original trauma. Being sensitive to the sequelae of disclosure and the client's D-R-C is essential for anyone involved in understanding and treating trauma.

Helping the Client Permit Themself to Identify an Experience as Traumatic

Clients may wrestle with calling an experience traumatic for many reasons, including (but not limited to) to avoid the six UNs of trauma and making it real. We help clients handle this phobic avoidance by making the acceptance of trauma manageable. We also educate clients about what objectively defines trauma, which allows them to recognize, name, and validate their own experience. Acknowledging trauma's effects makes healing and transformation possible.

Helping clients name an experience as traumatic can be complicated when their family or supportive others deny or downplay the reality and severity of traumatic events. Family members who act as bystanders to abuse are complicit with it. Acknowledging abuse may result in the bystander losing financial, material, and emotional support from the perpetrator. It may also lift dissociative barriers to their own victimization/perpetration history which they are not ready to handle.

I have worked with many families in which one parent had complete financial and physical dependence on the other. In one case, the parents of an upper-middle-class family were respected leaders in their church and on the school board. The mother, actively involved as a volunteer, did not earn money. Her husband and son, along with her nephews, had physically and sexually abused and tortured her three daughters over many years. She turned a blind eye to the abuse even when her daughters screamed and pled for their mother not to leave them in their father's, brother's, or cousins' care. The mother never accepted the terrible reality of her daughters' anguish and abuse because she feared losing the life and security she had. Born into abject poverty and an incest victim herself, the mother complicated her daughters' ability to define their experiences as traumatic.

Helping a client define something as traumatic or bordering on traumatic is especially important when working with victimizers. Victimizers often deny something is traumatic because taking responsibility for their perpetration may be so shameful and humiliating that it can feel annihilating. It can also result in initial or further prosecution and restrict visitation. When victimizers un/consciously weigh the consequences of admitting their violating behaviors, it affects how and whether their victims define their behavior as traumatic.

I witnessed this in my work with fathers who incested their children. "What if" therapy was a method by which I could be respectful of a victimizer's protective barriers while helping them take responsibility for their behaviors' effects on others. The stance involves articulating and holding both sides with the perpetrator. For example, I told one father, "I hear that what Carina said doesn't fit for you. Yet, you love your daughter and you said she seems afraid of you and doesn't want you to come near her. Since we agree your relationship with Carina is important—that you love and want to protect her—would it be okay if we imagined what it might be like for her if you had hurt her?"

We also need to help clients identify how and when they blur boundaries. This can prevent further escalation and violation. A colleague shared a case of a woman who absolutely delighted in motherhood and her 2½-year-old son, Barry. They shared long cuddle times before he went to sleep. They both enjoyed this intimate and relaxing time together, especially when Barry's father was away on business. When mom found herself falling asleep in Barry's toddler bed, she switched to bringing him into hers, so in case she fell asleep she could sleep more restfully. Over the weeks and months, the mother started caressing Barry at cuddle time, including more skin-to-skin contact. She taught Barry to touch her reciprocally in ways that soothed her.

My colleague shared that she felt a chill down her spine listening to these descriptions. What started as innocent and precious shifted into increased boundary violations. However, when my colleague tried to confront and name this concerning dynamic, Barry's mom spoke in absolutely glowing terms about Barry and their closeness, seeing nothing concerning. My colleague tried in vain to protect Barry and her client from the incestuous pattern that was developing, but the mother could not be disabused of her behaviors. My colleague called CPS, even though it caused a termination in her work with Barry's mother.

These examples highlight how important our role as trauma therapists is to clearly identify when a client who is a victim or victimizer denies something is traumatic because it is too ego-dystonic—whether shame-filled, intolerable, or may cause punitive or harsh consequences. A helpful rule of thumb is to prioritize safety. If life threat or danger is present, we need to call it a trauma, even if it causes ruptures in the therapy relationship.

What Isn't Traumatic?

Trauma's pervasiveness has become recognized locally and globally. Trauma has become part of our vernacular; professionals and laypeople name and describe things as "traumatic" and "causing PTSD" in everyday conversation. This probably follows from living with the effects of and media coverage about Covid-19, social injustice, racism, hate crimes, climate change/global warming, poverty, and war. Also, greater openness to talking about feelings and more readily seeking psychological help has added to trauma's recognition.

While concerns about calling everything "traumatic" have been voiced (Bennett, 2022), I believe the naming of so much as traumatic is a zeitgeist, reflecting a cultural and societal awareness of the reality and prevalence of all types of trauma. We can only hope that more resources will be devoted to education, prevention, intervention, and postvention. As therapists, we are on the frontlines of healing. We must remember that all therapists are trauma therapists to some extent, since everyone can and likely will be affected by trauma. Therefore, we need to open our awareness and seek training, education, and supervision to bring competence and skill to treat and heal the vulnerabilities that trauma exposes.

This leads us to the next chapter where we'll gain a more in-depth understanding of how trauma disturbs many facets of our functioning, internally and with others.

References

Baldwin, M. & Korn, D. (2021). *Every moment deserves respect: EMDR the proven trauma therapy with the power to heal.* New York: Workman Publishing.

Bennett, J. (2022, February 4). If everything is 'trauma,' is anything? *The New York Times.* https://www.nytimes.com/2022/02/04/opinion/caleb-love-bombing-gaslighting-trauma.html

Braun, B. D. (1988). The BASK model of dissociation. *Dissociation, 1*(1), 4–23.

Coburn, S., Grayson, A. M., & Sterenfeld, G. Z. (2022). Multigenerational cultural trauma considerations in dance/movement therapy. In R. Dieterich-Hartwell & A. M. Melsom (Eds.), *Dance/movement therapy for trauma survivors: Theoretical, clinical, and cultural perspectives* (pp. 248–269). New York: Routledge.

Danieli, Y. (Ed.) (1998). *International handbook of multigenerational legacies of trauma.* New York: Plenum Press.

Duchinsky, R. (2018). Disorganization, fear and attachment: Working towards clarification. *Infant Mental Health Journal, 39*(1), 17–29.

Farrell, D., Miller, P., & Nickerson, M. (2022, February, 18). *Moral trauma/injury – A philosophical, political, and clinical perspective through the lens of existential phenomenology: One day master class.* [Live Webinar]. EMDR Advanced Training and Distance Learning.

Feldman, R., Monakhov, M., Pratt, M., & Ebstein, R. P. (2016). Oxytocin pathway genes: Evolutionary ancient system impacting on human affiliation, sociality, and psychopathology. *Biological Psychiatry, 79*(3), 174–184. https://doi.org/10.1016/j.biopsych.2015.08.008

Fisher, J. (2017). *Healing the fragmented selves of trauma survivors: Overcoming self-alienation.* New York: Routledge.

Fonagy, P. (1995). Playing with reality: The development of psychic reality and its malfunction in borderline personalities. *International Journal of Psychoanalysis, 76,* 39–44.

Fosha, D. (2009). Emotion and recognition at work: Energy, vitality, pleasure, truth, desire and the emergent phenomenology of transformational experience. In D. Fosha, D. J. Siegel, & M. F. Solomon (Eds.), *The healing power of emotion: Affective neuroscience, development and clinical practice* (pp. 172–203). New York: Norton.

Fosha, D. (Ed.) (2021). *Undoing aloneness & the transformation of suffering into flourishing: AEDP 2.0.* Washington, DC: American Psychological Association.

Gendlin, E. T. (1981). *Focusing.* New York: Bantam Books.

Hays-Grudo, J. & Morris, A. S. (2020). The intergenerational transmission of ACEs and PACEs. In J. Hays-Grudo & A. S. Morris (Eds.), *Adverse and protective childhood experiences: A developmental perspective* (pp. 69–84). Washington, DC: American Psychological Association.

Hesse, E. & Main, M. (2006). Frightened, threatening, and dissociative parental behavior in low-risk samples: Description, discussion, and interpretations. *Development and Psychopathology, 18*(2), 309–343. https://doi.org/10.1017/S0954579406060172

Howell, E. (2005). *The dissociative mind.* New York: Routledge.

Lerner, R. M. (1991). Changing organism-context relations as the basic process of development: A developmental-contextual perspective. *Developmental Psychology, 27,* 27–32.

McCann, I. & Pearlman, L. A. (1990). Vicarious traumatization: A framework for understanding the psychological effects of working with victims. *Journal of Traumatic Stress, 3*(1), 131–149.

Nickerson, M. (2021, November). *Connection and belonging: A core human need and distinct category of NC/PCs.* Presentation at the 26th EMDR International Association Virtual Conference.

Shapiro, F. (2018). *Eye movement desensitization and reprocessing (EMDR) third edition: Basic principles, protocols and procedures.* New York: Guilford.

Siegel, D. J. (2020). *The developing mind: How relationships and the brain interact to shape who we are* (3rd ed.). New York: Guilford.

van der Kolk, B. A. (2014). *The body keeps the score: Brain, mind and body in the healing of trauma.* New York: Penguin.

Chapter 2

The Disturbance of Trauma

Dysregulation, Disintegration, and Disconnection

Since this book is meant to help therapists transform trauma with clients of all ages, we first must understand how trauma affects us at every level. This chapter provides an integrative yet broad theoretical overview of how trauma disturbs its victims to promote their survival. Through different examples, readers will understand how the mechanics of trauma present from a clinical perspective. This chapter lays the groundwork for how (and why!) integrating our playful spirit into trauma treatment will positively impact all our clients.

When trauma threatens us, we act to survive, minimize pain and suffering, and preserve who we are at our core. Our body and mind brilliantly deploy their conscious and unconscious arsenal of protections to prevent the death of our physical and metaphysical/spiritual life force—sometimes called our self-hood, soul, spirit, ultimate essence, truth, authenticity, connection to God, or sense of universal oneness. Throughout this chapter, I will refer to this self-hood as the (capitalized) Self (from Internal Family Systems [IFS] Schwartz & Sweezy, 2020), which is the "seat of consciousness" (Schwartz & Sweezy, 2020, p. 282), an inner experience of our inherent, undamaged, healing essence of our being, our birthright, imbued with spiritual qualities (Schwartz, 2019, 2023). By contrast, when the (uncapitalized) self is mentioned, it will refer to our self-constructed experience of being and relating to the world sometimes called self-identity (Siegel, 2007) or ego-identity (Taylor, 2021).

When trauma threatens us and ruptures our connection to our self identities or Self, a sequence of protective mechanisms or disturbances is triggered. This sequence looks like this (Figure 2.1).

While trauma's disturbances seem bad, they're in fact helpful and brilliant at enabling survival. However, when the trauma has passed and we are safe, the reverberations of being disturbed can linger, causing problems and thus the need for healing work.

Next, we will explore how each of these mechanisms disturbs overall functioning to help us survive trauma. Later, we will engage this knowledge through our playful approach to treat trauma and support meaningful change in our clients.

DOI: 10.4324/9781003509493-4

The Dysregulation of our Autonomic Nervous System

↓

The Disintegration of Brain Function

↓

The Disconnection of Relationship from Others and Self

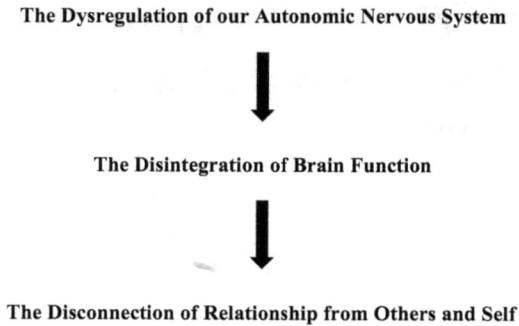

Figure 2.1 The trauma-triggered sequence of protective disturbances.

The Dysregulation of Our Autonomic Nervous System: Survival Protection #1

The autonomic nervous system (ANS) is the first line of defense in response to a traumatic trigger. Our ANS is our surveillance system, working around the clock to detect and register threats to our safety, life, or integrity.

Detecting Threat and Different ANS Pathways

The experience of danger or safety is a neural state; a pattern in the way neurons in our brain activate or fire, connect, and function. Through neuroception—a detection process that functions outside of our conscious awareness—our brains determine whether we are in a state of safety or danger. First, we begin to experience changes in affect, i.e., our basic emotions and mood with related bodily states and arousal that are nonconscious and unconditioned (Panksepp, 2009, pp. 1–2).[1] Next, our mind becomes consciously aware of the threat and our mind tells our nervous system what it already knows (Dana, 2018, p. 35). We call the autonomic state of danger and related experience of overwhelming affect and harm "trauma."

Our ANS constantly searches for and sends cues of safety or danger from our internal (bodily) and external environments to support our two wired-in needs: survival and connection (Dana, 2018, 2020). Co-regulating these two needs is a "biological imperative" (Porges, 2011). The dance of regulating these needs is choreographed by the ANS's slowing-down branch known as the parasympathetic nervous system (PNS) and the speeding-up branch, called the sympathetic nervous system (SNS). The vagus nerve, which runs from the stomach to the brain, is the main part of the PNS and has two branches, called the ventral vagus

---

1 Throughout this book ANS dysregulation assumes affect dysregulation, even if not mentioned explicitly.

> **Autonomic Nervous System (ANS):** surveillance system that neurocepts/unconsciously detects threat/risk
>
> The two branches of the ANS are:
>   **Sympathetic Nervous System (SNS):** Excites, speeds up
>   **Parasympathetic Nervous System (PNS):** Inhibits, slows down
>   The two parts of the vagus nerve contained in the PNS are:
>   • **Ventral Vagal (VV):** social engagement system—allows connection
>   • **Dorsal Vagal (DV):** shut down/faint/collapse, freeze, flop, dissociate

Figure 2.2 Outline of ANS branches, their acronyms, and functions.

(VV) and dorsal vagus (DV). You can use Figure 2.2 to help you remember the ANS branches and their functions.

Climbing up and down the ANS Ladder of Threat to Survival

When threat occurs, Polyvagal Theory (Porges, 2011) details three evolutionary pathways that are organized from most recent to primitive which promote survival: VV, SNS, and DV. All three pathways are active at all times (personal communication with Deb Dana, May 1, 2023), yet one tends to be dominant at any given moment depending on the level of threat to safety neurocepted by the ANS. Figure 2.3 depicts the ANS Ladder of Threat to Survival (based on the Polyvagal Ladder and the Personal Profile Map Template, Dana, 2018 and Elisabeth, 2020) and maps out how our ANS survival response changes depending on the perceived threat.

From Figure 2.3, you can see that when no survival threat exists, we neurocept safety. The VV pathway dominates, enabling social engagement as we are safe and connected. However, in the presence of fear or threat, the SNS excitatory pathway engages our flight/fight survival response. If the SNS is effective, we can mobilize into VV safety. If ineffective, we shift and drop into DV states whose inhibitory pathway enables survival through immobilization, shutdown, and collapse. We disconnect (from others and Self) and protect—and hopefully survive.

Regulating the ANS and the Heart with the Vagal Brake

As our ANS responds to threat, our heart rate gets faster or slower in response to SNS excitation and DV inhibition. Fortunately, our VV pathway keeps our heart rate suppressed (to around 72 beats per minute); without it, our heart would beat dangerously fast (Dana, 2018, p. 28). This function is known as the "vagal brake."

When we feel safe and connected, our vagal brake functions properly and consequently our internal organs are well-regulated, such as our heart and breathing rates, our vascular system, and our reflexes. However, during trauma—when our SNS engages flight/fight or we fall into DV protection and disconnection—our vagal brake does not function in a modulated way. If the SNS pathway takes over,

	Survival Strategy	Autonomic Nervous System (ANS) Branch	Did it Work?
Low	#1: Authentically connect with others	Ventral Vagus (VV)	Yes ➡ Danger over, I survived! No ➡ Go to #2
	#2: Escape, get away, or face the threat	Sympathetic Nervous System (SNS) Flight or Fight	Yes ➡ Danger ends. Return to #1 I survived! No ➡ Go to #3
	#3: Regulatory edge between: Can't flee/fight and submit/comply	Blended Freeze or Tonic Immobility	Yes ➡ Danger lessens/ends. Return to #2 or #1 I survived! No ➡ Go to #4a
	#4a: Hide my true Self or feelings but, if threat increases #4b: Shut down/collapse, disconnect, dissociate	Dorsal Vagus (DV) submit ⬇ DV collapse	Yes ➡ Danger lessens/ends. Return to #3, #2, or #1 I survived! No ➡ Go to #4b Yes ➡ Danger lessens/ends. Return to #4a, #3, #2, or #1 I survived! No ➡ Self disintegration
High			

Figure 2.3 The ANS Ladder of Threat to Survival (based on an adaptation of The Personal Profile Map Template, Dana, 2018, personal communication with Deb Dana on May 1, 2023, and; Elisabeth, 2020).

the brake is fully released and we move into hyperarousal (panic, fighting, or fleeing) as our breathing and heart rate increase. If the DV pathway takes charge, the brake gets slammed down and we move into hypoarousal (depression or dissociation) as our breathing and heart rates drop, causing us to submit and collapse. In short, the unmodulated vagal braking associated with trauma states dysregulates the digestive, pulmonary, cardiovascular systems, and reflexes (e.g., coughing, sneezing, swallowing, and vomiting) to help us get safe or keep us alive.

The Fusing of ANS States

ANS states can work and link together when safe or under threat. Let's see how to better identify this in our clients, which will later guide our playful interventions.

Safety

In the absence of threat, our safe and social VV pathways work together with mobilizing SNS and immobilizing DV pathways. For example, when playing tag, we connect with our friends (VV), while running away (SNS) from them to avoid getting tagged. In a restorative hatha yoga practice, our connection-oriented VV and immobilizing DV pathways engage together to help us rest and digest, relax and restore. We feel connected to our body, mind, and the yoga instructor (VV) while being still and calm (DV) as we breathe into our pose. Another example is having sex in which our socially engaged VV, speeding-up SNS, and slowing-down DV pathways work together in different rhythms.

Threat/Trauma

In a traumatized state, our ANS gets dysregulated, and we can experience "immobilization with fear" (Stanley, 2016). This means our slowing-down (DV) and speeding-up (SNS) responses get fused and confused with VV states (for a fuller understanding, see Stanley, 2016). You can see two examples below.

Ten-year-old Chris's mother repeatedly arrived home from work drunk, yelled at him, and beat him for not cleaning up and doing his homework well. Chris's SNS engaged as he fled to his room for protection and escape. Later, his intoxicated mother comforted Chris, dressing the wounds she inflicted, perhaps motivated by maternal instincts (VV states) or guilt (DV states). She then started cuddling him. Chris's VV engaged as he felt soothed.

As she calmed him with touch, she touched his genitals, which physiologically activated Chris's SNS—he got an erection. Upon this deeply disturbing realization, Chris dissociated and moved into a mental and physical state of collapse—indicating DV activation. Triggered by her DV state of shame, his mother then ran out of his room crying and started another drinking cycle linked with her SNS flight. Chris wanted to soothe his distressed mother but remained frozen by his profound upset at what happened between them. This complicated and confusing interaction caused Chris's ANS to become "immobilized with fear." This happens to many children whose parents both frighten or are frightened by them, or who both comfort and need comforting from their children. By contrast, Chris's mother drank (an SNS flight behavior) herself into a state of collapse (an alcohol-induced state of DV) which prevented her from repairing the relational rupture.

This paralyzing dynamic of fused ANS states also happens in adult relationships, as seen in cycles of intimate partner violence illustrated by the case of partners Mae Lynn and Arielle.

Mae Lynn welcomed Arielle home from another stressful day as CEO of a startup company. Mae Lynn, in her VV state, cooked Arielle's favorite meal, bought soothing bath salts for Arielle to use after dinner, and rented Arielle's favorite movie to watch before bed. However, Arielle blocked Mae Lynn's loving, supportive bids for connection. Arielle's SNS was still revving with frustration following an unsuccessful try at convincing the company's board of directors to grant her more authority (triggering inadequacy and DV states). During dinner, Mae Lynn accidentally spilled some wine she poured for Arielle, who screamed (SNS state) at her, "You idiot! You ruined the finish on this expensive table I bought!" Mae Lynn moved into DV disconnection, avoiding Arielle's eye contact as she sat down and became silent. Arielle then (with continued SNS activation) attacked Mae Lynn's protective mode, slamming her plate on the table, growling, "You think that's a turn-on, you getting all meek and quiet like that? You think I want to have sex with that?" Arielle then left the room and got dressed as if to leave the house—her escalating flight (SNS) behaviors. Wanting to soothe her fears of abandonment and shame (DV states), Mae Lynn mobilized herself (SNS activation) to reach and connect (VV state) with Arielle. This attempt at reconnection reflects Mae Lynn's linked VV, SNS, and DV states.

Arielle, still in a hijacked SNS state, reacted by shouting, "You want me to stay? You want me?" and proceeded to force herself sexually onto Mae Lynn, who disconnected from her body—a DV state. Mae Lynn's activated VV, SNS, and DV pathways got fused, as did Arielle's VV and SNS states. After leaving and cleaning up, Arielle felt shame, a DV state. She returned and asked Mae Lynn to join her to soak in the tub and watch the movie—VV connection linked with DV shame. As they spent time together, Arielle said in soft, loving tones, "You're the best thing in my life, Mae Lynn. I don't know what I would do without you by my side." Mae Lynn's VV state re-engaged as she consciously pushed away the trauma that just happened. Their bonding was toxic, linked with fear and shame.

Arielle and Mae Lynn show us how the biological imperative of connecting to survive overarches the absence of relational safety, whereby their SNS and DV states fused with VV states. Arielle and Mae Lynn each experienced fear without solution (Hesse & Main, 1999) in the painful dilemma to avoid rejection/abandonment and unbearable aloneness. Arielle's expression of rage and hurt (SNS states) caused harm to Mae Lynn, which raised Arielle's shame, guilt, and self-punishment (DV states). She distanced herself from Mae Lynn. Meanwhile, Mae Lynn felt caught between a rock and a hard place to experience relational safety with Arielle, who rapidly and unpredictably cycled through aggressive SNS states and passive/shame-filled DV ones. Mae Lynn's and Arielle's vagal brakes failed in tandem. Their cycles of dysregulated VV connection linked with SNS and DV states.

Tolerating States of Arousal

The more often trauma is experienced or relived in life or in mind (e.g., through flashbacks), the smaller a person's window for tolerating ANS arousal may become. The window of tolerance has an optimal zone of (ANS) affective arousal in which "various intensities of emotional arousal can be processed without disrupting the functioning of the system" (Siegel, 2020, p. 341). Below that zone is hypoarousal and above hyperarousal. This means not all states of hypoarousal or hyperarousal are intolerable and traumatic. We can comfortably experience extreme hyperarousal after winning the lottery by screaming and jumping with excitement. Similarly, we can deal with hypoarousal—like crying with deep sadness—after the sudden death of a kind neighbor.

Intolerable states of hypoarousal and hyperarousal link with fear and threat to life, integrity, or identity. States of immobilization with fear by definition lie outside of the window of tolerance and characterize trauma states. The more often we experience immobilization with fear, the less effective our vagal brake becomes at modulating autonomic and affective ups and downs. Our ability to handle all types of arousal diminishes. As trauma dysregulates our ANS and narrows our window of tolerance, other disturbances follow. Now, we will explore this next level of disturbance, which relates to our brain functioning.

The Disintegration of Our Brain Functioning: Survival Protection #2

The brain working with the ANS is the next line of defense in response to a traumatic trigger. Neurocepted threats also disrupt the way our brain processes trauma-related sensory information in an effort to increase chances of survival. Rather than detail neuroanatomy and trauma's impact on structures and functions (which are nicely detailed by Fisher, 2017 and van der Kolk, 2014), let's take a bird's-eye view and explore trauma's most clinically relevant and visible effects.

Trauma Impairs the Brain's "Going with the Flow" of Sensory Information

Trauma's high arousal states of fear alter how the brain processes and transmits trauma-related sensory information. As the brain prioritizes survival, literal neuroanatomical splits occur which disintegrate brain functioning (Siegel, 2020). The first split occurs in the vertical or up-and-down flow of information (think y-axis) from subcortical to cortical areas, causing disconnection from consciousness (Nani et al., 2019). From the top of the brain downward, trauma causes the prefrontal cortex (in the neocortex) to go offline. Next, it causes the emotional/limbic brain to become dysregulated and blare alarms (of the amygdala) indicating danger. Finally, at the bottom of the brain, the reptilian or survival brain comes to the rescue and takes charge to control autonomic (involuntary and automatic), essential bodily functions like heart rate, blood pressure, breathing, and temperature, which must be prioritized when faced with life threat. The reptilian brain is the only part of the brain evolutionarily equipped to help us survive overwhelming threats and functions from prenatal development onward. In summary, this split in vertical sensory processing prioritizes body survival over emotional regulation or thinking, planning, and organization.

The second trauma-induced split occurs in the horizontal flow of information (think x-axis) across the left and right hemispheres causing disconnection from affect and attention (Nani et al., 2019). In fact, when trauma happens, there is a left-to-right shift in hemispheric functioning (van der Kolk, 2014) because the right brain is both evolutionarily and developmentally better suited than the left to handle trauma. This split results in memories getting stuck in the right hemisphere and not benefitting from the left hemisphere's logic and language/narrative abilities to integrate sensory information. Also, owing to vertical splits, these right brain–encoded trauma memories are prevented from accessing the higher cortical brain centers which could provide mindful awareness for processing. This means our client's trauma memories get stored as unmetabolized, unintegrated, unconscious, symbolic, sensorimotor, and affective fragments, which lack meaning or a narrative. Herein lies the challenge: all therapists must bridge the hemispheric and cortical structural divides induced by trauma.

These splits have other major repercussions after the trauma has passed. Our post-trauma brain shifts toward left hemispheric dominance to cognitively protect ourselves from other internal or external threatening experiences. Our thinking and approach to life become rule-bound, rigid, either/or, formulaic, focused on parts thereby inhibiting the right brain's individualistic, creative, visionary, playful, wholistic thinking (Badenoch, 2017). Additionally, our ability to hold both/and, multiplicity, and handle dialectics becomes limited (Laub & Weiner, 2013).

An added challenge is when the disconnect between the cerebral hemispheres causes intrapsychic fragmentation and dissociation to emerge (Fisher, 2017; Lanius et al., 2014, p. 10). This means the once free-flowing, coordinated, and integrated processing of mental states may become discontinuous, disorganized, and incohesive.

Flow Problems and Different Dimensions of Consciousness

As trauma disrupts the continuous flow of sensory information in the brain, pervasive problems occur in our experience of consciousness, as it relates to awareness and states of mind, thought, body, sensations, emotions, time, and memory (Fosha & Lanius, 2019; Siegel, 2020; van der Kolk et al., 2019). Trauma impairs the functioning of our brain's default mode network (DMN) (Bergmann, 2022), which when resting allows us to daydream and get creatively lost in thought. However, when traumatized, our DMN leaves us feeling stuck in the past with no sense of the future (Fosha & Lanius, 2019), disturbing our ability to be fully integrated, embodied (Siegel, 2012, 2020), and present. As if this weren't enough, these disintegrative effects along the brain's pathways result in extreme experiences that are either dissociated/split off, or intense and full-on.

Let's further examine some of trauma's disintegrative effects on the brain to get a gist of how pervasive and interrelated they are.

Conscious Awareness and States

Trauma affects our consciousness or "awareness of being aware" (Siegel, 2020) in that we have trouble being an observer of our thoughts and sensorimotor and emotional experiences. When our conscious awareness is impaired, we can't mindfully distance ourselves to objectively and curiously observe triggering traumatic material. We can think of this impairment as the difference between watching a violent protest in a movie and feeling like we're in the middle of it. A diminished capacity for conscious awareness places us at greater risk of being flooded by intense affect and sensory material. Also, as we lack the ability to step back and reflect upon our knowledge, we cannot recognize our own experience or self-validate. We may become confused, struggling to discern what feels or is real to us and even mix up past and present.

Consequently, trauma challenges mindful dual awareness—the ability to notice the internal distress associated with trauma and the present safety (Laub & Weiner, 2013). Mindfulness is an empathic capacity of the observing self toward the experiencing self (Siegel, 2007). This means, although paramount for trauma processing and healing, traumatized clients cannot connect with their distress to allow self-validation, empathy, and compassion while distancing from it mindfully and nonjudgmentally.

Trauma's impact can also affect how our brain produces altered states of consciousness like dissociation (Fosha & Lanius, 2019; Frewen et al., 2023). Dimensions of consciousness like time (temporality), thought (narrative), body (embodiment), and emotions (affect) influence the presence of dissociative symptoms like flashbacks, hearing voices, depersonalization and derealization, numbing, and compartmentalization. Consequently, the experience of one's self is disintegrated while access to one's Self is blocked.

Body, Sensations, and Emotions

When trauma dysregulates our ANS, we may feel "hijacked" or "taken over" (Fisher, 2017; Ogden et al., 2006) by our sensations or emotions and become identified with them. Statements like "I am helpless" reflect hijacking, while "I feel helpless" or "a part of me feels helpless" reflects a conscious ability to observe, distance, and disidentify from the feeling.

Trauma can cause boundary problems like bodily and emotional contagion, where people have trouble telling where their body begins and ends (Fosha & Lanius, 2019). Traumatized individuals may overidentify with others' feelings and sensations and have trouble knowing if it's their own experience or the other's. For example, a Caucasian, female client of mine who would read racist Facebook posts attacking Black males, would cry, feel nauseous, stay in bed, and spend hours trying to reason with and "educate" racist commenters. Her trauma history of being physically abused and bullied caused her to overidentify with other persecuted victims. Together we termed this "uber-empathy." Her disproportionate level of empathy, care, and compassion for other victims prevented her from giving the same to herself and from daily functioning.

Trauma also affects how we experience physical sensations originating in the body. For example, trauma-linked sensations may become depersonalized, as when one's hand does not feel connected to oneself or look like one's own. Trauma can also cause sensations to be physiologically experienced with hyperarousal or hypoarousal.

Similarly, trauma can cause emotions to be numbed, split off/compartmentalized, or connected to significant negative affect. Even positive (receptive) affect tolerance is challenged (Fosha, 2021) when we have trauma histories marked by consistent dismissiveness, severe punishment, and shame.

Thoughts

Trauma affects our thoughts, causing "internal chaos" where a person is no longer the sole narrator of their experiences. They may hear voices and develop negative self-attributions (Fosha & Lanius, 2019). Sometimes these voices can be introjects of perpetrators. For example, Lisa, who was molested by a brother whom she loved, revered, and feared, was told by him, "You deserve what you get." Lisa was haunted by this voice for years, even after her brother died. Somehow, she needed to bring his narrative or explanation of her pain to fit with her own story, even though it caused deep suffering. This intrusive voice kept Lisa connected to him, even if ambivalently. Lisa's negative self-belief—*I am no good and deserve to be punished*—emerged as she tried to integrate the chaos of what happened and who she was.

Time and Memory

Trauma alters how the brain processes time, affecting how we *perceive* its passage. More specifically, during traumatic incidents, we most commonly experience things happening in slow motion. During a life-threatening situation, our amygdala (located in the limbic brain region) kicks into high gear, ensuring that all available brain resources attend to and remember the traumatic situation—this includes a secondary memory system, which helps these memories "stick" better (Eagleman, 2009). The brain functions as if it were recording the trauma in slow motion, allowing more information to get stored in an unusually short amount of time (Eagleman, 2009). This helps us better predict, prevent, and cope with another life threat, increasing our future chance of survival.

Trauma affects how memory is encoded, too. Trauma memories are stored implicitly or unconsciously as somatic, affective, and motor snippets or sound-bites, if you will, that signal key elements of the trauma the brain needs to remember for survival. Each person's brain encodes personally salient and relevant sensorimotor and affective features that signaled danger, creating a neural blueprint with "synaptic shadows" of the ways we adapted (van Nuys, 2013, p. 29). For example, in a one-time trauma, like a tire factory explosion, a survivor's brain might encode the loud booming noises, the chemical smells, the intense heat of the ensuing fire, and the sensation of leg muscles pumping in running to escape.

When the trauma is over, flashbacks or memory lapses can occur when the trauma-related neural network gets reactivated, dysregulating our ANS, present orientation, sense of continuity, and focus. The secondary memory system produces emotional, involuntary, recurrent, and intrusive flashback memories, which are experienced like rolling clips or constant loops (Eagelman, 2009). Flashbacks are triggered by sensorimotor and affective fragments, like the unexpected sound of an exploding firecracker triggering fear for a war survivor or the smell of a certain aftershave triggering nausea for an incest survivor.

Flashbacks connect us to "trauma time" (Wesselmann, 2014)—we experience the past trauma as if it is happening *now*. Since the amygdala can't tell time, it continues to ring its alarms despite the threat having passed. Therefore, trauma survivors remain "forever vigilant" (Wesselmann, 2014) or hypervigilant which interferes with their perception of being in the here-and-now.

A current disproportionate over or underreaction may indicate the activation of memory stuck in trauma time. Screaming, "Help and run for your life!" when a balloon pops at a birthday party, reflects an overreaction, while continuing to sit and read a book while the tornado siren sounds is an underreaction. Appropriate or proportionate responses calm us and resolve conflicts, while disproportionate reactions dysregulate us and leave conflicts unresolved.

Flow Problems and Self-Related Information Processing

Trauma-generated vertical splits between the brain's subcortical and higher cortical structures (see Fosha, 2021, and Yeung, 2021, for a more in-depth explanation) impact self-related processing. This is the unique way we each perceive and experience others (and the world) and ourselves by taking in personally relevant and salient information (Fosha, 2021: Fosha & Lanius, 2019). This individual process influences the sense of who we feel and believe ourselves to be, our sense of coherence and integration, and how we show up in life (Panksepp & Northoff, 2009; Siegel, 2020; Siegel & Drulis, 2023). It influences how we experience enjoyable and traumatic events. For example, Beethoven's Symphony No. 9 may bring one person to tears of joy and another to tears of anguish, while fireworks may delight one person and terrify another. Self-related processing accounts for why beauty is in the eye of the beholder and trauma is in the subjective experience of the victim (refer to Chapter 1).

The pervasive and repeated nature of chronic and complex relational trauma interferes with self-related affective-cognitive processes that give rise to our identity, agency, ownership of experience, behavioral coherence (Fosha, 2021, p. 387), values, empathy, clear boundaries, and ultimately our separateness and individuality (Siegel, 2012). Let's examine how this may manifest in our clients.

Personal Narrative

We consciously and unconsciously bring memories together to create our personal narrative that helps us make sense of who we are. Our personal story emerges from our adaptations to past experiences, genetics, epigenetics, toxic exposures (Siegel, 2012), and how our mind fits it all together. However, trauma-induced vertical and horizontal splits interfere with this self-integrative process, as do problems retrieving implicitly stored sensorimotor trauma memory fragments. Gaps in autobiographical memory occur. The "dis-integration" of neural information hinders access to important emotional, somatic, behavioral, and cognitive feedback about past life events critical to guiding future actions (Lamagna & Gleiser, 2007, p. 29), telling a coherent and full life story, and feeling a sense of continuity across time.

Gaps in our personal narrative leave us feeling incomplete, disturbed, yet sometimes curious about what's missing. Numerous clients have shared how, "I don't know why, but I just can't remember the first five years of my life." When asked what that's like, clients often respond, "I don't know. It's confusing… I feel like I'm missing part of who I am." Sometimes when clients are supported to sit with or make space for confusing and disconcerting feelings, affect creeps up. Some clients may surprise themselves by crying, feeling more disturbed, and asking spontaneously, "Do you think I'm blocking something? Do you think I was abused?" It is clinically important to leave open all possibilities for exploration.

Sense of Who We Are

Trauma challenges the emergence or maintenance of our integrated self or self-identity (Siegel, 2007) and our Self (Schwartz, 2019). Our top-down, cortically influenced self is self-constructed, based on our perceptions of continuity and coherence in how we see ourselves in relation to self and others (Siegel, 2007). By contrast, our Self reflects our deepest, intuitive sense of what is right for us, our truth sense, essence, deepest humanity (Schwartz, 2019, 2023).

Over time, survival adaptations may require us to sacrifice and disconnect from an integrated sense of who we are, including our mind, body, emotions, beliefs, morals, values, etc. For example, in relational trauma when others repeatedly fail to recognize what resonates with our personal rightness and truth, we don't feel seen and known for who we are. We become a shell of ourselves and disconnect from what is self-attuned, our felt core sense of truth (Fosha, 2005), authenticity, and "me-ness." This implies the more frequently we experience trauma, a greater discrepancy emerges between our identity of self and our Self. Therapy aims to align the two.

Sense of Who We Are with Others

When trauma disturbs consciousness along the dimensions of thought, body, sensation, emotion, memory, and narrative, the sense of being a coherent, separate self is severely challenged and possibly nonexistent. There is no sense of self others can reflect back (Fosha & Lanius, 2019). This impairs intersubjectivity, the experience of two people aware of self and other, sharing emotional attunement, attention, and intentions (Beebe et al., 2003). As Lanius says, "Without a sense of self there can be no other" (Fosha & Lanius, 2019). Trauma also challenges mentalization, the ability to hold another's mind in our mind or their heart in our heart (Fonagy et al., 2004). The healing relationship practices and grows these abilities.

Sense of Self in Relation to Trauma

Ironically, during traumatic experiences when survival is threatened, the sense of Self functions with agency, responsibility, and problem-solving efficacy to ensure we live. In other words, we are most connected to our Self when its existence is threatened. Trauma survival assumes there is a worthy Self in need of protection. In therapy, we mirror this exquisite irony and help our clients access, mobilize, and update this self-related process without fear or threat.

The Disconnection of Relationship from Others and Self: Survival Protection #3

Relationship disconnection is the final line of defense in response to a traumatic trigger. Relational disturbances occur with others and within oneself—which are called intrarelational, intrapersonal, or intrapsychic. These relational disturbances result from ANS dysregulation and brain disintegrative functioning and serve to protect our physical self, identity, and metaphysical Self from destruction.

While the literature often refers to disconnections—or ruptures in the attachment bond—in the infant-primary caregiver relationship, disconnects can occur to anyone, at any age, who regularly depends on another for comfort, support, care, or survival (Mikulincer & Shaver, 2016). Vulnerable dependents span the age spectrum from infants to the elderly and have caregivers whose skills, knowledge, experience, powers/influence, finances, physical, cognitive, and/ or mental strength/health are needed for comfort or survival. While childhood relational trauma affects the child's ANS, affect, and developing brain, those who experience adult-onset trauma are shaken to their once-solid core, threatening their sense of agency, continuity, physical cohesion, and affect (Boulanger, 2007; Felsen, 2017). Thus, we need to be aware of relational disconnections occurring to clients across the lifespan.

Disconnections—or threats of ruptured connections from those we depend on—require adaptations to enable our survival. Put simply, we cannot survive alone. Let's explore how, in the face of relational trauma, we shift from ruptured connections with caregivers to intrapsychic disconnections from our Self, others, and even the metaphysical (e.g., God or higher powers, spiritual belief systems) to fulfill our biological imperative—survival through connection.

Disconnection from Others: Relational Ruptures—A Threat to Survival

Ruptures in relationships are a daily part of life and not problematic in their own right. However, trauma occurs due to chronic disruptions of connection (Dana, 2020) in which ruptures are not repaired (Tronick & Gianino, 1986): caregivers neither effectively nor contingently soothe their dependent's distress, causing relational insecurity, affect dysregulation, and negative emotional states (Tronick, 1989).

Because dependents of all ages cannot survive alone, ruptures with their caregivers need repair. If caregivers cannot soothe the dependent's distress effectively, more responsibility falls on the dependent who must preserve their attachment to the caregiver to stay alive.

Repairing the Survival Threat through Re-connection and Co-regulation

Both caregivers (e.g., parents, teachers, spouses) and dependents (e.g., infants, children, or adults) are invested in repairing attachment and regulatory ruptures to ensure the dependent's regulatory well-being and survival. Strong connection decreases the chances the dependent will be abandoned and left in distress to meet their needs alone. It makes logical and evolutionary sense that caregivers who share genetics (e.g., birth parents, grandparents, children of ill or aging parents) or whose legacy can be continued (e.g., adoptive parents or spouses) have a strong stake in their dependents' survival. In other words, both caregivers and dependents have skin in the game and a role in helping the dependent be connected and soothed to not just survive but thrive.

The Regulatory Dance of Repair

Repair of relational ruptures occurs through a co-created, co-regulated affective dance which creates reciprocal autonomic flow and rhythm (Dana, 2018, p. 47). To identify the nature and quality of this relational, regulatory dance of repair, we need to ask, "Who is soothing whom?"

An attuned dance fostering security. In this circumstance, the dependent usually initiates the dance by signaling their needs. If the caregiver effectively soothes them, the dance is contingently attuned and coordinated: behavioral, emotional, and physiological synchronies (e.g., heartbeats and hormonal levels) emerge in the dyad (Feldman et al., 2011; Harel et al., 2011) as does positive affect (Tronick, 1989). A caregiving style that promotes interactive repair of regulatory ruptures and helps the dependent be and feel safe, seen, and soothed leads to attachment security (Siegel & Payne-Bryson, 2020). These caregivers effectively self-regulate prior to and while soothing their dependents.

Sometimes contextual factors might impair the expression of a caregiver's secure, relational style. An example could be a widowed parent who must work three jobs to pay for necessities, gives care to their terminally ill father, and has a short fuse due to lack of sleep. Chronic ANS dysregulation leaves them too drained—emotionally, physically, mentally, and even spiritually—to slow down, empathize with, and mentalize their dependent's experience. When in survival mode, securely attuned caregiving patterns may fall by the wayside.

A misattuned dance fostering insecurity. When the dependent's attachment and regulatory needs go unmet through caregiver misattunements, repair is incomplete and negative affect emerges, possibly resulting in more disconnection. Sometimes the caregiver's needs even supersede those of the dependent, and their needs initiate the repair dance. This, too, results in lots of missteps, uncoordinated moves, and unresolved ruptures. In these cases, attachment insecurity develops because the caregiver's style of relating and regulating is preoccupied, dismissive, or disorganized, causing the dependent's adaptations (unconsciously and automatically) to become anxious/ambivalent, avoidant, or disorganized, respectively (for reviews, see Mikulincer & Shaver 2016; Pando-Mars, 2017; and Wallin, 2007).

Caregivers with an insecure relational and behavioral style can pose a threat to their dependent's soothing and survival because repairs fail to meet the dependent's basic needs to feel and be safe, seen, and soothed. The caregiver's intention and attempts to soothe the dependent are often misattuned, co-opted by their own ANS and emotional distress which they insufficiently self-regulate. We might consider regulation as more caregiver than dependent-centric. Let's look at two examples with an infant and elderly woman.

Sydney vigorously rocks 2-month-old Elvie to quiet her because this worked with her older child. Sydney believes it's the right thing to do, yet Elvie prefers to be swaddled tightly and held close. Sydney's behaviors dysregulate Elvie's

ANS. The soothing fits Sydney's needs better than Elvie's. Repeated misattunements of this nature require Elvie to develop defensive adaptations to get contingently attuned care. First, she cries louder (SNS activation) and Elvie rocks
her harder. Eventually fatigued from screaming about her misattuned care, Elvie
moves into collapse (DV activation). Misreading Elvie's state, Sydney believes
she has successfully quieted Elvie. She continues to "do what she knows is best
for Elvie" for years, leaving Elvie feeling and being unseen and unsoothed.

Similarly, 58-year-old Roger tries to quiet his 85-year-old mother, whose
dementia-driven paranoia has her screaming that the Russian KGB is going to
kidnap Roger (whom she believes is 4 years old). For five years, Roger has
struggled with her increasing paranoia and hallucinations. He tries to speak
softly and hold eye-to-eye gaze to settle his mom, as her case manager taught
him. He reaches for his mom's arm, and she screams louder at him, "You mur-
derer!" She takes a swing at his face. This is the third episode in a week. Roger is
weary, yet reflexively protects himself and punches her. He starts yelling at her,
"You're crazy! You're ruining my life!" He collapses into tears, "Where did my
mother go?" His mother cries, too. Both become immobilized with fear, again.

In sum, the caregiver's relational and regulatory style influences whether the
dependent feels positive and safely connected, or negative and disconnected
with the threat unresolved. Let's briefly explore how the dependent adapts to
meet caregiving deficits.

The Insecurely Attached Dependent's Repair Efforts

Over time and in response to their caregivers' attuned and misattuned actions to
reconnect and regulate, dependents organize their behavior (Ainsworth, 1979)
and wire-in a corresponding blueprint of expectations called their internal working model (IWM) (Bowlby, 1969). The IWM helps dependents predict, "How
will my caregiver respond to my emotions and behaviors?" and accordingly
influences the dependent's ability to (1) feel—tolerate affect; (2) deal—handle ruptures; (3) relate—stay connected or related, especially when repairing
ruptures (Fosha, 2000); (4) balance proximity—have healthy boundaries for
closeness/distance; and (5) allow safety to explore/return—be comfortable
and secure with independence and dependence (Bowlby, 1988). Attachment-
oriented therapies focus on these dimensions while earning security to heal relational trauma.

Dependents may develop multiple caregiver-specific IWM's and relational
adaptations. This explains why children become so adept at playing each of their
parents differently. For example, 3-year-old Toni's mother is always fearful.
When around mom, Toni has learned to avoid jumping on the couch because
she gets panicky, screams, "Stop! You'll break your neck!", and remains agitated for a while after Toni has stopped jumping. Meanwhile, when at home
with his easy-going dad, Toni joyously bounces up and down on the couch

while dad watches and sometimes joins him. Over time, Toni, like all children, strings together these situational adaptations and develops a parent-specific style of behaving that promotes the greatest relational calm, connection, and self-protection. Older children, teens, and adults make these relationally-specific adaptations or adjustments, too.

However, when faced with chronic relational insecurity and dysregulation, a dependent's need for connection and protection may be threatened. To ensure their well-being and survival, dependents of all ages must do the best they can (consciously or not) with what they've got to repair ruptures and return to positive affect states (see Tronick, 1989). When caregivers can't effectively meet their needs, the insecurely attached dependents shift from relying on others to relying on themselves for regulation (Tronick, 1989).

Auto-regulation. From birth onward, dependents can auto-regulate or engage their unconscious, self-soothing ability to reduce internal arousal and block out external stimuli (Warner et al., 2020, p. 107). Auto-regulation can include rhythmic movements (like thumb-sucking, rocking, and leg-jiggling) or dissociation (disconnecting from mind, body, emotions, thoughts, sensation, and consciousness). Once soothed enough, the dependent may be less triggering to their caregiver's ANS. As a result, the caregiver's ANS returns to a VV state, allowing them to re-engage with and soothe (connect and protect) their dependent. This brilliant adaptation ensures the dependent is connected enough to survive.

Defensive exclusion. This is where the dependent filters out painful or distressing information about their caregiver's failed past efforts to soothe them, limiting the activation of the attachment system (Bowlby, 1980): they stay at arm's length to not get hurt. Consequently, the insecurely attached dependent doesn't signal their caregiver for needed soothing. This sacrifice leaves the dependent alone, holding unprocessed and dysregulated affects. On the upside, the dependent inadvertently prevents further dysregulation of their caregiver's ANS, enabling the insecure connection to remain intact. An unreliable and ineffective attachment is better than none.

Alienating others. Dependents sense when their caregiver feels or perceives threat by the presence of others (e.g., teachers, friends, neighbors, or members of the religious community) even when caring or helpful. Sometimes the caregiver fears their secrets (e.g., abusiveness, criminal behaviors) will be exposed and/or their inadequacies revealed. Dependents consciously and intuitively collude with keeping secrets and hide their caregivers' shameful behaviors to prevent harm to themselves and their caregiver. They "protect" their caregivers by alienating or pushing away "threatening" others, even if it means giving up their own genuinely healthy and attuned supports. Despite social isolation and withdrawal, dependents maintain the so-called peace in the relationship and preserve it.

Upside-down repair. Unlike healthy and attuned caregivers, deeply misattuned, abusive, and neglectful ones cannot consistently regulate their own ANS distress before soothing their dependents'. In these circumstances, the dependent (as if instinctively) becomes the soother, not the soothed, regulating the caregiver's ANS. In cases where the caregiver inappropriately solicits and takes the care and soothing offered by the dependent for themselves, I rename the caregiver a *care-taker* to more accurately reflect the direction of care—from the dependent to the depended-upon.

At first glance, this seems counterintuitive if not impossible. Yet even the youngest and oldest most vulnerable dependent can soothe their more powerful caregivers. Soothing may take the form of easing unease or bolstering security and confidence in an inadequate-feeling caregiver. It can even present as feeding a narcissistic caregiver's ego. For example, 9-year-old Glyceria swallows her distress about her best friend moving away, to comfort her father as he blame-shifts: "Glyssy, *I* am *truly* suffering. Your mother died. She was the love of my life and did everything. How does that compare to your situation?"

The dependent's upside-down attachment repair adaptations come at great cost to the dependent's physiological and psychic integrity. The dependent sacrifices authentic needs for regulation and connection, often struggling to feel, deal, or stay related, and develops dissociative coping mechanisms. Dependents may create and function from a false self to ensure their survival by staying connected. Appeasement (formerly known as Stockholm syndrome) reflects a more complex form of this survival adaptation as victims identify with their perpetrators and abandon their own identity, beliefs, and lifestyle and even soothe or grow to "love" their victimizers (Bailey et al., 2023).

Dependents also develop intrapsychic disconnections, which result in psychic fragmentation. The next section helps us understand this survival-supportive adaptation.

Disconnection from Our Self: Intrapsychic Ruptures to Promote Survival

Disconnecting from our authentic Self is an evolutionarily-driven, neurobiologically-wired-in adaptation present in each of us at any age and stage of brain development. This survival resource enables us to figure out, purposely or not, tailor-made ways to increase the odds of making it through trauma.

Disconnecting from Self is personally relevant, creative, and unique. It enables us to meet survival needs for connection, protection, and regulation as best as possible in the developmental-relational context in which the harm occurred. This piece of psychoeducation lays the groundwork for clients to embrace their symptoms and defenses—signals from trauma time indicating what needs attention and healing now (covered in Chapter 6). I like to emphasize to clients that adapting by disconnecting from their truth and rightness ironically helped them connect to any resources needed to protect their being, essence, or soul from destruction. Their survival enabled getting future support and healing.

Intrapsychic disconnection is supported by dissociation: a protective intra-psychic process that separates out of our awareness overwhelm (i.e., life threat) and related experiential content (e.g., somatosensory, emotional/affective, mental, energetic/spiritual) enabling us to address required life and developmental tasks (Fisher, 2017, pp. 20–22; Howell, 2005). Dissociation helps traumatic experiences be smaller and manageable through compartmentalizing, detaching, and/or forgetting (Warner et al., 2020, p. 13). This allows the traumatized person to split them off as "not me" which corresponds with intrapsychic fragmentation (Fisher, 2017).

Intrapersonal frameworks that map out how we disconnect to protect through dissociation include the Structural Dissociation Model of the Personality (SD) (van der Hart et al., 2006) and IFS (Schwartz, 2023; Schwartz & Sweezy, 2020). They offer neurobiologically informed and family systems–informed frameworks, respectively. They can be thought of as models of self-relatedness—an internal attachment system that regulates our affects, thoughts, perceptions, and behavior (Lamagna, 2011). These frameworks help us understand how intrapsychic parts serve to protect us from the six UNs of trauma (see Chapter 1) at the cost of disconnecting us from our full integrity and identity. While SD leans into the universality of evolutionary animal defenses, IFS aligns well with family systems and spirituality through the concept of our innate wise essence, or the Self.

Since inviting our playful spirit in treating trauma will include SD and IFS frameworks, a brief review of each with a clinical example follows and some similarities between them are noted.

Structural Dissociation Model of the Personality

The SD model is based on how the brain compartmentalizes overwhelming trauma by means of the neuroanatomical splits discussed earlier. The left-right horizontal split divides the two hemispheres: the left brain houses the "apparently normal part" of the personality (ANP), while the right holds the emotional parts (EPs) or trauma-related parts of the personality (van der Hart et al., 2006). The ANP is present-oriented and "goes on with normal life" (Fisher, 2017) "as if" nothing traumatic has happened—the disturbing material is "not (part of) me." It is phobic of EP trauma-linked, intense negative feelings, sensations, thoughts, and behaviors surfacing (Fisher, 2017, p. 68). However, trauma triggers are unavoidable and will activate the animal defense–based EP protectors of fight, flight, freeze/fear, submit/shame, and attach/cry for help (van der Hart et al., 2006). Consequently, the dissociatively split system is challenged with autonomic and behavioral disturbances as trauma-linked material moves into awareness. Chronic and complex trauma creates more dissociative splitting and the formation of subpersonalities with more ANPs and EPs (for more detail, see van der Hart et al., 2006).

For example, despite a childhood filled with abuse and neglect, Waylon, a 39-year-old advertising executive, led a fairly predictable and productive life. He lived alone, volunteered at a local soup kitchen, and was a community organizer for the local arts council—his ANP in action. A few times in the past year, Waylon found suspicious charges on his credit card and new kitchen utensils and items of clothing he didn't remember purchasing. He wasn't a drinker but found bottles of bourbon in the back of his closet. He also found numerous text messages from what he thought were random numbers, thanking him for "the wild night" and being "a great lay." Waylon became increasingly disturbed by these addictive (flight EP) behaviors, of which he had no recollection. The texts came from men and women; he believed he was unquestionably gay.

As more holes broke through his dissociative protective barriers, Waylon became anxious, paranoid, and felt he was going crazy (freeze/fear EP). As Waylon's ANP could no longer keep out these disturbing feelings and thoughts, his work performance declined and became erratic. His volunteerism ceased. He became withdrawn (submit/shame part EP). He was forced to confront that he was not who he thought himself to be and entered therapy.

Internal Family Systems

IFS Theory (Schwartz, 2023; Schwartz & Sweezy, 2020) explains that every human is born with a mind that is a dynamic system, with a mind and subminds—or parts of mind—that function like an internal family, so to speak. This framework embraces the healthy multiplicity of mind which consists of Self and protector parts known as *exiles, managers,* and *firefighters.*

Self is sheltered from destruction by various protectors (van der Kolk, 2014, p. 285). Self wisely and nonjudgmentally accepts and is equipped to lead all parts of mind and provides an internal healing environment. The Self has transpersonal unitive qualities (Fosha, 2021), the collective consciousness of humanity and the universe (Taylor, 2021), connecting us with our spirituality, soul, life force, and spirit of our being. When we are embodied in Self, all protector parts of mind are calm, aligned, and working cooperatively to support resilience, thriving, and even transcendence.

Exiles are protector parts stuck in trauma time holding unbearable trauma-related thoughts, feelings, urges, actions, sensations, and beliefs. Exiles get locked away (in the unconscious) with their burdensome trauma-laden material to best support present ANS regulation and brain integrative functioning. Nonetheless, they try desperately to get care and attention to be unburdened and updated (brought to the present). They are like dissociated EPs in SD.

The managers and firefighters work in different ways to protect the vulnerable exiles. Managers suppress exiled feelings, while firefighters distract from them (Schwartz & Sweezy, 2020, p. 151). Managers and firefighters work in polarized ways to keep the internal system regulated—the exiles quiet—to support survival. Managers work preemptively and proactively, functioning akin to the ANP in SD helping us go on with life's demands. Meanwhile, firefighters work reactively without regard for the consequences, functioning like hijacking EPs in SD. All IFS protectors seek to be witnessed, appreciated, and accepted for their efforts, and unburdened to allow the Self to wisely take charge and have us be who we always were meant to be.

For example, 25-year-old Savannah lived through a childhood of cult abuse and brainwashing in her church community. At age 16, she successfully ran away and found safety and anonymity in a homeless shelter for domestic violence. Her exiles sequestered her profound pain and vulnerability as Savannah's manager parts helped her develop a new life. She gave herself a new name, made up stories about being orphaned in a fire, got support to complete a GED, and earned a scholarship to an Ivy League college.

However, one day Savannah's marine biology professor started blurring boundaries with "my most capable student" and made sexual advances toward her. Savannah's exiles bubbled up. To distract Savannah from the emotional pain, her firefighter parts compelled her to start cutting her arms and legs. Since Savannah needed this course for her major and intended career as a marine biologist, her managers kept distracting her from the seriousness of the violations, reminding her she needed to focus on her future, the big picture, and that no one would believe her if she reported her professor. As the boundary blurring continued, Savannah noticed the professor giving her the highest grades in her section on her projects. She was unsure if this was her reward for silent compliance—a dynamic she had experienced in the cult. Owing to her managers and firefighters, Savannah found herself dissociating during each "office meeting" with the professor. Afterward, to prevent her exiles from breaking through, her firefighters engaged in ritualized cutting and pot smoking.

Both the SD and IFS frameworks help therapists and clients map and track intrapsychic adaptations and reveal clues and pathways toward deeper resolution.

The Interplay of Our Survival Protection Systems

The three survival protective systems reviewed interact according to the level of threat to life detected by our ANS. When survival threat is absent or low, our VV social engagement system predominates, brain functioning is integrative, and sensory information flows. We safely connect with others and our Self. There is intrarelational cooperation and coordination between the regulated protector parts of mind—whether ANP and EPs, or Self and exiles, managers, firefighters—to resolve any slight conflicts or ruptures. We are authentically embodied in Self and thrive.

As danger emerges—as in a relational misattunement or a fire that starts in our building—we mobilize into SNS states to fight or flee from the danger. During this ANS hyperarousal, splits in brain functioning and challenges to sensory information flow occur. We distance ourselves from others engaging protector parts like fight and flight EPs and managers to work harder to mitigate harm. We also move away from embodying our truth and acting from Self. Successfully ending the threat enables us to return to safety and connection as we have survived.

If the threat continues, we toggle between SNS and DV states of hyperarousal and hypoarousal. The brain continues to function with its divide-and-conquer strategy to promote survival. We increasingly disconnect from others as we grow more fearful about how to resolve the danger and interpersonal and intrapersonal conflicts. The fear/freeze EP protector activates endangering the ANP's functioning. Similarly, the distressed attach EP may desperately cling for help, or the submit/shame EP may take charge, hijacking the ANP. Trust in the Self's wisdom and leadership lessens, and firefighters threaten to shut down exiles that threaten to take over.

If life threat is inescapable—as in severe forms relational abuse or a tsunami— DV states of disconnect and protect engage as we move into immobilization with fear and eventually collapse. As a last resort to stay alive in this state of hypoarousal, our brain fully directs its energies into structures that support survival. We disconnect from others (especially if they pose the threat to life) and ANPs get hijacked by the submit (or collapse) EP. As exiles also fall into collapse, the resources of Self are inaccessible and disembodied.

And yet, the Self remains undamaged awaiting discovery through the healing relationship. Trauma therapists with clients of all ages aim to identify, seize, and transform the adaptive qualities of the three levels of trauma-induced disturbances in the ANS, brain, and relationship with others and Self.

Disturbances Preserve the Light within and Lead the Way Forward

This chapter has shown us how the disturbances caused by trauma seem troublesome at the surface, yet ironically are brilliant, evolutionarily-driven, all-encompassing survival adaptations. Dysregulated ANS and related affect, disintegrative brain functioning, and relational and intrapsychic disconnections work independently yet together to shroud our physical self and identity, plus our metaphysical Self in multiple layers of protective defenses. The trauma survivor's true Self, while inaccessible, remains static and intact, before, during, and after trauma, allowing their internal, eternal light to continue shining, even if only as a dim flicker. Herein lies the promise of trauma healing and transformation: in the safely connected healing relationship, we seek to access the innate life force housed in the Self of traumatized clients to transform the darkness, pain, hopelessness, and isolation of trauma into light, relief, hope, and connection.

The irony of finding adaptive value in trauma's disturbances leads our way forward to promoting deep, positive healing and change. Following this line of thinking, can we find something else that is incongruous and paradoxical to trauma that promotes healing? You got it, play—as an action, attitude, spirit, and mindset.

What we have learned in Part I will serve as the bedrock to understanding how engaging the spirit of play with our traumatized clients of all ages has the power to facilitate healing trauma's six UNs and disturbances—while making the process more fun, efficient, safe, and relational. As we move to Part II, we'll see how our playful mindset even supports transformational experiences. Part II explores what play is, the forms play takes across development, how it can be used in therapy across the age spectrum, and play's general powers.

References

Ainsworth, M. S. (1979). Infant-mother attachment. *American Psychologist, 34*(10), 932–937.

Badenoch, B. (2017). *The heart of trauma: Healing the embodied brain in the context of relationships.* New York: Norton.

Bailey, R., Dugard, J., Smith, S. F., & Porges, S. W. (2023). Appeasement: Replacing Stockholm syndrome as a definition of a survival strategy. *European Journal of Psychotraumatology, 14*(1). https://doi.org/10.1080/20008066.2022.2161038

Beebe, B., Rustin, J., Sorter, D., & Knoblauch, S. (2003). An expanded view of intersubjectivity in infancy and its application to psychoanalysis. *Psychoanalytic Dialogues, 13*(6), 805–841. https://doi.org/10.1080/10481881309348769

Bergmann, U. (2022, November 11). *Recent neural findings and why they matter: Featuring the hidden potential of the body scan practitioners.* [Live Webinar]. EMDR Advanced Training and Distance Learning. Beacon Live.

Boulanger, G. (2007). *Wounded by reality: Understanding and treating adult onset trauma.* New York: Psychology Press.

Bowlby, J. (1969). *Attachment and loss: Attachment* (Vol. 1). New York: Basic Books.

Bowlby, J. (1980). *Attachment and loss: Loss, sadness and depression* (Vol. 3). New York: Basic Books.

Bowlby, J. (1988). *A secure base: Parent-child attachment and healthy human development.* New York: Basic Books.

Dana, D. (2018). *The polyvagal theory in therapy: Engaging the rhythm of regulation.* New York: Norton.

Dana, D. (2020). *Polyvagal exercises for safety and connection: 50 client-centered practices.* New York: Norton.

Eagleman, D. M. (2009, June 23). *Brain time.* Edge.org. https://www.edge.org/conversation/brain-time

Elisabeth, J. (2020, March 5). Neuroception and the 3 Part Brain. Trauma Geek Blog. *Medium.* https://medium.com/age-of-awareness/neuroception-and-the-3-part-brain-b38f482c34b0

Feldman, R., Magori-Cohen, R., Galili, G., Singer, M., & Louzoun, Y. (2011). Mother and infant coordinate heart rhythms through episodes of interaction synchrony. *Infant Behavior & Development, 34*(4), 569–577. https://doi.org/10.1016/j.infbeh.2011.06.008

Felsen, I. (2017). Adult-onset trauma and intergenerational transmission: Integrating empirical data and psychoanalytic theory. *Psychoanalysis, Self and Context, 12*(1), 60–77.

Fisher, J. (2017). *Healing the fragmented selves of trauma survivors: Overcoming self-alienation.* New York: Routledge.

Fonagy, P., Gergely, G., Jurist, L. E., & Target, M. (2004). *Affect regulation, mentalization, and the development of the self.* New York: Other Press.

Fosha, D. (2000). *The transforming power of affect: A model for accelerated change.* New York: Basic Books.

Fosha, D. (2005). Emotion, true self, true other, core state: Toward a clinical theory of affective change process. *Psychoanalytic Review, 92*(4), 513–551.

Fosha, D. (Ed.) (2021). *Undoing aloneness and the transformation of suffering into flourishing: AEDP 2.0.* Washington, DC: American Psychological Association.

Fosha, D. & Lanius, R. (2019). *The neuroscience of trauma and its healing: The road back to the neurobiological core self.* AEDP Institute on Demand Seminar.

Frewen, P., Wong, S., & Lanius, R. (2023). The four-dimensional (4-D) model as a framework for understanding trauma-related dissociation. In M. J. Dorahy, S. N. Gold, & J. A. O'Neil (Eds.), *Dissociation and the dissociative disorders: Past, present, future* (2nd ed., pp. 327–340). New York: Routledge.

Harel, H., Gordon, I., Geva, R., & Feldman, R. (2011). Gaze behaviors of preterm and full-term infants in nonsocial and social contexts of increasing dynamics: Visual recognition, attention regulation, and gaze synchrony. *Infancy, 16*(1), 69–90. https://doi.org/10.1111/j.1532-7078.2010.00037.x

Hesse, E. & Main, M. (1999). Second-generation effects of unresolved trauma in nonmaltreating parents: Dissociated, frightened, and threatening parental behavior. *Psychoanalytic Inquiry, 19*(4), 481–540.

Howell, E. (2005). *The dissociative mind.* New York: Routledge.

Lamagna, J. (2011). Of the self, by the self, and for the self: An intra-relational perspective on intra-psychic attunement and psychological change. *Journal of Psychotherapy Integration, 21*(3), 280–307.

Lamagna, J. & Gleiser, K. A. (2007). Building a secure internal attachment: An intra-relational approach to ego strengthening and emotional processing with chronically traumatized clients. *Journal of Trauma and Dissociation, 8*(1), 25–52. https://doi.org/10.1300/J229v08n01_03

Lanius, U. F., Paulsen, S. L., & Corrigan, F. M. (Eds.) (2014). *Neurobiology and treatment of traumatic dissociation: Towards an embodied self.* New York: Springer.

Laub, B. & Weiner, N. (2013). A dialectical perspective of trauma processing. *International Journal of Integrative Psychology, 4*(2), 24–39.

Mikulincer, M. & Shaver, R. R. (2016). *Attachment in adulthood: Structure, dynamics, and change* (2nd ed.). New York: Guilford.

Nani, A., Manuello, J., Mancuso, L., Liloia, D., Costa, T., & Cauda, F. (2019). The neural correlates of consciousness and attention: Two sister processes of the brain. *Frontiers in Neuroscience, 13*, 1169. https://doi.org/10.3389/fnins.2019.01169

Ogden, P., Minton, K., & Pain, C. (2006). *Trauma and the body: A sensorimotor approach to psychotherapy.* New York: Norton.

Pando-Mars, K. (2017, January 12). *Tailoring AEDP interventions to attachment style.* [Online Transformance Talk sponsored by AEDP].

Panksepp, J. (2009). Brain emotional systems and qualities of mental life: From animal models of affect to implications for psychotherapeutics. In D. Fosha, D. J. Siegel, & M. F. Solomon (Eds.), *The healing power of emotion: Affective neuroscience, development and clinical practice* (pp. 1–26). New York: Norton.

Panksepp, J. & Northoff, G. (2009). The trans-species core SELF: The emergence of active cultural and neuro-ecological agents through self-related processing within subcortical-cortical midline networks. *Consciousness and Cognition: An International Journal, 18*(1), 193–215. https://doi.org/10.1016/j.concog.2008.03.002

Porges, S. W. (2011). *The polyvagal theory: Neurophysiological foundations of emotions, attachment, communication, and self-regulation.* New York: Norton.

Schwartz, R. C. (2019). *Internal Family Systems—What is Self?* https://www.youtube.com/watch?v=ldAfsoqg-cc&t=11s

Schwartz, R. C. (2023). *Introduction to Internal Family Systems.* Boulder, CO: Sounds True Adult.

Schwartz, R. C. & Sweezy, M. (2020). *Internal Family Systems* (2nd ed.). New York: Guilford.

Siegel, D. J. (2007). *The mindful brain: Reflection and attunement in the cultivation of well-being.* New York: Norton.

Siegel, D. J. (2012). A framework for cultivating integration: Happiness, mindfulness, neuroscience and self development. *PsychAlive.* https://www.psychalive.org/framework-cultivating-integration/

Siegel, D. J. (2020). *The developing mind: How relationships and the brain interact to shape who we are* (3rd ed.). New York: Guilford.

Siegel, D. J. & Drulis, C. (2023). An interpersonal neurobiology perspective on the mind and mental health: Personal, public, and planetary well-being. *Annals of General Psychiatry, 22*, 5. https://doi.org/10.1186/s12991-023-00434-5

Siegel, D. J. & Payne Bryson, T. (2020). *The power of showing up: How parental presence shapes who our kids become and how their brains get wired.* New York: Ballantine Books.

Stanley, S. (2016). *Relational and body-centered practices for healing trauma: Lifting the burdens of the past.* New York: Routledge.

Taylor, J. B. (2021). *Whole brain living: The anatomy of choice and the four characters that drive our life.* Carlsbad, CA: Hay House.

Tronick, E. Z. (1989). Emotions and emotional communication in infants. *American Psychologist, 44*(2), 112–199.

Tronick, E. Z. & Gianino, A. F. (1986). Interactive mismatch and repair: Challenges to the coping infant. *Zero to Three, 6*, 1–6.

van der Hart, O., Nijenhuis, E. R. S., & Steele, K. (2006). *The haunted self: Structural dissociation and the treatment of chronic traumatization.* New York: Norton.

van der Kolk, B. A. (2014). *The body keeps the score: Brain, mind and body in the healing of trauma.* New York: Penguin.

van der Kolk, B. A., d'Andrea, W., Lanius, R., & Sky, L. (2019). *How body experience impacts and alters the sense of self: Neuroscience research meets experiential inquiry and revisiting the "Corrective Emotional Experience": Creating deep imprints of safety and resonance using psychodramatic techniques.* [Presentation at 30th Annual International Trauma Conference, Boston, MA].

van Nuys, D. (2013, April–June). Dr. Daniel J. Siegel: A David van Nuys interview. *The International Journal of Neuropsychotherapy, 1.* https://www.shrinkrapradio.com/255.pdf

Wallin, D. J. (2007). *Attachment in psychotherapy.* New York: The Guilford Press.

Warner, E., Westcott, A., Cook, A., & Finn, H. (2020). *Transforming trauma in children and adolescents: An embodied approach to somatic regulation, trauma processing, and attachment-building.* Berkeley, CA: North Atlantic Books.

Wesselmann, D. (2014, April 4). *Trauma time.* https://debrawesselmann.com/2014/trauma-time/

Yeung, D. (2021). What went right?: What happens in the brain during AEDP's meta-therapeutic processing. In D. Fosha (Ed.), *Undoing aloneness and the transformation of suffering* (pp. 349–376). Washington, DC: American Psychological Association.

Part II

Play

Chapter 3

Play—The Who, What, When, Where, Why, and How of Play

In order for us to integrate the spirit of play into trauma treatment, we need to understand fully what we mean when we talk about "play." This chapter focuses on just that—what play is, how we know we're being playful, who's able to play, and how we can discern whether or not something is really "play." We'll grow our appreciation for how we intuitively *know* we're being playful at every level of our being—mentally, emotionally, physically, and spiritually.

What Is Play?

Play is an attitude or state of mind (Brown, 2009) or the spirit (Gross, 2018) that inspires our actions. This means that play is not the activity or behavior itself, but rather the "motivation and mental attitude" (Gray, 2013, p. 139) that informs how we show up alone or with others. Play is the free and joyful spirit in which we engage, connect with, and explore the world (Gross, 2018, p. 364). Play is not a noun, it is more of an adjective (Gray, 2013) or adverb. We are playful in how we move, breathe, and show up in our spirit or energy. That's why a play behavior, like playing catch, can have the playfulness sucked out of it if we show up with excessive rigidity, or a heavy, suffocating presence even if we continue to throw and catch a ball.

The play state of mind or spirit can be pure or blend multiple purposes and motivations (Gray, 2013, p. 140). For example, in pure play, we might splash in puddles just for fun. Alternatively, in blended play, we might purposefully clean a toilet bowl while singing and creating an explosion of sudsy bubbles. While we can play at all ages, children play purely more frequently than adults who must balance many demands and responsibilities. Having a playful mindset, spirit, or attitude allows us to engage in play to varying degrees no matter what the activity—including the activity of therapy. Each of us can uniquely engage our playful spirit with seven different types of play: attunement, body and movement/sensorimotor, object, social, imaginative and pretend, storytelling/narrative, and creative.

DOI: 10.4324/9781003509493-6

Before discussing these types of play, let's first figure out how we know we're being playful.

How Do We Know We're Being Playful?

We can tell we are engaging our playful spirit by the presence of certain characteristics (see Brown, 2008, 2009; Gray, 2013; Marks-Tarlow et al., 2018).

1. **We feel good.** Playfulness connects us with life-enlivening and life-enhancing states in our body, mind, emotions, and spirit. Playing releases our feel-good hormones, including endorphins, oxytocin, dopamine, and serotonin, which, respectively, help us feel pleasure/block pain, bond, feel rewarded, elevate mood, and improve sleep, learning, and memory (Edwards, 2016). Play is fun and pleasurable and helps us feel free, joyful, light, and sometimes euphoric. Whether spontaneous or more structured, play is innately fulfilling and rewarding. Playfulness allows us to more fully and deeply connect with positivity.
2. **We want to do more of it.** Because playing feels good and exciting and can rouse us from boredom, we willingly want more of it. Brown (2009) says, "Play is the essence of freedom, its own reward, its own reason for being" (pp. 17–18). It is no wonder that sometimes we don't want to stop playing and return to the responsibilities of daily life.
3. **We go with the flow.** When we are engaged playfully, we are focused on the activity and can get lost in it. We may lose track of or choose not to pay attention to time. Our only purpose and focus are to be present. We may become so absorbed in playing that our self-consciousness may decrease or fade into the background. While pure play is not goal-oriented, per se, it is driven by our internal needs and desires.
4. **We are more curious.** When we are playful, we access and nurture our curiosity and boundless imagination. We feel safe to discover and explore, improvise, and create.
5. **We connect with our Self.** When playing, we disconnect from stress and the seriousness of life. With life's demands put to the side, we are free to connect with our authenticity (Brown & Eberle, 2018), act with genuineness (Winnicott, 1989), and show up in ways that feel right to our core. Play is a portal to connect with our true self (Winnicott, 1960), Self (Schwartz & Sweezy, 2020), core self (Fosha, 2000), our essence, life force, and vitality.

Taken together, we see how being playful gives us an unmistakable experience of *knowing through feeling* in our mind, body, and spirit. Through playfulness, we tap into our drive to explore through curiosity, which connects us to the deepest expression of who we are. Who wouldn't want to have this experience in therapy or elsewhere?

Who Can Play?

So, who can play? Fortunately, children and certified play therapists are not the only ones who can be playful. Our brains—at any age—are wired to access and engage our playful spirit.

We Are All Wired to Play: Our Brain's PLAY Circuitry

Play is part of the shared human experience across culture, gender, social, political, and religious backgrounds. In fact, Jaak Panksepp (1998) discovered that we are all literally wired to play, which is why we all can engage a playful spirit no matter our age or developmental stage. When Panksepp mapped the mammal's noncognitive (subcortical) brain, he found seven hard-wired emotional-motivational circuits which help us learn and adapt to changes in our internal or external environments (Davis & Montag, 2019). These universal emotional-motivational circuits are SEEKING, LUST, RAGE, FEAR, CARE, PANIC/GRIEF/ Separation Distress, and, yes, PLAY.

All animals have the primary emotional circuits of SEEKING, LUST, RAGE, and FEAR. Only the more socially oriented mammals (including humans) developed motivational systems of CARE to nurture their offspring, PANIC/GRIEF/ Separation Distress to maintain social contact and bonding, and PLAY to enable social joy and limit-setting through physical activity (Davis & Montag, 2019).

During development different circuits serve different roles. In the first few weeks of a baby's life, the SEEKING circuit gathers information (e.g., through taste, hearing, touch, smell, and movements of the head, lips, and limbs). Meanwhile, during the first 6 months of the infant's life, the caregiver's PLAY circuitry is engaged through attunement play (discussed in Chapter 4) to facilitate bonding that sets the stage for all other forms of play. The baby might respond with emerging smiles and cooing. After 6 months of life, the baby's PLAY circuitry comes online and initiates the curiosity-driven SEEKING system (Ogden & Fisher, 2007). With their PLAY circuitry fully engaged, true joy and laughter are seen and shared by baby (Ogden & Fisher, 2007) and caregiver. Engaging the PLAY circuit with clients of all ages capitalizes on these hard-wired evolutionary, survival-enhancing, and attachment-promoting powers. The PLAY emotional-motivational circuit enables playful action when safety (Gross, 2018, p. 370) and connection (Dana, 2020) are present. The PLAY circuit holds a key role in forming social connection, learning the relational "rules of the road," expanding knowledge, and experiencing joy (Panksepp, 1998, p. 281).

Our Playing Brains Grow in the Same Way

While each of our brains has a PLAY circuit, its wiring and expression are unique, affected by our individual developmental-relational-contextual factors.

Yet even with these individual different influences, all of our brains grow by following a common neurodevelopmental sequence (Perry, 2014). Physically, our brains grow from the bottom up—from the reptilian brainstem, to the limbic system/emotional midbrain, up to the neocortex. They also grow from the right hemisphere to left and from the inside out to where the outermost layers of the cortex have the most recently developed cells. We all share the same evolving sequence of play organized around the brain's neurological development (Chapman, 2014; Prendiville & Howard, 2017). From birth forward, this sequence includes attunement, body and movement/sensorimotor, object, social, imaginative and pretend, storytelling/narrative, and creative play (see Brown, 2009, discussed thoroughly in Chapter 4).

Broadly speaking, when the lower, reptilian, right-brain stem structures develop, play is attunement and sensorimotor based. When the emotional midbrain develops, play can use art media to express emotions. As the lower cortical structures develop, symbolic play emerges. And as the higher prefrontal cortex grows, more creative, integrative play develops (Chapman, 2014).

Owing to its universal, wired-in circuitry, and shared neurodevelopmental sequencing, play is widely applicable, accessible, and "central to who we are throughout our lives" (Badenoch & Kestly, 2014). Since play "can transcend differences in ethnicity, language, or other aspects of culture" (Schaefer & Drewes, 2014, p. 1), people of all ages and backgrounds with various developmental and physical abilities can be playful given appropriate support and nurturance. We can be playful in most settings—home, therapy, school, work, hospitals, during times of peace or war, with others, or by ourselves. Play is also portable—wherever we go, we can tap into our playfulness and engage our PLAY circuitry. We can give credit to the fact that each of us once was a child or is still a child at heart. In other words, all humans can be playful, including therapists who treat adults and never took a play therapy course!

We can express ourselves playfully at any stage of neurodevelopment, regardless of age or trauma history to facilitate growth and healing. Some clients may need to learn to play for the first time. Playfulness helps therapists naturally drop into right brain-to-right brain connection and communicate with our clients in neurodevelopmentally relevant and attuned ways (Perry, 2006). Specifically, through neurodevelopmentally sensitive right brain–focused playfulness, we can reach the preverbally traumatized parts of child, teenage, and adult clients (Warner et al., 2020) stuck in the right hemisphere. Neurodevelopmentally sensitive playfulness in the context of a professional therapy relationship can help clients with early trauma histories of pervasive neglect (e.g., orphans) which may have impaired brain structure growth and functioning (discussed in Child Welfare Information Gateway, 2015; Ohashi et al., 2019; Teicher, 2022). Clients with severe cognitive, physical/medical (e.g., paraplegia, trauma brain injury, blindness, and deafness), relational, or functional limitations (e.g., severe autism, psychosis), or cultural/religious oppression can also benefit from neurodevelopmentally sensitive play.

At a minimum, we can introduce attunement-based playfulness (discussed later in this chapter) with these clients using sensorimotor channels. All therapists can feel reassured that we can reach all clients with playfulness that is attuned and neurodevelopmentally sensitive.

Different Ways to Play across Our Development and in Therapy

Now, we'll unpack the seven types of play that emerge across our development. Let's remember that all types of play can overlap and work cumulatively and synergistically. We'll look at the general features/characteristics of each type of play, and how we can engage them in a clinical setting with clients of all ages. As you read along, notice which types of play you most resonate with and do. Bring curiosity to how you might stretch your play comfort zone and use your imagination to envision what that might look like in practice.

Attunement Play

Attunement play can be thought of as the "mother of all play" as it is the earliest type of play and sets the stage for all other forms of relational play across the age and ability spectrum. Attunement play starts in utero (Lohre, 2017; Skove, 2015; Wilson, 2020), continues fiercely through a baby's first year, and is present throughout our lifetime. In utero and prior to 6 months, attunement play is initiated by the caregiver since the baby lacks control over their movements and cannot yet speak or initiate. After 6 months of age, both the baby and their caregiver can initiate attunement play.

Attunement play centers on making contact with someone in ways that leave them feeling tuned in to safely. In attunement play, we can use a melodic voice, eye gaze, light touch, and coordinated and rhythmic breathing to promote a sense of being and feeling safe and seen.

After assessing boundaries and comfort levels with a pregnant client, therapists can model prenatal attunement play by speaking to the growing fetus. I've joked when speaking close to my client's pregnant belly, saying, "Hello, growing little one. You are the youngest client I've ever had in my practice. I'm impressed!" I love when my clients say their baby kicks in response. I might ask the expectant mother, "Could you tell if that was a happy kick or *leave me alone, I'm only here because she brought me?*"

As a therapist, we might use attunement play with a 5-month-old by gazing eye to eye while smiling and saying, "I see you. You're a little bundle of joy." Or in a sing-songy voice we might coo, "You're sooooo sweet and sooooo adorable." However, therapists need to repeatedly check in with clients, particularly if they had early relational trauma because they may feel jealous, unseen, ignored, and even upstaged by their infant getting the therapist's attention. Therapists need to mindfully offer balanced attention and celebration. If attuning to the infant causes misattunements with the parent client, we have a fertile area to explore and unfold relationally.

Attunement play with adults can look very similar to that with little ones. Thirty-two-year-old Sarayah was hijacked by the pain of yet another cruel and biting paternal rejection. Her eyes were downcast as she cried, wailing with violent heaves. I very carefully moved my chair toward her, saying gently and very slowly, "Sarayah? . . . Sarayah? . . . I'm here . . . Yes, I'm here with you." I moved my head side to side trying to make eye contact. She remained disconnected. I moved my hand to my heart center, saying quietly and slowly, with deep exhales, "Ooooh, ooooh, oooh." I modeled a slower breathing pace to co-regulate hers. Soon her breathing slowed. I acknowledged it. "Yes, that's it . . . Yeah . . . Yeah." I then crossed my arms and started stroking them, as if I were holding and stroking her.

To bring her into connection, I said, "I'm here with you. Yes, yes. Ooooh, Sarayah. I see you." She started looking up and I intentionally slowed my arm strokes, exaggerating them. Eventually, I just firmly held my arms and rocked them side to side. Sarayah looked up and cocked her head to the side. "Yes," I reassured her, "I'm here with you, holding all you need me to hold." We sat together, quietly. First, she glanced at me and then averted my gaze. After her eyes darted away and returned multiple times to mine, we shared and held a mutual gaze. I smiled with closed lips and nodded. She mirrored me, fully returning to connection with me.

Sensorimotor Play

Sensorimotor play—also called body and movement play—is just that: playing with body sensations and movement. Similar to attunement play, it starts in utero. A mother who pokes her belly to make her fetus kick in response is a form of sensorimotor play. After birth, caregivers guide and move a young baby's body for them and touch them with soft tickles, rocking, close and protective holding. As babies develop motor control and coordinate their movements, they can play by more intentionally moving their legs, arms, feet, hands, fingers, and mouth, allowing them to explore their personal body and external worlds. Body and movement play continues throughout life as in dance or exercise and may include object play (e.g., basketball) as motor coordination grows.

Tracking and making explicit eye gaze and movement are a marvelous use of sensorimotor play with all ages. For example, when reflecting to 17-year-old Larry that his father left him feeling shamed and inadequate, he dramatically rolled his eyes. I commented, "I saw your eyes roll. That was a big one! I guess part of you really didn't agree with or like what I said?" After exploring this further, I learned that his eye-roll was more of a big *Duh, isn't it obvious?* Later when I repeated how Larry's father raised his shameful and inadequate feelings,

Larry just shot me a look. I met his gaze, mirrored back the same look, and said, "Duh, Monica." Then, I rolled my eyes, mockingly hit my head with my hand and said, "I guess I didn't need to be a rocket scientist to figure this one out, huh?" Getting a smirk and head nod from Larry meant he acknowledged me seeing him and teasing myself. By naming, mirroring, and playing with his movements, I invited Larry to notice his own bodily experience. Together we dropped down into what our bodies felt to sensorily track and explicitly explore the hurt. Body and movement play guided Larry to more deeply connect with and share his vulnerability and shame. Using sensorimotor play, Larry and I each gained access to and insight into a previously unverbalizable, unconscious experience.

Object Play

Object play emerges at 6 months of age and continues across our lifetime as we play with all kinds of objects in our environment. The objects of play do not need to be designated toys like balls or dolls, nor do they need to be used in only one way. Play objects may be a box to drum on, cups to fill and empty in a tub of water, bubble wrap to jump on, or toilet paper to wrap around ourselves.

In therapy with children, we can play hide and seek with an object (e.g., a little doll or car) or a child's full body self to metaphorically address themes of in/visibility that engage the child's choice and control. For example, when 6-year-old Sonya hides under a blanket in full view of the therapist, the therapist plays along and wonders out loud, "Where did Sonya go? She was here just a minute ago. She's a great hider!" This self-as-object play helps a child develop mastery and control over being seen.

Adult clients may hide without initiating the seek. This may not reflect play but a defense, like shame, inadequacy, and a wish to remain unseen. My clients with body image issues have put pillows and even stuffed animals on their stomachs or laps as a protective barrier. After growing safety and deep trust in the client-therapist relationship, I slowly introduced playfulness. I suggested clients experiment with putting their barrier up or down, to one side or the other, to see if it feels more or less helpful. Eventually across sessions, clients have moved their pillow barrier consciously or unconsciously, reflecting changes in their protector parts' degree of guardedness. I've explicitly tracked and playfully explored this shift and paradoxically asked, "The pillow hasn't been on your lap in weeks: do you miss it or does it miss you?" We can encourage intrarelational processing with protector parts from these types of queries (see Chapter 11).

When playing catch with objects like pillows, tissues, or balls, we help clients re-orient to the present and shift out of dissociative states (Knipe, 2007, p. 202). We can further encourage states of safety and connection (VV states see Chapter 2) by including others, like a spouse or family members to join in the play. As therapists guide clients how hard or soft, fast or slow, to throw or roll a ball to us (or others), we help them increase their ability to empathize and mentalize; this supports them to safely respect physical boundaries of others and the space they're in. It also playfully serves to modulate and regulate behavior and affect. Pillow or foam sword fights with clients of all ages can be fun and similarly practice nervous system and affect modulation, empathy and mentalization, safe versus unsafe aggression.

Social Play

Social play refers to a sequence of developing social skills starting around age 2, when the left hemisphere comes online, allowing toddlers to communicate more verbally. Three types of social play occur in succession. They are parallel play, around age 2, associative play, between 3 and 4, and cooperative play, after age 4 or 5 and continuing throughout the lifespan.

Parallel play emerges first and characterizes how 2-year-olds play alongside or near, but not with others—in other words, in parallel with them. This play is more egocentric than social because children are not yet able to think about someone else's feelings, wants, and needs and therefore they cannot share. Therapists introduce parallel play to clients of all ages who have not yet mastered social play, do not trust others to share space and things, or fiercely protect their boundaries. To play in a parallel way, we give a client separate space and possibly their own supplies. For example, we can draw or make a craft independently with separate supplies, and sit side by side interacting minimally or not all with our client. Over time, we can safely start to engage our client with contact statements that encourage interaction.

Associative play emerges when children shift from playing next to others to engaging with others minimally in a related play activity (i.e., on monkey bars or at a kitchen set). At this stage, the child's egocentrism wanes and they start to show interest in what others are doing, talk to others, and use the same toys without losing focus on their own play. In the spirit of social play, therapists can braid lanyards, especially with pre-teen and teenage clients, which keep the client engrossed in their personal creation while being curious about and relating to the other's. Therapists can address the client's mastery and creativity. The play may soften and distract defenses, allowing discussion of important topics to emerge.

In cooperative social play, children want to play together, share a common interest in an activity, and work together toward a common goal. Cooperative play can be structured as in team sports or unstructured as in a treasure hunt. It can be, but isn't necessarily, competitive. Therapists who play in-office basketball with a makeshift or real ball and hoop introduce cooperative and competitive play. Playing board games like checkers, chess, or Connect-4 can bring safe competition between client and therapist. While therapists may naturally get lost in the play, they must stay mindful and grounded in their role, ensuring their actions and comments are goal-oriented, supporting the objectives of therapy like client mastery, trust, cooperation, or positive affect and affect tolerance.

Therapists can use mindful and intentional language to safely lead the client from parallel to associative to cooperative social play, increasing their client's tolerance of and capacity for positive affect. Specifically, when commenting about the client's play, like drawing a tree, the therapist might proceed as follows:

1. Speak of the object not the person. "Those leaves are bright and colorful" (parallel play—no social connection).
2. Explicitly reference the person using non-evaluative language. "You draw such bright and colorful leaves" (associative play—hint of connection and sharing positivity).
3. Directly refer to the client's positive influence or mastery in the play. "You draw those leaves so carefully and well, and with such detail." "Would it be okay if I try to draw it like you?" (associative play—social connection grows as client is seen as subject and master of a skill from which therapist would like to learn. Players are still separate).
4. Finally, engage the client, their skill, and wish to play together. "Would you help me draw it like you did?" or "Can we draw a leaf together?" (cooperative play—social engagement and cooperation while leaving the client feeling positive in the role of leader or master).

Imaginative and Pretend Play

Imaginative and pretend play starts around 14–18 months and wanes dramatically around ages 10–12 years when children become more focused on socializing, structured play, and games with rules. Imaginative or pretend play is make-believe or "as if" play, when children and adults take on and experiment with a certain role or character. Imaginative and pretend play can be reality- or fantasy-based, alone or with others. Solitary imaginative play can be with an imaginary friend that can be invisible or embodied in an object like a stuffed animal. Daydreaming is another type of solitary imaginative play. Social pretend play includes others, with or without imaginary friends or objects, and can be creative physically and verbally (as in storytelling).

Imaginative and pretend play is fostered in the therapy room by offering time for free play with open-ended materials like paper, Play-Doh, "dress up" clothes, or opportunities for spontaneous storytelling. When a child or adult's mind is supported to roam free, their imagination and creativity grow. Pretend play lessens as early childhood moves into adolescence when teens think more theoretically, hypothetically, abstractly, and use reason and logic. As a result, when teenagers notice inconsistencies in their worlds of make-believe, they may abandon this play preferring to engage in real-life social interactions, more rule-bound games, and screen time. As teenagers shift away from overt imaginary and pretend play, they may move toward inward, quiet, imaginative play like daydreaming.

Thanks to pretend play, children who are supported to roam freely in all therapy settings—even those without toys—will transform the mundane into imaginative themes worthy of therapeutic exploration. Patty, a 5-year-old transgender client, played hide and seek under chairs and a desk to introduce themes of wanting to hide their body from the world and not wanting to see their own genitalia because it induced too much gender dysphoria. Meanwhile, 3-year-old Liana used those same chairs and desk to show me how she tried to hide and dissociate from witnessing her parents' drug abuse, domestic violence, and getting sexually abused by her father. Ten-year-old Elizabeth crawled under my desk and cornered herself in. When she allowed me to do the same in the opposite corner, a somatic countertransference emerged, helping me grasp how hiding and cornering herself kept Elizabeth safe when her auditory psychotic symptoms emerged.

We also can welcome our adult clients' imaginative use of the office space and objects with playful respect and curiosity. I said to 30-year-old Tiffany, wedged into the corner of the couch, "You look quite supported in the corner of the couch. How does it feel? Would you like to adjust yourself to feel even more supported? Would you like to use the pillow?" Tiffany pushed herself further into the corner with her feet and legs and placed a pillow on her lap. I invited Tiffany to slow down, breath, "Notice, what's that like?" and "Allow your imagination to bring your creativity to what you notice."

Tiffany said, "I feel like I am well protected in a fortress right now." And off we went, playing with her fantasy of the medieval fortress she had erected. When I offered Tiffany more pillows, she laughed, shook her head sideways, and said, "No thanks. I think I'm good with the alligator-filled moat, closed drawbridge, and knights with lances standing guard."

If clients feel held and safe in a trusted therapy relationship and space, one of the most powerful ways to engage imaginative and pretend play is by using the powerful prompt: "Just imagine." Through one's imagination, far-off worlds and real-life possibilities can be explored for the fun of it and linked back to therapy themes. When possible, I like to include movement with make-believe play to promote embodiment of the positive affective experience.

When 43-year-old Ashley talked about her fear and rage at her always-bordering-on-inappropriate and power-hungry boss, she blurted, "I wish I could kick that asshole in the balls!"

"Imagine that," I replied. Coming to the edge of my seat, with my eyes wide, I said excitedly, "Go for it!"

Ashley and I further developed and unfolded the imagined play scene. Her initial timid kick and run evolved into a roundhouse kick, with Ashley firmly standing her ground and growing into a full-size Hulk. Imagining her boss looking at her, Ashley said in a deeply resonant voice, with her finger up in his face,

"You think that hurt? Just try it again and I will not only go to HR and file a sexual harassment claim, I'm also going to call your wife and tell her what a skeevy, perv you are!" The power, joy, and delight Ashley felt helped her navigate ways to handle her boss with stronger boundaries and clarity.

Storytelling and Narrative Play

Storytelling and narrative play start preverbally and can be solitary or social. It can be verbal, visual, or nonverbal, as in writing, drawing, dance, and movement. Preverbal babies can listen to stories, while toddlers through adults love telling or listening to fantasy or reality-based stories or writing and illustrating them. Watching movies and reading books is also a form of storytelling and narrative play, which requires left hemisphere–based receptive and expressive language skills, which come online around age 2.

World play is a more fully developed, complex, and elaborated imagination-infused form of narrative play (Root-Bernstein, 2014). It can start age around age 2 but is more commonly associated with middle childhood and moves into adulthood (Root-Bernstein, 2014). While pretend or imaginative play is short term (i.e., minutes to hours), world play can last days, weeks, months, or years (Krisch, 2018). The scope and scale of world-play dwarfs pretend play; imaginary societies or worlds are created that may have their own geography, art, history, political or religious institutions, language, social conventions, cultures, religions, etc., and characters have specific beliefs and emotions. The American Girl Doll, *Game of Thrones,* or the fantasy game Dungeons and Dragons are examples of world play.

Humor can be thought of as another type of storytelling play, although it is present as early as infancy and toddlerhood. Humor includes anything people say or do which is perceived as funny and makes people laugh (Martin & Ford, 2018, p. 3). Early forms of humor are expressed in less elaborate forms, like sensorimotor-based attunement play with babies (e.g., making funny noises, goofy faces, or tickling), object and social play with young children (e.g., sitting on a whoopee cushion), and imaginative or pretend play (e.g., dressing up and speaking like a loathed teacher, saying ridiculous things like, "You have three minutes to finish all twenty pages of homework or you'll miss lunch, recess, and you won't be able to go home!"). As children grow into storytelling-narrative play, humor becomes increasingly varied and moves from nonverbal to more complex verbal and written forms.

From around age four onward, children experiment with jokes and puns using wordplay. An example might be a knock-knock joke, "Knock, knock. Who's there? Atch. Atch who? Bless you" (as if it was a sneeze). Older children, teenagers, and adults have a more extensive vocabulary, understand syntax and semantics, can write, read, and speak more fluently which allows them to enjoy more complex forms of humor. They can think abstractly or use out-of-the-box thinking to discover unpredictable responses. An example of a corny riddle for young teens might be, "What do fish in high school worry about? Shellfishteem." Developmentally, more advanced nonverbal or verbal, written or watched forms of humor include double-entendres, sarcasm, dark/gallows, self-deprecating, surreal or absurd, improvisational, and bathroom or potty.

In therapy, storytelling can take different forms and serve different purposes. The therapist or client can tell a story directly or use objects like a doll, figure, hand, pencil, etc. to gain distance from the affective intensity. Journaling can help clients problem-solve or promote self-related processing that brings meaning and coherence to their life story and identity. Hand gestures can be used for storytelling, too. Gestures reflect and constitute thought and hold knowledge of what our brains are not yet conscious (Kestly, 2018, p. 122).

Some of my clients call me a "hand reader" because I track and try to read and interpret their hand movements. I joke that because I am a Jewish New Yorker, I have learned to talk with my hands and hand read, too. I encourage clients to notice their own hand movements and notice the story being told. Often clients are amazed that their hands express what they haven't yet consciously thought of or felt hesitant to express. As they language their hand (and other body-part) movements, stories unfold.

Therapists can tell clients very brief stories about other clients who faced similar challenges and found resolution. Always, but especially when working in a small, tight-knit community, changing identifying characteristics and preserving confidentiality is paramount. Hearing these stories helps clients feel less alone and more hopeful. Often clients have said, "Even though I know I can't meet these other clients, I feel like we'd understand and support each other. Ever think about starting a group?" Wisely sharing appropriate stories from a therapist's own life can serve this same purpose and help clients feel even more connected to the therapist, less alone, and know that therapists are humans like them.

Clients can be encouraged to create stories through words, songs, poetry, drawing, and movement during and between sessions. Whether clients share out loud or ask the therapist to read or hear their stories, therapists can follow up with unfolding the narrative, sharing how the story affected them, and what it was like for the client to create and share it with the therapist. Metaprocessing storytelling can further deepen its reparative and transformative qualities (see Chapter 9).

Three of my teenage clients wrote novels about dystopian societies that took years to create. Each world-play story drew directly from their life histories and what they witnessed in the world around them. Interestingly, each of these clients initially hesitated to share their elaborate, private worlds, fearing their shadow or dark sides would be exposed and judged. Once trusting that their sharing would be safe, these clients revealed their characters' inner and external conflicts and details of their complex worlds, including maps, family trees, songs, poetry, and political and religious institutions. Sometimes therapy involved brainstorming ideas to support client creativity or deepen plot conflicts, role-playing with the sinister sides of characters, and problem-solving stuck points and inconsistencies in the narrative. Feeling respected, admired, and supported in their narrative world play deepened these teenagers' therapeutic alliance with me.

Finally, humor as a form of narrative play is one of my most enjoyed forms of playfulness in therapy and can be used creatively but judiciously. We can make the subject or recipient of the humorous intervention ourselves, the client, someone else, or the client-therapist relationship itself. The therapist or client can deliver the humorous remark. As a rule of thumb, the closer the humor targets the client or those close to them, the greater the potential for ANS and affect dysregulation. The risk for dysregulation seems lowest when the therapist self-deprecates, higher when we poke fun at their loved ones, and highest when we directly poke fun at the client. Puns that are objective, silly, and not directed at anyone seem most neutral, while sarcasm about the client may cause hurt, shame, and feeling deeply misunderstood.

For example, my adult client Asna and I sarcastically applauded her mother's increased affect tolerance when Asna refused to date yet another Muslim male of her mother's choice. Historically, Asna's mother turned on the guilt saying she'd become gravely ill if Asna dated and married out of the faith. I sarcastically joked, "Wow, this time mom only threatened to have a panic attack instead of her usual heart attack and stroke that would leave her paralyzed and mute!" Asna and I playfully rejoiced at her mom's growth.

Creative Play

As with all forms of play, creative play is intrinsically motivated, can occur alone or with others, and stems from pretend or imaginative play. Creative play can take place in free, open-ended play or rule-bound contexts. Creative play is blended with other forms of play—attunement, body and movement, object, social, storytelling/narrative, or pretend/imaginative. In creative play, objects whether toys or everyday materials are used in new, unique or unusual ways and are a form of self-expression. Creative play brings inventiveness and imagination to everything from creating rhythms, music, a dance, or painting, to writing scholarly journal articles or developing a new structure for an organization to run most efficiently. Creative play involves innovative thinking, experimentation, experiential learning—in part through trial and error—in an iterative process (Resnick, 2007).

Supporting our clients' creative, playful self-expression in session through music, role-playing, sculpting, painting, photography, dance, etc. can be fruitful and fun. The possibilities are endless. Rashti, a 53-year-old client, lost her career and role as primary breadwinner following a traumatic brain injury. During her rehabilitation, Rashti rediscovered her love of guitar, singing, and found a new hobby, videography. Rashti shared her videos in session, explaining her use of special effects, different techniques, and subject matter. Her progress was visible, as was her improved self-confidence. She found excitement, challenge, and joy in videography. Eventually, her friends, neighbors, and family members saw Rashti's talents and requested that she video their family milestone events. They were so pleased with her skill that they paid her, although she did not charge. As Rashti became very skilled, therapy became a place to solidify her new part-time career, set a fee that reflected her value, and help her contribute financially to her family.

Therapists can safely discuss and process how clients engage in sex play alone and with others, as it too can be a form of creative self-expression, foster personal identity and confidence, and impact closeness and distance in relationships. Therapists can process the impasses and satisfaction creative sex play produces. While still a taboo and uncomfortable topic for some clients and therapists alike, we need to know when to seek supervision/consultation or refer our client for consultation if our strong religious, cultural, or personal beliefs block our clients' safe exploration. Especially when working with survivors of sexual abuse, therapists hold a key role to help clients develop and explore safe physical boundaries, reciprocally give and receive pleasure, and become educated about healthy sexual development, impulses, and exploratory behaviors. Our clients' early sexual encounters may raise questions about their gender identity and identity as sexual beings. When prepubescents and teenagers enter stages of emerging sexuality and desire, they actively explore and seek to understand their bodies, how they are changing, what makes them feel pleasure versus pain, safe versus uncomfortable or afraid. Clients who wish to creatively explore sex can benefit immensely from supportive and grounded therapists who openly welcome discussion and curiosity, while emphasizing safety and consensual behaviors.

Danni, a 17-year-old girl, was initially timid and hesitant as she discussed her feelings about JoJo. Aside from self-questioning and shame about being attracted to a same-gendered peer, Danni felt "fucked up" for having sexual fantasies about ways she wanted to share her body with JoJo. I supported Danni to feel safe, validate her own truth, and find ways to communicate openly and sincerely with JoJo. Danni and my nonjudgmental discussions enabled the young couple to safely and mutually discover enjoyable and creative sex play that was attuned, fulfilling, and fun. Danni's sexual self-esteem spilled over into her growing confidence as a young woman who felt self-attuned, empowered, appropriately boundaried, and less inhibited.

We can also use creative play to safely experiment with altered states of consciousness in controlled and boundaried ways, which may enhance artistic, scientific, literary, or musical creativity. High school, college, and postgraduate-aged clients have talked about appreciating the textures and depths of music, connecting more deeply with literature, dancing more freely, writing with renewed creative juices, or feeling sillier and laughing more while high on marijuana. Drinking to get buzzed can leave some people feeling more relaxed and uninhibited.

Therapists who work with these artistic clients, especially those under the age of 18, must balance providing an open, welcoming, safe, and confidential environment, while assessing whether the experimentation is safe, crossing a line, or dangerous. Minors who experiment sexually can fall into this tricky zone, too. While substance experimentation can include self-exploration, independence-seeking behaviors, and different ways to self-express, it may bleed into getting high for therapeutic purposes, escaping or numbing uncomfortable emotions, memories, thoughts, or responsibilities. I give clients examples of internationally known performers and artists who have used cocaine, alcohol, and marijuana to inspire their work yet became addicted, harming themselves and others. This illustrates how using recreational substances to enhance creative play can be a slippery slope into concerning and even destructive behaviors.

Any of the seven types of developmental play can be infused in therapy playfully, creatively, and in endless ways. Welcoming the array of play into therapy facilitates us and our clients to reach insights through accessing nonverbally-encoded information (in the right hemisphere) related to developmental limitations or medical, relational, or emotional trauma. When we learn what our clients' preferred and neurodevelopmentally-attuned types of play are, we can create tailored and attuned interventions which yield endless opportunities for growth and fun.

Where Are We on the Play Continuum?

Tapping into our playful spirit means we feel and know that we are being playful. As therapists, we must take this self-awareness an extra step. We need to be mindful and discerning to ensure that our own and others' playfulness has not moved out of states of safety and connection into something questionable, uncomfortable, or even detrimental (e.g., fear-based arousal or protection and disconnection, see Chapter 2). While playfulness can be expressed in different ways across our lives and engender wonderful feelings, play can also turn into something bad. Play exists along a continuum of quantity and quality, which can be influenced by age.

Generally speaking, as we mature, we spend less of our awake time engaged in free, unstructured play because we become more physically, emotionally, and cognitively capable of taking on responsibilities. As children develop, they are assigned more homework, get involved in more structured extracurricular activities (e.g., religious school, competitive sports), community involvement (i.e., volunteer activities), and are given more family responsibilities (e.g., cleaning their room, cooking, or doing laundry). Adults, especially those who are caregivers for young children or elderly relatives, often complain there is no time for fun and are stressed by an overabundance of responsibilities. Older adults, especially those with good physical health and financial means, who have fewer responsibilities, often return to playing, which can look like painting, tennis, and exploration through travel. We need to be sensitive how to support each client to gain a balanced connection to their playful spirit.

Balancing Play Quantity and Quality

Quantity of Play: Too Much, Too Little, or Just Right?

While the need to play exists across the lifespan, it's important to have a sense of how much play is too much or too little. Too little time in unstructured free play for children can hamper cognitive, social, and emotional development and problem-solving. Consequently, limited time playing freely reduces self-empowerment and resiliency (Gray, 2013), hampers brain development and plasticity (Panksepp & Biven, 2012; Siviy, 2016), and even contributes to the emergence of ADHD symptoms (Panksepp, 2007). For adults, consequences of play deprivation include increased stress, pessimism, escapism to temporary maladaptive fixes, a sense of victimization, decreased life satisfaction, and a drop in curious and explorative problem-solving (Brown, 2014).

Therefore, reserving or carving out time to enrich, nurture, and enliven our mood, energy, or spirit is a necessary practice. Married couples or co-parents going on dates (e.g., to ice-skate or explore their favorite hiking spot), children putting down their screens and schoolwork to engage in a game of manhunt with their neighbors, or adults taking time to listen and dance to a favorite song, crochet, blow bubbles into the wind, or build a birdhouse are examples of taking time to play.

By contrast, too much play can interfere with taking on necessary responsibilities and handling emotional challenges and uncomfortable situations. This can include anything from building elaborate model train worlds to playing on five sports teams. Discovering a healthy-enough balance of how much play to include in our lives is challenging yet necessary.

Quality of Play: Free and Easy, Uh-Oh, or Toxic?

In addition to the time we spend in play activities, the quality of play can range from life-affirming and joy-filled, to restorative and relaxing, to life-limiting and toxic. Nine-year-old Jesse started playing her video game to get a break from how "tired my brain is from doing homework." She found the game relaxing and distracting. However, over the course of three weeks, Jesse started lying about finishing her homework to play her game. She began neglecting her school work, spent less time studying for tests, and snuck any opportunity she could to play her videogame. Jesse loved achieving new challenging levels in the game and getting more adept at using her players' powers to get higher scores. In bed, she thought about new strategies to earn more points and unlock more levels and powers. One day, unbeknownst to her parents, Jesse took their credit card and entered its information on the gaming site to purchase additional powers for her characters and unlock different worlds. Jesse got increasingly absorbed in her game and spent less time with friends and family.

When Jesse's parents asked her to stop playing and come to dinner, clean up, or get ready for bed, Jesse became angry, irritable, and refused to stop playing. Fights between Jesse and her parents erupted daily. Her parents started limiting Jesse's screen time; she nagged them incessantly for more time. After learning she had stolen their card to purchase more game options, Jesse's parents took away her device and completely ended her screen time. Jesse became withdrawn and cranky. She isolated. She tried to find the confiscated device, but after discovering it, she realized they had changed the password and she threw it on the floor, shattering the screen.

Jesse shows us how her everyday solitary play with videogames shifted along the play continuum from a state of relaxation to excitement and life-affirming to life-limiting and addictive, as she couldn't function easily without it.

Other types of play that can easily move from life-affirming to life-limiting are creative sex play and altered states. The pretend/imaginative play of daydreaming is a less obvious example of unhealthy play. A child who struggles socially, perhaps because they are bullied or lack the needed skills and practice to make friends, may increasingly get lost in their thoughts or inner world stories, which provide them calm and satisfaction. They may prefer to isolate, stare off for long periods of time, not attend to their schoolwork, and become even more uneasy with peers.

We could apply the general rule of thumb that all play, like most things, needs to be engaged in moderation. And it is true that we humans need to experience play and work, joy and sorrow, freedom and structure, challenge and ease. However, knowing where play falls on the continuum of quality and quantity is more nuanced. In fact, I teach parents about *uh-oh* play: play that seems positive, safe, and life-enhancing, but could cross over at any moment to *uh-oh* states of concern, and then to ones that are dangerous, life-limiting, and potentially toxic or traumatic.

Even my work with adults requires exploration into whether play behaviors are *uh-oh* or possibly concerning, as happened with one of my adult female clients who engaged in BDSM (i.e., bondage and discipline, dominance and submission, sadism and masochism), with her partner. While dating, she and her partner enjoyed the erotic edges of BDSM play, but after they married, her history of sexual trauma emerged and these same once energizing and fun behaviors with her spouse became uncomfortable and eventually retraumatizing. While the initial forays into BDSM sex play felt freeing, my client needed further work to rescript her old sexual abuse themes to prevent this play from becoming a reenactment.

*Is This Really Being Playful? Questions to Guide the Player
and Play Observer*

As discussed earlier in this chapter, we know we're being playful because we feel good, want to do more of it, go with the flow, explore and are curious, and connect with our true Self. Sometimes, though, when we are being playful a niggling or discomfort emerges. As the player, we pay attention to this and "trust our gut" to determine whether something's off. We often give this advice to children and teenagers to help them discern whether play is really playful. We remind them to "listen to your inner voice," or to notice, "what is your gut feeling or letting you know?"

However, it may be hard for children and teens to discern and articulate what their discomfort in playful situations is about or means. This is especially true in new and unfamiliar situations. Similarly, the play observer, whether parent, teacher, caregiver, or even play therapist, may have trouble discerning whether others are being playful. For example, when someone is sarcastic, it might be unclear whether they were being playful or intentionally insulting someone. This dilemma applies to adults too, who frequently struggle to discern whether emails and texts are intended as playful or hurtful.

We can guide clients of all ages how to discern whether or not play is really playful and safe by asking the following questions:

1. What is the **context** of the play? Is it a natural, free-flowing form of self-expression, curiosity, exploration, or experimentation? Is it an effort to avoid the discomfort (e.g., of emotions, behaviors, responsibilities, or thoughts) of completing something? Is it driven by a need to defend against something?
2. How much **choice, control**, and appropriate **responsibility** does the player have/take when engaging in the play, and how does it affect me and/or others?
3. What does the play **mean** to the player? What is the **purpose** of the play?
4. How **frequently** is this play occurring? Is it too often, infrequent, or just the right amount?
5. What is the **duration** of this play when it occurs? Is it too long, too short, or just right?
6. What is the **intensity** of the play? Is the player consumed in a healthy or unhealthy way? Can they stop playing easily? With some persuasion? Or with a lot of drama or conflict?
7. What **feelings** get evoked in others observing this player play? (for example, does it feel light, tense, deadly serious, inviting, cathartic, defended, etc.?)
8. How does playing this way **affect** life? Is it benefitting or putting strain and stress on relationships with or responsibilities to self and others?

Clearly Crossing the Line: Post-Traumatic Play

We can appreciate that all types of everyday play can cross the line and shift from promoting states of freedom, curiosity, and safety, to states of fear, threat, or danger, as seen when children roughhouse or when they draw a picture that evokes fears of suicide or homicide. Post-traumatic play often holds this energy of crossing the line, moving into an unhealthy zone, which lacks the free, easy, and light-spirited feel of everyday play (Terr, 1981). Post-traumatic play feels rigid, grim, and monotonous, can be very literal and anxiety-producing, can be dangerous, and has a contagious quality, affecting others in disturbing ways (Gil, 2017, pp. 11–12). It can harm others or oneself. The felt sense quality of engaging in post-traumatic play is clearly negative, yucky, somewhat or deeply uncomfortable. It is not the least bit joyful or fun.

Post-traumatic play is driven by an effort to repair something that has been ruptured. It uses all the senses to externalize painful or frightening thoughts and feelings through symbol, metaphor, and story (Gil, 2017, p. 13) with the intention of *restoring personal power and control* (Terr, 1981). Post-traumatic play behaviors are intense, repetitive, lack flow, reflect avoidance and negative affect like sadness, despair, anxiety, fear, anger, and have themes of traumatic reenactments (victimization), death/loss/threat, and parentification, among others (Myers et al., 2011; Tobin, 2021). However, not all post-traumatic play is the same.

Dynamic post-traumatic play. Just as everyday play holds growth-promoting qualities, *dynamic* post-traumatic play embodies a positive and natural reparative strategy. In dynamic post-traumatic play, a child repeats or replays the traumatic elements of an experience where negative emotions like anxiety and fear are released and mastery over the trauma occurs (Gil, 2017). Five-year-old Julie, who witnessed her mother's near-lethal Covid-19 experience, kept burying her dolly under the sofa pillows, saying, "She's not doing well." This was a line she probably overheard adults around her say euphemistically as they discussed Julie's mother's health status. Julie walked away from the sofa but kept returning to check on dolly. Julie placed a blanket, a baby bottle, and candy that looked like medicine/pills under the pillow with dolly. Julie would first run, then walk away from, and eventually hover around the sofa. After repeating this sequence countless times, Julie pulled out her dolly and announced, "She's okay and wants to play Candyland with me now." Julie propped dolly up in a small chair across from her, set up the Candyland game, and smiled ear to ear as she and dolly chatted about the game. Julie even won the game and consoled dolly that she'd probably win next time.

Julie needed to dynamically work through her fears and uncertainty about her mother's well-being. She gained mastery of this scary scenario by being the one in charge of putting dolly "away" or out of sight—in contrast to how others had not allowed Julie to see her mom. Through dynamic post-traumatic play, Julie also had a role in helping dolly recover even though dolly was not directly in her view or reach. Finally, Julie was able to resolve her fears about dolly not getting better as she joyfully engaged with her in the Candyland game. Julie's ability to beat dolly in the game seemed to reflect the security that dolly was no longer vulnerable and Julie could defeat her and still look forward to a rematch with healthy dolly.

Toxic post-traumatic play. By contrast, *toxic* post-traumatic play can be dissociative, lacks a here-and-now quality, and shows up as compulsive repetition of the traumatic elements, causing re-traumatization. Without direct intervention, there is little to no relief of negative affect or gaining of mastery or control over the trauma (Gil, 2017, pp. 12–13). The energy behind toxic post-traumatic play is painful and shame-based, leaving others who engage in the play feeling the same. My early work engaging in play therapy with traumatized child clients left me feeling lousy, drained, shell-shocked, confused, agitated, and holding a pit in my stomach. These somatosensory countertransferences in play with traumatized children also showed up in my traditional talk therapy experiences with traumatized adults. The resounding theme with traumatized clients of all ages was that trauma-induced ruptures had not been sufficiently or completely repaired. Consequently, the themes of trauma repeated and looped, which makes toxic post-traumatic play easier to identify.

Post-traumatic play can include any of the seven types of everyday play: attunement, object, social, metaphor/symbolic, pretend/imaginative, storytelling/narrative, and creative. Through the play, there is an effort toward mastery and undoing what has been done where "magically" one can change from victim to victimizer. As clients have shown or said, "It's better to hurt others or myself before I'm hurt," reflecting their control over being or causing hurt, rather than being the helpless victim. Let's now systematically look at examples of how the seven types of play can show up as toxic play.

Toxic post-traumatic attunement play can appear as conscious or unconscious sensorimotor misattunements. Three-year-old Henry, who had been neglected, struggled in sensorimotor ways with other children: he was unable to hold eye contact, touched them in ways that were either too hard or not firm enough, spoke inaudibly, and seemed to ignore others speaking to him. Other children learned to avoid Henry because he was so misattuned to them on the most basic levels of touch, sound, and sight.

An example of toxic post-traumatic object play was shown by Tanya, a 1½-year-old little girl whose father had repeatedly penetrated her digitally and with objects. Tanya's mother brought Tanya to her first session with her pet dog, Scooby. Tanya tried to penetrate Scooby's anus with her finger. She thought it was funny when Scooby tried to get away and she chased him, thinking this was "a game." Loyal Scooby, like Tanya, eventually became submissive to his loved human.

Toxic social post-traumatic play is commonly seen in different forms of social play like bullying where safety, cooperation, a sense of belonging, being seen and heard, are all violated intentionally. Ten-year-old Darron, whose alcoholic father shamed, mocked, and beat him up mercilessly during drinking binges, would pick on smaller boys at school, making fun of their athletic skills and saying, "You worthless piece of shit," "You don't know what you're doing," or "You suck."

Ernesto demonstrated toxic post-traumatic pretend and imaginative play when animating his superhero action figures Wonder Woman and Batman. He repeatedly made Batman scream at Wonder Woman, saying things like, "Why didn't you kill the Joker?" "You never get the job done right!" "I can't trust you!" Ernesto often made Batman throw Wonder Woman into walls or across the room. Ernesto was a witness to horrific domestic violence.

Toxic post-traumatic play that blends social, storytelling-narrative, and creative types is seen when 10-year-old Lola, one of eight children, spent time with her much beloved Uncle Gus. Ever since toddlerhood, Lola loved how Uncle Gus doted on her, telling her completely engrossing and interactive stories, and bought Lola her favorite snacks, forbidden by her parents. Lola was unaware that Gus's stories, attention, and provision of "secret treats" were mechanisms to groom her. Uncle Gus sprinkled in tickles and touches that ever so gradually pushed Lola's boundaries of physical comfort. He also cajoled Lola to tickle and touch him in return. If Lola didn't comply with his touches or requests to be touched, Gus would threaten to stop giving her the "secret treats" or storytelling, thereby stopping Lola from getting special attention and adoration. Storytelling had changed from a joy and intrigued-filled special bonding time between Lola and Uncle Gus, to a tool of manipulation whereby Gus used his power and control to exploit Lola's affections, loyalty, shame, and fears.

I share the example of Uncle Gus to demonstrate that while toxic post-traumatic play has been described in children, adults engage in it too. Adults externalize the pain and trauma of earlier losses, betrayals, bullying, and sexual and other abuses by perpetrating others and themselves in similar ways they were harmed. These post-traumatic play behaviors might have first appeared during childhood in games with friends, written stories, or doll-play. If inadvertently enabled, dismissed, or unresolved through therapy, this post-traumatic play may develop into sometimes criminal, retraumatizing behaviors. Toxic abusive and/or criminal adult behavior can be conceived as childhood toxic post-traumatic play grown up and run amuck.

Playful Is a State of Mind, a Spirit of Being

This chapter has defined play's universality and its different types that emerge across development. It has provided guideposts to help us discern the quality and quantity of play that slips us out of a zone of genuine playfulness into something questionable or possibly toxic and destructive. Most importantly, I hope this chapter has grown your appreciation that all of us can engage playfully in life and in therapy. Play is really a state of mind, a spirit, an attitude to bring to our life as a whole, and to our practice as healing professionals, more specifically. This playful spirit is enlivening and therapeutic. It's one of those things in life that not only tastes good but also is good for us! Playfulness is powerful.

The next two chapters will put to rest possible left brain–based skepticism that engaging a playful spirit is not academically grounded. We'll explore developmental, therapeutic, and trauma-related superpowers of play. You will learn how engaging your playful spirit makes scientific sense, is necessary in trauma healing and transformation specifically—and healing work in general—and is just plain fun and energizing.

References

Badenoch, B. & Kestly, T. A. (2014). Exploring the neuroscience of healing play at every age. In D. A. Crenshaw & A. L. Stewart (Eds.), *Play therapy: A comprehensive guide to theory and practice* (pp. 524–538). New York: Guilford.

Brown, S. (2008, May). Play is more than just fun. [Video] TED Talk. https://www.ted.com/talks/stuart_brown_play_is_more_than_just_fun?language=en

Brown, S. (2009). *Play: How it shapes the brain, opens the imagination, and invigorates the soul.* New York: Avery.

Brown, S. (2014). The consequences of play deprivation, *Scholarpedia, 9*(5), 30449.

Brown, S. & Eberle, M. (2018). A closer look at play. In T. Marks-Tarlow, M. Solomon, & D. Siegel (Eds.), *Play and creativity in psychotherapy* (pp. 21–38). New York: Norton.

Chapman, L. (2014). *Neurobiologically informed trauma therapy with children and adolescents: Understanding mechanisms of change.* New York: Norton.

Child Welfare Information Gateway (2015). *Understanding the effects of maltreatment on brain development.* Washington, DC: U.S. Department of health and Human Services, Children's Bureau.

Dana, D. (2020). *Polyvagal exercises for safety and connection: 50 client-centered practices.* New York: Norton.

Davis, K. L. & Montag, C. (2019). Selected principles of Pankseppian affective neuroscience. *Frontiers in Neuroscience, 17.* https://doi.org/10.3389/fnins.2018.01025

Edwards, D. (2016, June 23). Play and the feel good hormones. *Primal Play.* https://www.primalplay.com/blog/play-and-the-feel-good-hormones

Fosha, D. (2000). *The transforming power of affect: A model for accelerated change.* New York: Basic Books.

Gil, E. (2017). *Posttraumatic play in children: What clinicians need to know.* New York: Guilford.

Gray, P. (2013). *Free to learn: Why unleashing the instinct to play will make our children happier, more self-reliant, and better students for life.* New York: Basic Books.

Gross, S. (2018). The power of optimism. In T. Marks-Tarlow, M. Solomon, & D. J. Siegel, (Eds.), *Play and creativity in psychotherapy* (pp. 359–375). New York: Norton.

Kestly, T. (2018). A cross-cultural and cross-disciplinary perspective of play. In T. Marks-Tarlow, M. Solomon & D. Siegel (Eds.), *Play and creativity in psychotherapy* (pp. 110–127). New York: Norton.

Knipe, J. (2007). Loving eyes: Procedures to therapeutically reverse dissociative processes while preserving emotional safety. In C. Forgash & M. Copeley (Eds.), *Healing the heart of trauma and dissociation with EMDR and ego state therapy* (pp. 181–226). New York: Springer.

Krisch, J. A. (2018, January 24). Brilliant kids visit (and create) imaginary worlds. *Parenting: Fatherly.* https://www.fatherly.com/parenting/creative-children-imaginary-world-genius

Lohre, S. B. (2017). *Attune with baby: An innovative attunement program for parents and families with integrated evaluation.* [Dissertation Antioch University Seattle]. https://aura.antioch.edu/etds/350

Marks-Tarlow, T., Solomon, M., & Siegel, D. (Eds.) (2018). *Play and creativity in psychotherapy.* New York: Norton.

Martin, R. A. & Ford, T. E. (2018). *The psychology of humor: An integrative approach* (2nd ed.). San Diego, CA: Academic Press.

Myers, C. E., Bratton, S. C., Hagen, C., & Findling, J. H. (2011). Development of the Trauma Play Scale: Comparison of children manifesting a history of interpersonal trauma with a normative sample. *International Journal of Play Therapy, 20*(2), 66–78. https://doi.org/10.1037/a0022667

Ogden, P. & Fisher, J. (2007). The movements of play: Restoring spontaneity and flexibility in traumatized individuals. *Sensorimotor Psychotherapy Institute (SPI) Newsletter, 1*(1), 2–8.

Ohashi, K., Anderson, C. M., Bolger, E. A., Khan, A., McGreenery, C. E., & Teicher, M. H. (2019). Susceptibility or resilience to maltreatment can be explained by specific differences in brain network architecture. *Biological Psychiatry, 85*(8), 690–702. https://doi.org/10.1016/j.biopsych.2018.10.016

Panksepp, J. (1998). *Affective neuroscience: The foundation of human and animal emotions.* New York: Oxford University Press.

Panksepp, J. (2007). Can PLAY diminish ADHD and facilitate the construction of the social brain? *Journal of the Canadian Academy of Child and Adolescent Psychiatry, 16*(2), 57–66.

Panksepp, J. & Biven, L. (2012). *The archaeology of mind: Neuroevolutionary origins of human emotions.* New York: Norton.

Perry, B. D. (2006). The neurosequential model of therapeutics: Applying principles of neuroscience to clinical work with traumatized and maltreated children. In N. B. Webb (Ed.), *Working with traumatized youth in child welfare* (pp. 27–52). New York: Guilford.

Perry, B. D. (2014). The neurosequential model of therapeutics: Application of a developmentally sensitive and neurobiology-informed approach to clinical problem solving in maltreated children. In K. Brandt, B. D. Perry, S. Seligman, & E. Tronick (Eds.), *Infant and early childhood mental health: Core concepts and clinical practice* (pp. 21–53). Washington, DC: American Psychiatric Publishing.

Prendiville, E. & Howard, J. (Eds.) (2017). *Creative psychotherapy: Applying the principles of neurobiology to play and expressive arts-based practice.* New York: Routledge.

Resnick, M. (2007). *All I really need to know (about creative thinking) I learned (by studying how children learn) in kindergarten.* https://web.media.mit.edu/~mres/papers/kindergarten-learning-approach.pdf.

Root-Bernstein, M. (2014). *Inventing imaginary worlds: From childhood play to adult creativity across the arts and sciences.* Plymouth: Rowman & Littlefield Education.

Schaefer, C. E. & Drewes, A. A. (2014). The therapeutic powers of play and play therapy. In C. E. Schaefer & A. A. Drewes (Eds.), *The therapeutic powers of play: 20 core agents of change* (2nd ed., pp. 1–15). Hoboken, NJ: Wiley.

Schwartz, R. C. & Sweezy, M. (2020). *Internal Family Systems* (2nd ed.). New York: Guilford.

Skove, E. (2015, December 15). Teaching babies in the womb: How fetal experiences can impact your baby. *Motherly.* https://www.mother.ly/lifestyle/teaching-babies-in-the-womb

Siviy, S. M. (2016). A brain motivated to play: Insights into the neurobiology of playfulness. *Behaviour, 153*(6–7), 819–844.

Teicher, M. H. (2022, March 26). *Effects of childhood maltreatment on brain development and psychopathology.* Online presentation Resonance Summit: Harnessing the Healing Power of Connection.

Terr, L. (1981). Forbidden games: Post-traumatic child's play. *Journal of the American Academy of Child Psychiatry, 20,* 741–760.

Tobin, G. K. (2021). *Development of the Posttraumatic Play Screening.* [Dissertation, Georgia State University]. https://scholarworks.gsu.edu/cps_diss/153

Warner, E., Westcott, A, Cook, A., & Finn, H. (2020). *Transforming trauma in children and adolescents: An embodied approach to somatic regulation, trauma processing, and attachment-building.* Berkeley, CA: North Atlantic Books.

Wilson, M. (2020). *Creating attunement in utero: Dance/movement therapy for women who are incarcerated while pregnant.* [Thesis Lesley University]. https://digitalcommons.lesley.edu/expressive_theses/330/

Winnicott, D. W. (1960). Ego distortion in terms of true and false self. In D. W. Winnicott (Ed.), *The maturational processes and the facilitating environment: Studies in the theory of emotional development* (pp. 140–152). New York: International Universities Press.

Winnicott, D. W. (1989). *D. W. Winnicott: Psycho-analytic explorations* (C. Winnicott, R. Shepherd, & M. Davis, Eds.). Cambridge, MA: Harvard University Press.

Chapter 4

The Incredible Powers of Play

Play is truly incredible. It's not only fun and energizing; it's also packed with different and important functions that support our physical, emotional, and relational development throughout our lives. Alongside this, play has amazing therapeutic powers that promote healing, change, and growth in and out of therapy.

This chapter will explore these incredible developmental and therapeutic powers, or functions, that play holds for everyone. We can use this knowledge to guide our playful, therapeutic attitude to best attune to our traumatized clients and address their unmet developmental needs. Although this chapter is not prescriptive, it will give us the lay of the land of play's powers to inspire and inform our relational work with clients of all ages.

The Developmental Powers of Play

Play is absolutely essential for healthy growth and development. As Brown and Eberle poignantly state, "We are built to play, and built through PLAY" (Brown & Eberle, 2018, p. 38) referring to our wired-in PLAY circuitry (see Chapter 3). Play is nutritive helping our brain and mind grow (Gross, 2018; Kestly, 2014; Perry, 2006) at any age across our lifetime (Valkanova et al., 2014). Whenever we engage our PLAY circuitry alone, but especially with others, new neuronal connections and networks are established. This enables higher level cortical functions such as learning, memory, planning, organization, problem-solving, and innovation (Gross, 2018; Kestly, 2014; Pellis et al., 2014, p. 91; Perry et al., 2000). Additionally, the PLAY emotional-motivational system supports neural integration and neural organization (Kestly, 2014; Panksepp & Biven, 2012; Prendiville & Howard, 2017).

As trauma therapists, we need to keep in mind that clients with early trauma histories may not have fully benefitted from the developmental powers of play. Those who have suffered a lack of opportunities to play because of neglect, maltreatment, malnutrition, lack of stimulation, cultural values, or traumatic environments (e.g., war) have been shown to have impaired brain growth and development, deficits in emotional, social, cognitive, and behavioral areas of

DOI: 10.4324/9781003509493-7

functioning, and limited curiosity, learning, and exploration (Child Welfare Information Gateway, 2015; Pellis et al., 2014; Teicher et al., 2020). Being relationally attuned and playful with our traumatized clients gives them opportunities to fill in these gaps in all spheres of living.

We'll now explore how the seven types of play (discussed in Chapter 3) have powers to promote social, emotional, and cognitive growth at each stage of our development. The powers listed are not exhaustive, and future advances in neuroscience research will likely reveal yet-undiscovered ways play promotes our cognitive, emotional, and social development.

The Powers of Attunement Play

Attunement play is centered around "tuning in" to the baby using right brain–based sensorimotor language. Attunement refines the biological and/or contextual (e.g., adoption or fostering) attachment by promoting emotional bonding in relationship. Specifically, psychobiological attunement to the infant's internal states, not to their overt behaviors (Schore, 2019, p. 9), strengthens the caregiver-infant bond. When a caregiver attunes to their baby, brain waves (Schore, 2021), facial expressions and body postures (Chartrand & Bargh, 1999), hormones (Feldman et al., 2013, 2016), and heartbeat rhythms (Feldman et al., 2011) synchronize.

Communicating and playing with preverbal babies uses primary process language, such as body movement, posturing and gesturing, facial expression, voice inflection, sequence, rhythm, tone, and pitch of spoken words, with a strong reliance on visual-facial, auditory-prosodic, tactile-proprioceptive channels (Fisher, 2017; Prenn, 2011; Schore, 2021). Examples include a soft gaze, smiles, an open-mouthed "aaahhh" and "ooooh," clapping hands, and leaning in with interest. Primary process communications are replete with mirroring and imitative behaviors, as when adults with babies or with foreign-language speakers consciously and unconsciously match the tone, pitch, pacing, depth of emotion, and rhythm. Mirroring helps validate the other person, join with them, and be on the same page (Blum, 2015; Prenn, 2011). Primary process sensorimotor communication and mirroring comprise the language of attachment (Winnicott, 1971) and attunement.

Attunement play helps grow the bond between the infant and caregiver as it supports the baby to feel and be safe, seen, soothed, and secure (Siegel & Payne Bryson, 2020). These tenets of a secure attachment are practiced as the caregiver plays with the baby and repeatedly awaits cues—smiles, coos, bubble blowing, or babbling—to affirm their baby is engaged, regulated, and enjoying their connection. Attunement play helps caregivers learn what fits the baby's regulatory and attachment needs, enabling them to earn the title "good enough mother (or caregiver)" (Winnicott, 1971). Consequently, caregivers feel, and are, effective and protective which regulates their nervous systems, too.

The interactive, relational practices of attunement play exercise autonomic nervous system (ANS) co-regulation as the caregiver and infant move together to calm/downregulate or energize/upregulate activation (Badenoch & Kestly, 2014; Dana, 2018; Gil, 2017; Marks-Tarlow, 2012). Across development and practiced through all subsequent types of play, this co-regulatory dance helps the baby learn to self-regulate and soothe. In turn, self-regulation and affect tolerance grow, which increases self-worth, resilience, inquisitive and explorative capacities, and promotes a healthier internal working model (Bowlby, 1969). Attunement play lays the foundation for reciprocal, attuned socialization, empathy, mentalization, and intersubjectivity (Kestly, 2014; Marks-Tarlow et al., 2018) and promotes feeling important and valued, and a sense of belonging.

The Powers of Sensorimotor Play

Sensorimotor play—which includes body movement and sensation—lays building blocks for social and emotional abilities, such as reading others' body language and communicating. Caregivers teach babies to wave, give high fives, or clap to encourage babies to interact with others. Some parents teach babies sign language to encourage meaningful and intentional communication of needs like hunger or thirst. As the infant grows, they purposefully learn body language— eye gazing, facial gestures, touching, pointing, pushing, pulling, reaching, grasping, yielding—to communicate their needs or wants, get support, and establish boundaries.

As babies grow into children, sensorimotor play supports coordination, balance, fine motor skills (e.g., pouring or drawing), gross motor skills (e.g., throwing or running), and spatial awareness of themselves in relationship to the world around them. Sensorimotor play can be expressed in solitude as children explore their own bodies visually or through smell, taste, and touch (like self-soothing or stimulation), helping them gain a sense of their physical boundaries and sensory comfort and preferences. It also helps build skills underlying cognitive development like eye coordination for reading, eye-hand coordination for writing and typing, and their integration for athletics, playing music, dancing, and working with others. Engaging in sensorimotor play also promotes overall fitness.

The Powers of Object Play

Object play serves a myriad of developmental roles. It helps children learn the function of objects, how to develop and use tools, and problem-solve. Therefore, it's sometimes called "functional play" (Smilansky & Shefatya, 2004). Before 6 months of age, when little ones cannot yet successfully grasp and manipulate objects, they observe others to learn about their uses and functions. After 6 months, when babies and children play freely with objects, they find new and different uses for them. This is a part of creative play. Adults who bend the rules about objects may find new and creative uses for them, and this flexibility can help adults problem-solve. Without a hammer, we might think to use a boot or a block to put a nail in the wall. The ability to use an object in non-conventional ways is a form of symbolic play and has adaptive functions throughout life. Those on the autism spectrum may lack this developmental skill (Lee et al., 2021).

Object play also helps 4–12-month-olds learn object permanence—the concept that a concrete object isn't actually gone when it can't be seen, touched, or sensed. Caregivers hide an object in a box or a under cloth and a baby learns to find it. This is precursor to the hide-and-seek game, which requires a little one to move and hide their own body or objects out of others' view so they can be searched for and found. Object permanence is a developmental milestone that underlies and leads to the emergence of object constancy (from ages 2 to 3).

Object constancy refers to the child's ability to understand that the emotional connection with their caregiver remains intact even when out of sight. It also refers to the child's capacity to have positive, loving feelings toward the caregiver even if they behaved in unsatisfying ways to the child (or vice versa). This is an internalized sense of emotional permanence and constancy that enables the child to hold both the positive and negative sides of an attachment—which is of paramount importance during social play. Object constancy enables a child to experience a stable and intact emotional attachment, preventing feelings of abandonment despite setbacks, disagreements, and conflicts. Separation anxiety, which develops around 6 to 8 months, is related to mastering the object constancy milestone. Problems with separation in later years (after age 3) may point to clients' unresolved object constancy issues.

Object play also ushers in the use of a transitional object. This is an object that provides soothing and security to a little one, allowing them to shift from their caregiver as a primary source of soothing to an object they can control. With a secure transitional object base, little ones and sometimes adults (e.g., college-bound teenagers or adults moving to a new home) can feel safe, comfortable, and regulated enough to explore, learn, and grow with curiosity. Drawing from attunement and sensorimotor play, little ones use sensory cues (i.e., touch/sensation/texture, taste, sound, sight, and scent) to explore and choose which object will serve this important role. The toddler's independent exercise of personal choice, responsibility, and control is a huge developmental accomplishment. They choose what their preferred comfort object will be, take responsibility to access it, and manipulate the object (e.g., stroking, sniffing, squeezing, hugging, and kissing) to regulate their nervous system.

Transitional objects may also function as objects of play. They offer comfort, joy, and delight, promote curiosity in their own right, and provide a secure base to help little ones explore their world. A toddler might grab their blankie, hug it, nap with it, and drag it alongside as they walk. Minutes later, they might ask their mommy to make it into a cape to help them fly around the house. An adult might have a Hamsa (a symbolic hand-shaped amulet) which they wear as jewelry and play with in their hand or put by their mouth to soothe.

Object play simultaneously nurtures the child's receptive and expressive language skills. Caregivers make dolls or puppets "talk" and encourage their child to talk back and grow their expressive vocabulary. Caregivers may creatively use their hand, a block, or a banana to teach communication. For example, a father might say, "Hello. You want to speak with Shayna? Hold on, here she is," handing the banana to Shayna.

Through object play, adults teach little ones the basics of social cooperation through turn-taking, sharing, and reciprocity even before the toddler formally engages in social play with peers. Object play offers toddlers opportunities to learn social etiquette like saying "please" and "thank you" and lays the groundwork for social interactions like taking turns around coveted objects, like a colorful dinosaur.

Object play helps develop physical strength, balance, and coordination. Formal and informal toys encourage skills like pushing (e.g., a mini shopping cart, lawnmower that blows bubbles), pulling (e.g., a wagon or wooden dog on a string), or self-propelled movement (e.g., crawling through a cardboard tunnel or climbing onto a big pillow tower and jumping off). Object play also encourages fine and gross motor development, eye-hand coordination, depth perception, and spatial awareness through using art supplies and everyday objects in nature (e.g., rocks or leaves) or at home (e.g., tissues or dried pasta).

The Powers of Social Play

Each type of social play serves different purposes to help the growing child navigate their relationships.

Parallel play. In parallel play, toddlers play side by side and do not interact with or influence others. They are content in their solo play while tolerating others' presence, as seen when two children build towers side by side, unaffected by the other's activity. Caregivers hold important roles to lay the foundation for empathy and mentalization as they repetitively supervise and guide toddlers to practice turn-taking, sharing, and cooperation. At this stage of social play, caregivers soothe the toddler's hurts and helplessness when their playmate plays unfairly (e.g., doesn't share or takes, hides, or breaks their toy) or does not listen to them. Caregivers validate and soothe, while modeling and assisting the little child to repair social and emotional ruptures. Caregivers also teach toddlers how to develop boundaries, guiding them to leave their favorite object or toy (e.g., their blankie or race car) in a safe place to not lose it and to prevent others from taking or breaking it.

Associative play. Children engaged in associative play show interest in others and their play and use early forms of socializing. For example, a child will notice their peer building an impressively tall tower of blocks and start to build their own tall tower. As the skills of sharing space, respecting boundaries, and cooperation evolve, caregivers still supervise and guide but can become less involved. At this stage, caregivers may not intervene directly but review the skill sets to help the child soothe themselves, repair ruptures, and establish/ re-establish boundaries in their play with others. If the child's efforts fall short, the caregiver encourages them in the presence of their playmate. If the child's efforts are still ineffective, the caregiver may take charge to resolve the social and emotional dysregulation and rupture.

Cooperative play. Cooperative social play further develops turn-taking, reciprocity, healthy boundaries, empathy, mentalization, trust, and social norms as children work together collaboratively to strategize and problem-solve. These interpersonal skills promote lifelong success in relationships with friends, co-workers, teammates, and family members.

Cooperative play further enhances communication as children listen to and learn from their peers and adults, expand their vocabulary, and refine their articulation to be better understood. Communication skills grow more when children at this stage of social play development guide younger (i.e., 2-year-old) children how to play and follow rules of simple board games or sports. By participating in organized and unstructured small and large group play, kids learn to speak in ways they are seen and heard and reciprocate the same with others—a very important lifelong skill.

Cooperative social play from elementary school years onward promotes strategic problem-solving, especially in sports. For example, in a game of kickball, children will discuss where the weakest defense is and try to kick the ball in that direction, hoping to get someone on base or score a run. As children play cooperatively, they learn to collaboratively evaluate risks and assess each player's strengths and weaknesses to increase their chances of winning the game. Cooperative play, like kickball, integrates learning and following rules, developing sportsmanship, and the ability to compromise and resolve conflicts (e.g., a bad call by the umpire, an unfair lineup change by the coach, or an opposing team's intimidation tactics).

Children learn to collaborate, cooperate, and develop independent skill mastery and interdependence in noncompetitive cooperative play. For example, when dancing *The Nutcracker*, one's mastery of the dance techniques, timing of movements, and sharing the stage (e.g., not upstaging others) affects the other dancers and vice versa. Holding awareness of how our behavior affects others is an essential social skill for appropriate responsibility-taking. Cooperative play also helps empathy develop as children learn to recognize and respond to others' feelings and perspectives, show affection, and offer support and care to others.

In summary, social play helps build pro-social brains, allowing us to interact, cooperate, share, respond appropriately, develop and navigate complex social systems and power hierarchies, and practice aggression and submissiveness

(Panksepp & Biven, 2012; Pellis et al., 2014). Through social play, we role-play, develop, and practice new skills and competencies, and develop mastery, which enhance survival and offer trauma survivors new ways to cope and thrive.

The Powers of Imaginative and Pretend Play

Imaginative and pretend play emerges early and continues through life. We'll briefly examine solitary and social forms of pretend play and how they support growth.

In solitary pretend play with an imaginary friend, children experiment with social and emotional skills like empathizing, noticing and supporting others' needs and preferences, appreciating similarities (e.g., "he's just like me") and welcoming differences, negotiating conflicts, and acting politely. Play with imaginary friends helps children develop language skills, enhance school performance (Fahmy, 2009), and problem-solve.

Daydreaming helps us imagine real-life situations for which we lack experience and make up stories that parallel them to fill in the gaps. When we imagine situations, we trigger our mirror neurons (discussed in Chapter 8) to fire, which help us feel the emotions and sensations "as if" we are engaging in the actual activity (Agnati et al., 2013). Daydreaming gives us practice to understand and process information and complex emotions, organize strategies to handle imagined events, and self-reflect (Singer & Singer, 1990). Daydreaming in children is associated with better creativity, healthy social adjustment, and good school performance. It's an antidote to boredom and an alternative to socializing (Singer & Singer, 1990) with real others. Too much daydreaming, however, can lead to isolation and/or difficulties dealing with the challenges of real life and people.

Whether solitary or with others, reality or fantasy-based, imaginative and pretend play allows people of all ages to experiment with new experiences, broaden their horizons, and develop a more context-based way of communicating. Particularly, in reality-based imaginative play, children gain familiarity with novel or scary situations that may arise (e.g., their first day of school) and rehearse solutions to everyday and possible problems which can calm anxieties. Through pretend play, children create memories and images which they can access when similar real-life scenarios emerge. Pretend play helps kids gain understanding of science, the world in which they live, and important world events.

Imaginary and pretend play supports children to grow language and communication skills. They build their vocabulary in context- and situation-relevant ways to better express their comfort levels and needs in ways they are heard and understood. Particularly when playing pretend with others, children learn the how different people may react differently to the same words and play themes. Kids subsequently gain experience repairing ruptures, speaking and acting in more thoughtful and attuned ways, and tailoring their behavior to the context and people they are with. This experience helps kids and grown-ups become cognitively and socially flexible and develop compassion and mentalization skills.

Physical pretend play aids the coordination of gross and fine motor skills and physical fitness. For example, as children act like firefighters, they climb up and down ladders, zip down poles, and swish down slides all while holding a garden hose and directing water at a target. Playing dress up or dressing up dolls helps children grow their hand-to-eye coordination as they zip, button, roll up sleeves and pant legs, and fold and unfold clothes and costumes. Physical pretend free play also teaches children how to safely engage in rough and tumble. For example, when two children become villains and fight each other to achieve world domination, they are supporting frontal lobe development, which helps them self-regulate behaviors, put a check on impulses, discern boundaries of physical safety, and differentiate fantasy from reality.

The creativity and inventiveness that spring out of all types of imaginative and pretend play enhance the growth of children's and adult's self-esteem, confidence, and self-awareness as they safely experiment with and test boundaries of what is possible. In pretend play, anyone can be anything they want to be; in the world of imagination, anything is possible, and dreams can come true. These become freeing and empowering metaphors for each of us to continue guiding our exploration, imagination, curiosity, and creativity.

The Powers of Storytelling and Narrative Play

When caregivers read or tell stories to preverbal babies, they use attunement and sensorimotor play to help develop receptive and expressive language skills and an interest in reading and storytelling. At this stage, storytelling can occur through books that are highly visual (vivid and contrasting colors), tactile (soft, rough, smooth, and hard pages), and auditory (crinkly, squeaky, rhythmic, and melodic). Narrative play with babies is heavily relational, animated, and mainly driven by the teller to connect and entertain.

As we grow older, we still enjoy others telling us stories. Favorite past-times for some include sitting at their grandparent's side and learning about what their parents were like as little kids. Sitting around a campfire and hearing scary stories is a treat for many. Adults love being told stories through movies or TV series. The vast imaginative and pretend play elements woven into plots are entertaining and sometimes suspenseful, causing some to binge many episodes in one sitting. While it lacks the direct relational bonding element babies derive from being told stories, watching shows with others or discussing them brings connection and commonality. People of all ages love being entertained and transported to different times and places through story.

Three-year-olds can learn the basic elements—the beginning, middle, and end—of storytelling. Little children can develop simple themes, characters, setting, point of view, plot, conflict, and resolution. Storytelling builds expressive language, communication, and grammar skills. As children grow, their characters become more complex and have internal and external conflicts. Plots become more elaborate, nuanced, and laced with conflicts that shift from concrete (e.g., finding the lost puppy) to abstract (e.g., morality). Storytellers play with dramatic action and pacing, the use of symbolism, metaphors, suspense, mystery, intrigue, horror, and humor, to name a few. Storytelling-narrative play helps people distinguish fantasy from reality, grow symbolic and metaphorical communication, and understand themselves and how others live and solve problems.

Storytelling-narrative play continues throughout life and, with practice, can become increasingly creative, engaging, and parlayed into a writing and speaking career. Storytelling-narrative play also can be nonverbal even in adulthood. This may include, but is not limited to, performing music, dance, painting, sand play, clay sculpting, or drawing. In fact, through expressive arts therapies, people tell stories, narrate and figure out solutions to their problems, work through trauma, and express themselves, their needs, and their identity (Malchiodi, 2023). Themes and narratives emerge from nondirective play in the ways objects are used or the body moves. These nonverbal expressions hold meaningful metaphors to guide therapeutic work.

Part of storytelling-narrative play is world play (see Chapter 3), in which the participant develops a complex and deeply felt relationship with their subjective universe. This relationship enhances the ability to empathize and mentalize, think integratively, plan, organize, problem-solve, and analyze complexity. World players engage in cognitive and aesthetic exercises relevant to lifelong creativity (Root-Bernstein, 2013). The creation of a soothing alternative reality can serve as a great escape from real-life pain.

Humor, another wing of storytelling-narrative play, has regulating and dysregulating effects on our nervous system. In physical or slapstick humor, there are both. As we witness someone else become physically vulnerable, perhaps while watching *America's Funniest Home Videos*, our anticipation builds as we wonder what might happen to them. This activation is followed by a release as we laugh and shout, "Oh no!" or, "Ouch!" We may even find ourselves feeling empathic and inadvertently protect the body parts that the witnessed victim injured. In this way, we are developing our interoceptive empathic connection through attunement and mirroring (discussed further in Chapter 8).

Humor can also lower the emotional, physiological, cognitive, and spiritual discomfort of the most horrific traumas. Viktor Frankl, a Holocaust survivor of Auschwitz, said humor served as one of the "soul's weapons" he and others used to transcend despair and fight for preservation (Frankl, 1959, p. 43). Similarly, gallows and black humor can serve as "an index of strength or morale on the part of oppressed peoples" (Force, 2016). It reflects resilience and hope in the soothing of deep suffering. An adult, who as a child experienced chronic abandonments by his parents, shared this gallows humor example: "Today I decided to go visit my childhood home. I asked the residents if I could come inside because I was feeling nostalgic, but they refused and slammed the door in my face. My parents are the worst."

Humor can also raise autonomic dysregulation, emotional discomfort, and even violate boundaries of appropriateness. Because of this, the humorist—whether comedian or therapist—must be aware of their audience to determine how their jokes will land. They must also be evaluative, empathic, and practice mentalization.

Finally, humor can be used in therapy to lessen defenses and promote resiliency. It can strengthen the therapeutic alliance by fostering a sense of trust and belonging, make the therapist seem more "real," and cause change through right brain-to-right brain relational implicit knowing (Valentine & Gabbard, 2014). Appropriately timed and boundaried humor can shift regulatory edges of comfort, help clients laugh about topics that previously evoked tension and tears, and release tension.

The Powers of Creative Play

In early childhood, when little ones are supported to be safely explorative, they play creatively and learn about familiar and new objects, relationships, roles, their world, and new and unusual ways to engage all these categories. In early adolescence, creative play is infused with theoretical, hypothetical, and counterfactual thinking, abstract logic and reasoning, strategizing, planning, and applying concepts across situations and contexts. Limitless possibilities and novel ideas appear that promote functioning, solutions, and progress. Creative play helps us take risks and express ourselves in new ways. It helps us handle dialectics and paradoxes, like learning to follow the rules while finding ways to improvise or use our imagination (British Council, 2021). When resolving dialectics using creative play, functionally diverse brain regions are activated, synergistically integrating their functions (Brown, 2009) and facilitating divergent thinking processes (Bateson, 2014).

Through creative role-playing at any age, we practice taking on new identities. A child can play dress up and act like mommy going to work, while an adult can play dress up in a Broadway play or in sex play with their partner. Through role-play, we develop empathy, compassion, understanding for the person we are trying to be, and expand our identity. This is what method actors do when immersing themselves in a role; they creatively try on another identity by living the way the character would in how they eat, sleep, dress, move, etc. When teenagers dress, talk, walk, and sing like their favorite singer or actor, they are expanding their identifications and imagination and experimenting with trying on their future self.

We can engage in creative play through sexual and erotic exploration. Sex play refers to healthy sexual behaviors which involve private parts (i.e., genitals, breasts, buttocks) and are appropriately boundaried and exploratory, starting in childhood/adolescence continuing throughout adulthood. When sex is playful, it is creative—it embodies a free, spontaneous, explorative, curious quality. It can bring physiological arousal, release, and laughter, and we want to engage in it again and again. Creative sex play can include all developmental play types: attunement, body and movement, object play (e.g., sex toys), social play or solitary play (as in masturbation), imaginative or pretend and storytelling/narrative (as when people include "dress up" and role-play). We can creatively play in sexual ways that are implicit or explicit. An implicit, symbolic form is when we text someone a squirting eggplant or peach emoji. A verbal form that includes metaphor and innuendo is when we say, "It feels so hot in here. I'm getting wet and sweaty." Attunement play is one of the hallmarks of what makes sex play healthy and normative as opposed to unhealthy or abusive (which will be explored in the next section). Creative sex play can have rules, as in BDSM where people consensually experiment with control and power, role-play, and fantasy around themes of bondage and discipline, dominance and submission, sadism and masochism.

In sum, when we engage creative play, we embody the spirit of play. We lean into and borrow from all developmental types of play and their powers, enabling growth in all areas of life.

Play's Therapeutic Powers for Clients of All Ages

In addition to promoting healthy development across all spheres of life and living, play offers a wide array of powers therapists can mine to be holistically helpful to clients of all ages.

Playful Relationships Promote Safety and Resiliency

All of us can relate to how the presence of a consistent, accessible, unconditionally nurturing, loving, and supportive other provides refuge in a world filled with trauma and isolation. Clients have shared how playing in these relationships made a lifelong impression that elevated their joy, warmth, and reassurance. They felt held and protected while bubbled in a safe world with a caring, playful other. Some of my clients' playful memories include cooking with their grandmother; sitting and listening to stories on their grandfather's lap; shooting hoops at the Boys and Girls Club with older peers; stroking their dog for hours; or being listened to and talking about their future dreams with their babysitter. Clients explained how these loving, playful relationships helped "get them through" dark, hopeless, helpless, and pain-filled years.

Protective playful relationships can also mitigate the effects of trauma. In a study of adults who experienced four or more adverse childhood experiences, negative outcomes to their well-being were prevented and mitigated due to engaging in play and expressive arts in the context of nurturing relationships

(Pliske et al., 2021). Specifically, these supportive and nurturing relationships were with adult community members (e.g., teachers, coaches, or spiritual/religious mentors), not mental health professionals. The participants used play for stress management, self-expression, catharsis, abreaction, indirect learning and teaching through metaphor, self-esteem, creative problem-solving, positive and multifaceted identity formation, gaining a sense of control, and experiencing positive emotions (Pliske et al., 2021, p. 255). In the context of safe relationships, "the therapeutic powers of play provided a gateway to effect change" or "posttraumatic growth" (Pliske et al., 2021, p. 255).

Play also promotes resiliency. Because play includes a certain randomness and uncertainty, it creates opportunities to reinforce successful ways of relating and problem-solving and expands coping skills (Seymour, 2015, p. 35). Being playful increases creativity, imagination, intuition, and thinking out of the box and allows us to envision a future different from the present or past (Malchiodi, 2023), which is the "essence of resilience" (Marks-Tarlow et al., 2018, p. 156). Play helps our nervous system become resilient (Kestly, 2018, pp. 124–126) as we learn to deal with activated sympathetic nervous system and parasympathetic dorsal vagal ANS states in the context of safe connection or ventral vagal states (see Chapter 2). Play helps us embody the three tenets underlying the definition of resiliency, including the ability to (1) adapt flexibly to change; (2) connect socially or bond, which manages stress, provides protection, and allows collaboration; and (3) make meaning of suffering (Feldman, 2020, pp. 135–137). Through play, particularly with others, we grow and deepen our sense of self and agency to confidently manage what life sends our way.

Play Has Healing Powers for Clients of All Ages

It is encouraging to know that all safe playful relationships can be protective while promoting well-being and resiliency. As healing professionals, it is also affirming to learn that play has *healing* powers, powers that function as the agents and mechanisms underlying change and transformation (Drewes & Schaefer, 2016; Gil, 1991, 2010; Peabody & Schaefer, 2019; Schaefer, 1993; Schaefer & Drewes, 2014). Schaefer and Drewes (2014) defined 20 therapeutic or healing powers of play and further classified them into four categories based on the treatment goals they support which include fostering emotional wellness, enhancing social relationships, increasing personal strengths, and facilitating communication. Figure 4.1 summarizes Schaefer & Drewes' (2014) findings by showing which therapeutic power of play supports each treatment goal.

In therapy, these reparative or therapeutic play powers can:

1. Help change client's dysfunctional thoughts, feelings, and/or behaviors (Peabody & Schaefer, 2019);

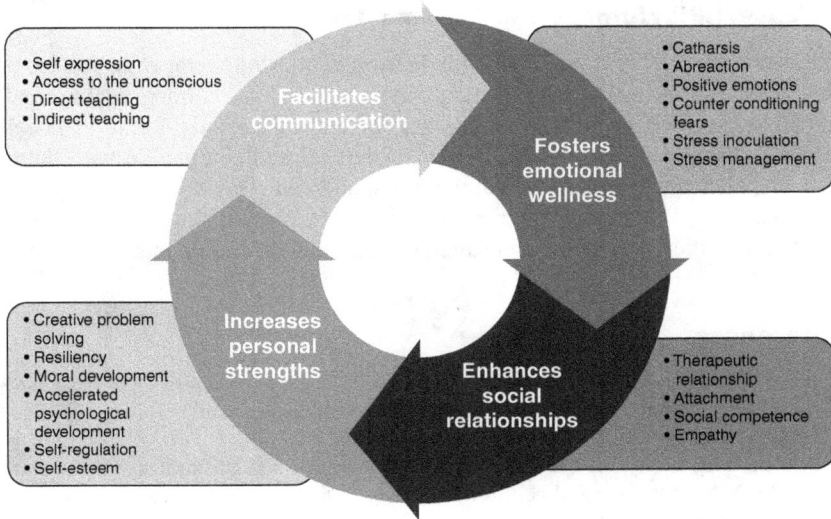

- Self expression
- Access to the unconscious
- Direct teaching
- Indirect teaching

Facilitates communication

Fosters emotional wellness

- Catharsis
- Abreaction
- Positive emotions
- Counter conditioning fears
- Stress inoculation
- Stress management

- Creative problem solving
- Resiliency
- Moral development
- Accelerated psychological development
- Self-regulation
- Self-esteem

Increases personal strengths

Enhances social relationships

- Therapeutic relationship
- Attachment
- Social competence
- Empathy

Figure 4.1 The 20 therapeutic powers of play. Graphic adapted and reprinted with permission from the Association for Play Therapy, *Play Therapy*™, *14*(3) from the September 2019 issue. Original graphic from Dr. Judi Parson, Deakin University, Melbourne, Australia.

2. Initiate, facilitate, or strengthen the therapeutic effect (Drewes & Schaefer, 2016, p. 36; Shen & Masek, 2023); and
3. Lead to positive treatment outcomes (Peabody & Schaefer, 2019, p. 5).

Whether acting as the agent of change in and of itself (Schaefer & Drewes, 2014, p. 2; Shen et al., 2023) or as a nonspecific factor in therapeutic effectiveness (Marks-Tarlow, 2012, p. 352), play is powerful.

While play's mechanisms of therapeutic change are often discussed in relation to play therapy with children, many authors support play's relevance and efficacy in treating adults (Badenboch & Kestly, 2014; Fisher, 2017; Homeyer & Morrison, 2008; Malchiodi, 2023; Marks-Tarlow, 2012; Marks-Tarlow et al., 2018; Olson-Morrison, 2017; Schaefer, 2003; Shen & Masek, 2023). Across the life cycle, playing naturally maintains emotional balance and connection with others (Seymour, 2016, p. 12), which is especially relevant for the therapist-client relationship. We can tap into the therapeutic powers of play with clients across the age spectrum as part of myriad treatment modalities while working through a lens of many theories.

A Teaser: Playfulness and Trauma Treatment

In this chapter, we've learned how the developmental and therapeutic powers of play are numerous and vast, reaching across age, ability, culture, background, and all levels of cognitive, emotional, and physical functioning. Relational healing work using playfulness also is transtheoretical and compatible with therapists and clients who are open to dipping into and exploring their creativity. The next chapter will convince any reader who is still skeptical how the powers of play are specifically relevant and suited to treat trauma with clients of all ages.

References

Agnati, L. F., Guidolin, D., Battistin, L., Pagnoni, G., & Fuxe, K. (2013). The neurobiology of imagination: Possible role of interaction-dominant dynamics and default mode network. *Frontiers in Psychology, 4,* Article 296, 1–17.

Badenoch, B. & Kestly, T. A. (2014). Exploring the neuroscience of healing play at every age. In D. A. Crenshaw & A. L. Stewart (Eds.), *Play therapy: A comprehensive guide to theory and practice* (pp. 524–538). New York: the Guilford Press.

Bateson, P. (2014). Play, playfulness, creativity and innovation. *Animal Behavior and Cognition, 1*(2), 99–112.

Blum, M. C. (2015). Embodied mirroring: A relational, body-to-body technique promoting movement in therapy. *Journal of Psychotherapy Integration, 25*(2), 115–127.

Bowlby, J. (1969). *Attachment: Attachment and loss* (Vol. 1). New York: Basic Books.

British Council (2021). *Defining creative play: Literature review, part 2 of 3.* https://www.britishcouncil.org/programmes/creative-play/defining-creative-play-literature-review-part-2

Brown, S. (2009). *Play: How it shapes the brain, opens the imagination, and invigorates the soul.* New York: Avery.

Brown, S. & Eberle, M. (2018). A closer look at play. In T. Marks-Tarlow, M. Solomon, & D. Siegel (Eds.), *Play and creativity in psychotherapy* (pp. 21–38). New York: Norton.

Chartrand, T. L. & Bargh, J. A. (1999). The chameleon effect: The perception-behavior link and social interaction. *Journal of Personality and Social Psychology, 76*(6), 893–910.

Child Welfare Information Gateway (2015). *Understanding the effects of maltreatment on brain development.* Washington, DC: U.S. Department of health and Human Services, Children's Bureau.

Dana, D. (2018). *The polyvagal theory in therapy: Engaging the rhythm of regulation.* New York: Norton.

Drewes, A. A. & Schaefer, C. E. (2016). The therapeutic powers of play. In K. J. O'Connor, C. E. Schaefer, & L. D. Braverman (Eds.), *Handbook of play therapy* (2nd ed.) (pp. 35–62). Hoboken, NJ: John Wiley.

Fahmy, M. (2009 August, 12). *Make-believe friends make kids' language skills better: Study.* Reuters.com. https://www.reuters.com/article/lifestyleMolt/idUSTRE57B1UB20090812

Feldman, R. (2020). What is resilience: An affiliative neuroscience approach. *World Psychiatry, 19*(2), 132–150.

Feldman, R., Gordon, I., Influs, M., Gutbir, T., & Ebstein, R. P. (2013). Parental oxytocin and early caregiving jointly shape children's oxytocin response and social reciprocity. *Neuropsychopharmacology, 37*(8), 1154–1162.

Feldman, R., Magori-Cohen, R., Galili, G., Singer, M., & Louzoun, Y. (2011). Mother and infant coordinate heart rhythms through episodes of interaction synchrony. *Infant Behavior & Development, 34*(4), 569–577. https://doi.org/10.1016/j.infbeh.2011.06.008

Feldman, R., Monakhov, M., Pratt, M., & Ebstein, R. P. (2016). Oxytocin pathway genes: Evolutionary ancient system impacting on human affiliation, sociality, and psychopathology. *Biological Psychiatry, 79*(3), 174–184. https://doi.org/10.1016/j.biopsych.2015.08.008

Fisher, J. (2017). *Healing the fragmented selves of trauma survivors: Overcoming self-alienation.* New York: Routledge.

Force, N. (2016, May 17). *Humor as weapon, shield and psychological salve.* PsychCentral. https://psychcentral.com/lib/humor-as-weapon-shield-and-psychological-salve

Frankl, V. E. (1959). *Man's search for meaning.* Boston, MA: Beacon Press.

Gil, E. (1991). *The healing power of play: Working with abused children.* New York: Guilford.

Gil, E. (2010). *Working with children to heal interpersonal trauma: The power of play.* New York: Guilford.

Gil, E. (2017). *Posttraumatic play in children: What clinicians need to know.* New York: Guilford.

Gross, S. (2018). The power of optimism. In T. Marks-Tarlow, M. Solomon, & D. J. Siegel (Eds.), *Play and creativity in psychotherapy* (pp. 359–375). New York: Norton.

Kestly, T. (2018). A cross-cultural and cross-disciplinary perspective of play. In T. Marks-Tarlow, M. Solomon, & D. Siegel (Eds.), *Play and creativity in* psychotherapy (pp. 110–127). New York: Norton.

Kestly, T. A. (2014). *The interpersonal neurobiology of play: Brain-building interventions for emotional well-being.* New York: Norton.

Lee, G. T., Qu, K., Hu, X., Jin, N., & Huang, J. (2021). Arranging play activities with missing items to increase object-substitution symbolic play in children with autism spectrum disorder. *Disability and Rehabilitation, 43*(22), 3199–3211. https://doi.org/10.1080/09638288.2020.1734107

Malchiodi, C. A. (Ed.) (2023). *Handbook of expressive arts therapy.* New York: Guilford.

Marks-Tarlow, T. (2012). The play of psychotherapy. *American Journal of Play, 4*(3), 352–377.

Marks-Tarlow, T., Solomon, M., & Siegel, D. (Eds.) (2018). *Play and creativity in psychotherapy.* New York: Norton.

Olson-Morrison, D. (2017). Integrative play therapy with adults with complex trauma: A developmentally-informed approach. *International Journal of Play Therapy, 26*(3), 172–183.

Panksepp, J. & Biven, L. (2012). *The archaeology of mind: Neuroevolutionary origins of human emotions.* New York: Norton.

Peabody, M. A. & Schaefer, C. E. (2019). The therapeutic powers of play: The heart and soul of play therapy. *Playtherapy*, *14*(3), 4–6.

Pellis, S. M., Pellis, V. C., & Himmler, B. T. (2014). How play makes for a more adaptable brain: A comparable and neural perspective. *American Journal of Play*, *7*(1), 73–98.

Perry, B. D. (2006). The neurosequential model of therapeutics: Applying principles of neuroscience to clinical work with traumatized and maltreated children. In N. B. Webb (Ed.), *Working with traumatized youth in child welfare* (pp. 27–52). New York: Guilford.

Perry, B. D., Hogan, L., & Marlin, S. J. (2000). Curiosity, pleasure and play: A neurodevelopmental perspective. *Advocate*, *9*, 9–12.

Pliske, M. M., Stauffer, S. D., & Werner-Lin, A. (2021). Healing from adverse childhood experiences through therapeutic powers of play: "I can do it with my hands". *International Journal of Play Therapy*, *30*(4), 244–258.

Prendiville, E. & Howard, J. (Eds.) (2017). *Creative psychotherapy: Applying the principles of neurobiology to play and expressive arts-based practice*. New York: Routledge.

Prenn, N. (2011). Mind the gap: AEDP interventions translating attachment theory into clinical practice. *Journal of Psychotherapy Integration*, *21*(3), 308–329.

Root-Bernstein, M. (2013). Worldplay as creative practice and educational strategy. In L. Book & D. P. Phillips (Eds.), *Creativity and entrpreneurship: Changing currents in education and public-life* (pp. 55–65). Cheltenham: Edward Elgar Publishing.

Schaefer, C. E. (2003). *Play therapy with adults*. Hoboken, NJ: John Wiley.

Schaefer, C. E. (Ed.) (1993). *The therapeutic powers of play*. Northvale, NJ: Jason Aronson.

Schaefer, C. E. & Drewes, A. A. (2014). *The therapeutic powers of play: 20 core agents of change* (2nd ed.). Hoboken, NJ: John Wiley.

Schore, A. N. (2021). The interpersonal neurobiology of intersubjectivity. *Frontiers in Psychology*, *12*, Article 648616. https://www.frontiersin.org/journals/psychology/articles/10.3389/fpsyg.2021.648616/full

Schore, A. N. (2019). *The development of the unconscious mind*. New York: Norton.

Seymour, J. W. (2015). Resilience-enhancing factors in play therapy. In D. A. Crenshaw, R. Brooks, & S. Goldstein (Eds.), *Play therapy interventions to enhance resilience (creative arts and play therapy)* (pp. 32–51). New York: Guilford.

Seymour, J. W. (2016). An introduction to the field of play therapy. In K. J. O'Connor, C. E. Schaefer, & L. D. Braverman (Eds.), *Handbook of play therapy* (2nd ed., pp. 3–15). Hoboken, NJ: John Wiley.

Shen, X. & Masek, L. (2023). The playful mediator, moderator, or outcome? An integrative review of the roles of play and playfulness in adult-centered psychological interventions for mental health. *The Journal of Positive Psychology*, 1–14. https://doi.org/10.1080/17439760.2023.2288955

Siegel, D. J. & Payne Bryson, T. (2020). *The power of showing up: How parental presence shapes who our kids become and how their brains get wired*. New York: Ballantine Books.

Singer, D. G. & Singer, J. L. (1990). *The house of make-believe: Children's play and the developing imagination*. Cambridge, MA: Harvard University Press.

Smilansky, S. & Shefatya, L. (2004). *Facilitating play: A medium for promoting cognitive, social-emotional and academic development in young children*. Gaithersburg, MD: Psychosocial & Educational Publications.

Teicher, M. H., Ohashi, K., & Khan, A. (2020). Additional insights into the relationship between brain network architecture and susceptibility and resilience to the psychiatric sequelae of childhood maltreatment. *Adversity and Resilience Science*, *1*, 49–64. https://doi.org/10.1007/s42844-020-00002-w

Valentine, L. & Gabbard, G. O. (2014). Can the use of humor in psychotherapy be taught? *Academic Psychiatry, 38*(1), 75–81.

Valkanova, V., Rodriguez, R. E., & Ebmeier, K. P. (2014). Mind over matter—What do we know about neuroplasticity in adults? *International Psychogeriatrics*, *26*(6), 891–909. https://doi.org/10.1017/S1041610213002482

Winnicott, D. W. (1971). *Playing and reality*. London: Tavistock.

Part III

How Play Meets Trauma and Trauma Welcomes Play

Chapter 5

Play's Relationship to Trauma Treatment

In Chapter 4, we learned about the powers of play across development and, generally, as a curative factor in therapy for clients of every age. In this chapter, we'll focus on play's specific powers relevant to helping therapists treat and heal trauma. We'll explore play's "superpowers"—scientifically supported mechanisms of action specifically suited to treat and transform trauma. By the end of this chapter, we will have all the evidence needed to validate the importance of integrating a playful spirit into trauma therapy. Then we'll be ready to apply the lessons found in the rest of this book about how to bring playfulness into our clinical work with traumatized clients.

Play and Trauma Coming Together in the Right Hemisphere

As we have read in previous chapters, the right hemisphere houses the problem—trauma memories. Ironically and fortunately it also houses its solution—relational healing. As play lives in the right brain too, it offers a powerful relational tool for trauma treatment and transformation.

Wired for Playful Trauma Healing

Is it a coincidence that playfulness and trauma memories are both housed in the right hemisphere? No. It's part of how brilliantly animals are designed. We are wired to heal from the get-go (Fosha, 2021). Just like our bodies fight off infections and form scabs over cuts, our brains, specifically the right hemisphere (and reptilian brain), have a mechanism for healing trauma.

Why is the right brain the residence of play and trauma? The right hemisphere is engaged from cradle to grave—actually, even in utero. By contrast, the left hemisphere comes online around age 2, when language develops. More importantly, even when the left brain is developmentally engaged, it goes offline again during trauma. There is a tilt to right brain functioning (van der Kolk, 2014), since it's always on and at the ready—neuronally speaking. Because trauma can

DOI: 10.4324/9781003509493-9

occur at any time in life, only the right brain can be counted on as always available and ready to protect life. Similarly, attachment and relationality, which exist before we have words until we die, live in the "always-on" right hemisphere. Play is relational, occurring in relationship with self, others, the larger world, or higher powers, and offers the relational bridge within the right hemisphere to trauma memories which disconnect us from these relationships.

Coincidentally and brilliantly, the relational work of psychotherapeutic change lives in the right hemisphere (Schore, 2010, 2022). Right-brain structures are responsible for:

1. Memory: implicit, affective, and pre-symbolic/preverbal relations;
2. Attachment: implicit and relational knowledge;
3. Communication: nonverbal/implicit, emotional, relational, and unconscious; and
4. Affect regulation: unconscious.

Is it any wonder that play and trauma states take up right-brain real estate? Each appreciates location, location, location.

Where Pain and Promise Reside

So here we have it: the right hemisphere is the place where the pain of trauma and the promise of relational healing live together. The particulars of play offer unique relational possibilities and promise for healing and transformation. Let's spell out the problem and the two-part solution to work effectively with trauma:

The problem: For people of all ages, trauma gets encoded automatically and implicitly in the right brain where it remains stuck as nonverbal, sensorimotor, and affect-filled memory fragments lacking a cohesive narrative.

The solution: Part 1. Healing trauma memories and symptoms is relational. Therapy aims to use right brain–mediated mechanisms of relationality to heal by creating relational safety and security; working with right brain–based relational dynamics like transference, countertransference, projective identification, gut feelings, felt-sense experience, intuitive knowing, and clinical intuition (Gendlin, 1981; Marks-Tarlow et al., 2018); and by using implicit, nonconscious, face-to-face, and nonverbal exchanges (Schore, 2010, 2022).

The solution: Part 2. Healing must benefit clients of all ages' developmental and cognitive levels, so it needs to speak a right brain–based language that fits everyone and is flexible. Many particular qualities of engaging playfulness relationally meet that need.

In essence, the right hemisphere allows all humans, at any age or cognitive level, to survive and heal trauma, whenever it happens. It therefore follows that engaging our right hemisphere is *necessary* for all trauma healing, which is relational. By using right brain–based playful relationality that privileges positivity (Fosha, 2000), therapists can help clients experience connection in safe ways and access particular advantages to healing trauma (discussed in the following section). Finally, engaging left-brain work (e.g., completing and rescripting the trauma narrative and meaning-making) can further deepen and integrate the trauma repair work if clients are developmentally and cognitively capable and their context allows (Rothschild, 2021).

Why Relational Playfulness Leads the Way to Heal Trauma

When we bring a playful mindset and action to trauma treatment, we facilitate and possibly expedite the healing process in a number of ways. Let's examine why playfulness is particularly suited to treat and heal trauma. I will use the word "play" throughout this section to refer to a playful mindset, action, spirit, and relational approach.

Play, Like Other Bottom-Up Approaches, Has a Proven Track Record

For many decades, play, dance, music, and creative therapies with traumatized children have capitalized on right-brain healing mechanisms. Only more recently, in the late 1990s, have adult trauma therapies come to the right-brain party and started integrating right-brain mechanisms. For example, Eye Movement Desensitization and Reprocessing, Sensorimotor Psychotherapy, Somatic Experiencing, Dance Movement Psychotherapy, Hakomi, Mindfulness, and Accelerated Experiential Dynamic Psychotherapy (AEDP) have emphasized the need to include the body, nonverbals, sensation, and movement in trauma treatment. Using right brain–based playfulness and creativity in adult therapy is increasingly accepted and encouraged (Marks-Tarlow et al., 2018). Explicitly integrating right brain–based spirituality has been supported in adult trauma therapy (Pargament, 2007; Stanley, 2016), though not yet with children, per se.

Right brain–reliant approaches like play (e.g., Gil, 2010 or Warner et al., 2020), creative (e.g., expressive arts therapies, see Malchiodi, 2023), and bottom-up therapies (e.g., Sensorimotor Psychotherapy [Ogden et al., 2006] or AEDP [Fosha, 2000]) facilitate the most direct and efficient access to encoded trauma memories: they target the original trauma through its bodily held sensation, affect, and movement fragments. These approaches unfold the memory fragments and their neuronally linked negative or disturbing emotions, sensations, movements, and cognitions, revealing positive, calming, or life-affirming ones. They promote right and left brain integrative functioning to develop a coherent, meaningful narrative.

Similarly, when we are simply playful with clients without fully engaging a bottom-up therapy approach, we still can access affective and sensorimotor expressions of trauma. Even those of us who are not full-on play and creative arts therapists can cull the fruits of the right brain. Examples might include when a therapist appropriately smiles and giggles, integrates levity or sarcasm, shares embarrassing and self-effacing stories, sings, and dances, or uses objects playfully with clients (i.e., tossing a pillow). These right brain-to-right brain communications promote an automatic, unconscious, implicit relational knowing of the other and foster attunement, clinical intuition, and creativity (Marks-Tarlow, 2018; Schore, 2011, 2022), which are particularly needed to navigate trauma. Playfulness helps us stay in this right-brain space, enriching the texture of the work, supporting innovation and openness, and allowing the hidden content of trauma memories to be revealed and articulated as they move into explicit awareness. A playful holding environment feels supportive and reassuring to both therapist and client as they move forward processing pain and celebrating successes.

Play Meets Our Clients Where They Are Developmentally

Right brain engagement through playfulness allows therapists to access trauma memories in clients of all developmental and cognitive levels of functioning. When working with adult victims of early complex trauma and attachment insecurity, we need to meet them where they are developmentally (Olson-Morrison, 2017). Adults whose younger parts or states of mind hold memories of early abuse may not understand or process material at an adult cognitive level. Effectively resolving early trauma requires therapists to work with preverbal or child parts through right-hemisphere language and allows for neurodevelopmental sensitivity (Perry, 2014; Warner et al., 2020).

Play Efficiently Directs Us to the Storage Site of Trauma Memories

Using a relationally playful spirit with our traumatized clients helps us safely access and connect with encoded unmetabolized trauma memories in the right hemisphere. Playful relational language and action are the right hemisphere's native "tongue" naturally facilitating and possibly expediting access to the attuned processing of implicitly encoded trauma memories. Our attuned playful approach becomes an important part of healing work assisting affect and nervous system regulation, the flow and integration of memory and overall brain functioning, and developing secure attachment to others and the Self.

Play "Speaks Right-Brain Language"

Playfulness and trauma memories speak right-brain language, though with a different dialect. Play's dialect is affectively and autonomically positive, light, and engaging; trauma's dialect is negative, heavy, disconnecting, and distancing. Fortunately, both play and trauma can connect through the following shared aspects of language: sensorimotor communication, primary process language, symbols, and metaphors. Yet, play's language of laughter and joy, not spoken by trauma, enables trauma states to shift.

Sensorimotor

Sensorimotor play uses the brain's sensory (e.g., sight, sound, touch, taste, smell) and motor pathways and finds its home in the right hemisphere and the reptilian part of the brain. "Playing out" the traumatic event physically in sensorimotor play assists the brain in moving the memory from the nonverbal parts—amygdala, thalamus, hippocampus, or brainstem—to the frontal lobes (Homeyer & Morrison, 2008, p. 211). This facilitates integrating and creating a meaningful narrative.

For example, Sal, age 48, used sensorimotor play when he took a stuffed bear, which represented his younger self, wrapped it securely in his arms, stroked its fur, and rocked it to reassure his vulnerable child part that he was now safe. He could then verbalize his memories of his abusive mother.

Primary Process

Primary process language characterizes how we communicate and play with pre-verbal babies and animals. It includes our body movements, postures, gestures, facial expressions, voice inflection, rhythm, pacing, tone, word sequencing, and pitch and emotional tone. Primary process language is heavily dependent on visual-facial, auditory-prosodic, and tactile-proprioceptive channels see (Fisher, 2017; Prenn, 2011 and Chapter 4). Mirroring and imitation are central components of primary process language and hold key roles in attachment formation (Winnicott, 1971) and attunement (Blum, 2015; Prenn, 2011).

For example, in a relational, playful use of embodied mirroring (Blum, 2015) with 52-year-old Gail, a rape survivor, I mirrored Gail's breathing, posture, and gaze as she recalled the traumatic memory. Collaboratively through mirroring her movements and using a soft, slow-paced voice, holding eye gaze, and saying, "I'm here with you," I supported Gail to somatically unfold a memory of being isolated, drugged, and overpowered into an act of triumph (Ogden, 2019) in which she freed herself and made the perpetrator run away. The embodied mirroring practice helped Gail have a new experience (see Chapter 13 for a fuller description).

Symbols and Metaphors

Symbolic and metaphorical play refers to how we use our bodies and objects to express emotions, wants, or needs and tell stories. For example, encoded trauma memories can find expression through object play (i.e., using sand or dolls).

Manny, a 39-year-old client who suffered severe humiliation and physical abuse by his birth mother for his first 15 years, found great empowerment through symbolic object play with toys in my office. He selected a 2-foot-long toy alligator to represent what his mother felt like to him when he was a child. When asked how he preferred to represent his mom in the present, he picked a tiny plastic ant. As he noticed both alligator and ant, his felt sense of strength and maturity grew. He smiled broadly, knowing he now physically overpowered her in height and force.

Laughter and Joy

Unlike the other right brain–based languages, the laughter- and joy-promoting forms of playfulness (like humor) lean into lean into right brain–based creativity and spontaneity while relying on the synergy of both sides of the brain. Laughter and joy are mutually incompatible with trauma states and therefore challenge trauma as they bathe us in positivity. They are incompatible with states of immobilization with fear and encourage connection and exploration (detailed in the section on play's superpowers).

The language of laughter can include many different forms of play like object (i.e., a whoopee cushion) or narrative and creative (i.e., telling a joke). Laughter and joy lessen defenses, promote resiliency, and strengthen the therapeutic alliance by fostering a sense of trust and belonging, making the therapist seem more "real," and causing change through right brain-to-right brain, relational, implicit knowing (Valentine & Gabbard, 2014). Appropriately timed and boundaried sarcasm can shift regulatory edges of comfort and help clients laugh about topics that previously evoked tension and tears.

For example, Emily and I appreciated her pastor father's increased affect regulation through my sarcasm, "Wow, dad has made progress. This time he only told you to leave the house instead of his usual threat to excommunicate you and mourn your journey into hell!" With mirrored eye-rolls, we both acknowledged his growth.

In sum, the right brain–based language and relational process of play are accessible through the lifespan and allow us "to speak the unspeakable," making what seems "unmanageable manageable" (McCarthy, 2007, p. 31). We've learned how play is a developmentally flexible, verbal and nonverbal relational language, process, attitude, and spirit. When used in a trauma-informed way, it can facilitate accessing and working with trauma memories.

To complete our exploration of why we need to invite a playful spirit into trauma treatment, we will next gain a detailed, academically supported understanding of how play's powers are actually "superpowers." Once secure in this knowledge, we will be ready to bring theory into practice.

Play's Superpowers: Meeting the Specific Needs of Trauma Treatment

Play states[1] possess a number of mechanisms of action that we can engage intentionally to target and help shift and transform trauma states. I call these mechanisms of action "superpowers." In contrast to the therapeutic powers of play (discussed in Chapter 4), which refer to general and descriptive properties, play's superpowers are "super" because they: (1) are relevant to clients of all ages, backgrounds, and abilities; (2) can be used by all healing professionals regardless of their theoretical orientation or modality of practice; (3) gain strength in relationship—especially in the context of intentional healing relationships (e.g., therapy); and (4) have a strong theoretical and research foundation that demonstrates they are themselves agents of and vehicles for change in therapy and trauma treatment. While therapeutic powers may overlap with the superpowers of play, only the latter are steeped in the deep theory and research on which trauma-treatment modalities are based.

This section reviews and synthesizes adult trauma theories to define the mechanisms of action undergirding play's superpowers that make them effective in challenging, shifting, healing, and transforming trauma states for clients of all ages. The review deepens our understanding of different problems trauma presents in treatment and the solution play offers as it turbocharges healing efficacy—while, of course, making the process more fun. The superpowers overlap and interact, yet for clarity, I discuss them as distinct to highlight their specific contribution.

Superpower #1: Mobilizing Brain Circuitry and ANS Pathways

The Trauma Problem: Danger/Life Threat and Immobilization

Our brain has different emotional-affective-motivational circuits (Panksepp, 1998, 2011a, 2011b) that turn on when our autonomic nervous system (ANS) detects danger versus safety. Danger or life-threatening trauma states activate our RAGE (anger), FEAR (anxiety), PANIC/GRIEF (Separation Distress), and SEEKING (survival) circuits (Panksepp, 2011b, p. 1798). Once activated in the face of danger, these circuits result in immobilization as we disconnect and protect—dropping into dorsal vagal (DV) states of shutdown, collapse, or dissociation. DV activation downregulates all actions (i.e., including heart rate, breathing, digestion) to enable survival (Dana, 2018). Connecting with clients whose danger-activated brain circuits and ANS pathways are "on" is really difficult because their neurobiology and nervous system are engaged to do one thing: survive the neurocepted threat (for a review see Chapter 2). In trauma states, the SEEKING circuit is geared only to enable survival.

---

1 I use the term "state" to refer to the wired-in sensorimotor experiences, mood, and thoughts evoked by behavior.

The Play Solution: Safety and Mobilization

Fortunately, one brain circuit when activated promotes thriving: the PLAY circuit. The PLAY circuit is associated with social joy and laughter and helps us acquire social knowledge and pick up subtle social interactions we need to thrive (Panksepp, 2011b, p. 1800). The PLAY circuit is activated in tandem with CARE (nurturance), sometimes LUST (sexual excitement), and SEEKING (explorative, expectancy, reward, "go-get it") circuits. The SEEKING circuit helps us become explorative to find opportunities for reward and thriving when we are safe and connected.

For the PLAY circuit to be activated, our ANS must neurocept safety, which engages our ventral vagal (VV) or social engagement system branch. In safe relationships, especially in therapy, we create safety and connection with clients to quiet the activation of the PANIC/GRIEF/Separation Distress and activate CARE circuits. In the presence of relational safety, when FEAR and RAGE circuits are activated, they mobilize us. By contrast, the danger of trauma initially activates FEAR and RAGE circuits to mobilize us into safety, but when ineffective, we become immobilized. The safety of play engages the sympathetic nervous system (SNS) branch of our ANS to upregulate actions, helping a person successfully master the challenge. For example, in a game of manhunt—a tag game played in the dark—PLAY, FEAR, and RAGE circuits are activated, motivating a person to escape being caught. Brain circuits work in tandem with VV and SNS pathways to complete an action pattern that provides a resolution to the challenge.

Therefore, *the strength of this superpower of playfulness lives in how it activates mutually exclusive brain circuits* (see Kestly, 2014; Panksepp, 1998) *and ANS pathways* compared with trauma. Play states enable us to experience safety, mobilizing us to thrive, while trauma states exist in the experience of danger, immobilizing us to survive. I intentionally use the word "experience" to qualify that even if the context is objectively safe, we can experience the opposite (see Chapter 1). This experiential dynamic presents itself with clients with chronic, complex relational trauma histories.

Just like we can't live on love alone, therapists cannot solely rely on their CARE circuitry to safely engage their relationally traumatized clients. Historically, such trauma survivors were harmed and even met with a life threat when dependent upon and vulnerable with their abusive or neglectful caregivers (i.e., reactive attachment disorder or interpersonal violence). Autonomically, VV connection and immobilizing fear SNS and DV pathways fused or intertwined (Dana, 2018; Kestly, 2016; Stanley, 2016). At the brain circuitry level, the caregiver's behaviors activated their dependent's CARE circuits alongside those of RAGE, FEAR, PANIC/GRIEF/Separation Distress, and SEEKING for survival. To prevent potential relational harm, clients learned to erect walls to protect against unsafe care and connection. Therefore, a therapist's CARE circuitry may evoke their relational memory history, triggering the cascade of related ANS pathway and brain circuitry activation. Similarly, because the client lacks a neural blueprint for safe connection, their brain reacts to the therapist's unfamiliar type of care and compassion as if it is dangerous.

By intentionally engaging the neuronal and autonomic superpowers of play, therapists can "co-opt the primitive neural mechanisms of immobilization in the service of learning how to manage pleasurable low-arousal behaviors ... that require immobilization without fear" (Kestly 2016, p. 21, explaining Porges). Wise and attuned playfulness with our relationally triggered clients can override their hijacking trauma state, activate the VV and SNS pathways of the ANS, and turn on the CARE and mobilizing FEAR (and RAGE) circuits while quieting the activation of the PANIC/GRIEF/Separation Distress circuit.

Superpower #1 Case Example: When Sam sat, dissociated and shutdown, hijacked in his DV state, I sat quietly with him. I knew not to make contact statements that would trigger CARE circuits and their trauma-related brain and ANS protective reactions. I continued to sit patiently and quietly, being mindful of my breath. Then, my stomach grumbled audibly. I saw Sam's eyes move askance and then look downward again. As if on cue, my stomach made an even louder sound. It was as if my stomach was trying to shift the relational stuckness. I grabbed the opportunity.

I giggled and said, "I'm sorry Sam. I think my stomach just farted." He looked up and slightly smirked. I said, "Be glad I didn't eat beans for lunch. Then you'd be hearing *and* smelling real farts!" Sam shook his head side to side (SNS mobilization). Self-deprecatingly I joked, "Sam, I told you my style may not be like that of other therapists." (He had had nine before me.) He reestablished eye-to-eye gaze (VV state) and said, "You're right, Monica. It's not. But it's okay" (Hints of CARE circuitry).

Then his stomach made a gurgly noise. You can't make this up! I laughed and said, "Awww, your stomach is talking to my stomach!" (invoking PLAY, CARE, and SEEKING to explore circuitry).

Sam said, "Ya, sure. Wait till you hear what my ass has to say!" (VV pathway and PLAY circuitry).

I belly laughed and asked, "Should I get the Febreeze (air freshener)?"

He laughed and said, "No worries, I didn't have beans either." (More social engagement with PLAY and protective CARE circuitry).

Before moving on to the next superpower, we need to remember that, for some clients, PLAY circuitry has sometimes been fused with immobilizing DV states, as occurs with grooming play by a sexual perpetrator and their child victim. Grooming does not embody safety or play's true essence. It might feel good physiologically and grow attachment, yet it exploits and manipulates power in the inequitable victim/victimizer relational dynamic. The desire to do more of it is driven by an effort to undo personal victimization/powerlessness. A victim's PLAY circuitry probably shuts off when grooming behaviors cross the line from safe to threatening. We must distinguish when play is safe or not since engaging clients playfully can trigger trauma-related brain circuitry and ANS pathways. Therapists must remain mindful, attuned, and discerning to ensure that using their playful spirit will be wise and harness its superpower properties.

Superpower #2: Exercising/Strengthening the ANS and Affect Tolerance

The Trauma Problem: A Weakened ANS Shrinks Affect Tolerance

As we just reviewed, in trauma states our ANS neurocepts danger. If shifting from the VV to SNS fight/flight branch of the ANS does not resolve the life threat—as is often the case for many trauma survivors—the primitive, DV pathway becomes dominant. We disconnect and protect (Dana, 2018; Kestly, 2016; Porges, 2011) ourselves from harm, death, or dysregulating discomfort. DV states of immobilization-with-fear work with activated FEAR and RAGE, PANIC/GRIEF/Separation Distress circuitry. Low-arousal behaviors emerge to manage harm. DV states are experienced as immobilization with fear in isolation and cause "fright without solution" (Hesse & Main, 2006), seen in examples of disorganized attachment and being alone when a big T trauma hits like a tsunami.

With only enough energy to support survival, exploration is usurped by survival SEEKING circuitry and our ANS becomes impaired from effective vagal braking because the VV branch is not in charge (see Chapter 2). In trauma states when we face danger, time is of the essence. Our vagal brake gets slammed or released rapidly, without modulation. Chronic trauma causes our vagal brake to lose tone and to not function properly; regulatory problems arise for organs involved with digestion, respiration, and cardiovascular and reflex systems. Our braking becomes hair triggered, causing rapid and dramatic ANS responses.

In addition, and related, trauma states constrict our window of affect tolerance (WOT) (Siegel, 2020b), which means our ANS becomes more rigid, challenging a person to effectively and flexibly neurally navigate SNS and DV activation. Put simply, impaired affective self-regulation arises from disintegrative brain functioning, an overwhelmed ANS marked by poor vagal braking tone, and leaving our WOT. Chronically traumatized individuals may have nervous systems that react in confused, under, or overreactive ways. Relatively benign situations may hijack a person or cause them to lose their cool, as when the wind slams a door shut and they jump and scream "help." Life-endangering events may leave a person calm or unfazed, like when a person stays inert in the middle of a frozen lake as the ice below them cracks. People may approach dangerous situations and avoid safe, satisfying ones.

The Play Solution: An Exercised/Strengthened ANS Grows Affect Tolerance

In contrast to trauma states, play engages the VV pathway, allows us to mobilize in the face of fear, and helps increase vagal braking tone. In fact, play is a complex "neural exercise" in which our ANS gets triggered and learns to neurocept alternating states of danger and safety (Porges, 2015) in which we, respectively, apply and release our vagal brake. For example, in the manhunt game, the ANS applies the vagal brake to slow down our heart rate, breathing, and digestion, as we quietly wait for the threat of *it*—the person trying to find and imprison us—to pass us by undetected. When safe, and *it* has gone far away, the ANS releases the vagal brake, energizing us and speeding up our heart rate, breathing, and digestion so we can run, release our friend from "jail," and return to calm (a safe and connected VV state). In life, vagal brake release can also help us learn, grow, and thrive.

Through play, we practice applying and releasing our vagal brake in response to autonomic triggers (e.g., to our VV, SNS, or DV systems) of different intensity, duration, and frequency. Our vagal brake gains tone, like a muscle, strengthening our ANS's flexibility through its actions on the heart (Dana, 2018, p. 28). Toned vagal braking means we can apply the brake in nuanced ways to gradually press down or release it to ease how rapidly we slow down or speed up our ANS responses. We know that the wilder we play, the greater the chance someone will get hurt or break something—which shocks us and forces our vagal brake to slam down. Balancing playful excitement without being too rough is the neural exercise we all need to practice across the lifespan with somatic, emotional, and cognitive activities, especially competitive ones.

In contrast to trauma states, in play, we maintain social engagement (VV states). Through reciprocal dynamic interactions (Porges, 2009) we co-regulate and tolerate a greater range of nervous system activation intensity and shifts between different neural states. Our WOT for nervous system arousal expands. Through playfulness in the context of a safe, therapeutic, healing relationship, play's superpowers lessen and unblend fear states. States of high arousal or immobility grow vagal brake flexibility in response to activation and increase the WOT. Play truly is a superpower in healing trauma because it helps clients ride the regulatory edges of the WOT in states of connection (VV) and mobilization (SNS), where the greatest brain and relational change occurs (Schore, 2011, p. 85). Play lives in the space between what we know and what we don't, helping us straddle arousal and comfort while seamlessly joining security and thrill (Brown & Eberle, 2018, p. 31). Engaging our PLAY circuitry fuels play's superpowers as it strengthens and exercises our vagal braking skills and expands our WOT.

Superpower #2 Case Example: During one session, 35-year-old Jacob accidentally knocked over a lamp with his wild arm gestures as he expressed anger and hurt at his wife's insensitivity. He froze and his eyes widened. Jacob said imploringly, "Oh no, Dr. Blum. I'm so, so, sorry. I'll pay for any damages."

After picking up the intact lamp and returning it on the side table, I reassured him, "Jacob, everything's fine. Nothing is broken. I'm not angry with you. Mistakes happen. How are *you* feeling?"

Jacob hesitatingly looked up at me while scanning my body language. With uncertainty he shrugged saying, "I'm okay. But are you sure? I'll pay." Across his life, Jacob had paid a great price for his angry outbursts.

With a very calm voice, I answered, "All is fine." I shook my head and made broad arm gestures saying emphatically, "You don't need to pay a thing." I was somatically modeling big, safe movements and speaking.

Then, I ironically said to Jacob, "Would you do that again?" He looked at me puzzled. I clarified, "Show me again how upset you feel with your arms." Jacob double-checked that he heard me correctly. I nodded with encouragement. With hesitation, Jacob took a breath and expressed his upset with more contained movements. We playfully experimented with Jacob intentionally using bigger and smaller arm gestures to express his level of upset without causing destruction. This practice helped Jacob exercise his vagal brake with SNS activation while staying in VV connection and expanding his WOT.

Superpower #3: Building Relational Co-Regulation and Security

Interpersonal Neurobiology (see Siegel, 2020b) helps us understand play's third superpower of building affective co-regulation and earning attachment security. In relationships, implicit right brain-to-right brain communication is always present and happens below the level of awareness—similar to wireless communication (Vaisvaser, 2021). The right brain-to-right brain process is bi-directional (Hopenwasser, 2016), meaning the therapist's brain can mirror the client's and vice versa. When two brains mirror each other, owing to mirror neurons, they activate and coordinate in resonant and synchronized ways (Feldman, 2007, 2020), accounting for empathy, attunement, and prosocial feelings (Gallese, 2009, 2010; Iacoboni, 2007; Lenzi et al., 2009).

In therapy, right brain-to-right brain mirroring fosters the emergence of a common field, sometimes called the intersubjective space or the analytic third (Ogden, 1994). In it, both client and therapist connect to a shared affective, cognitive, or somatic experience and yet are separate. From this co-created relational field springs forth the therapist's somatic, affective, or cognitive countertransferences (Blum, 2015) and projective identifications, the client's transferences, and relational enactments (Maroda, 1998). We explicitly and relationally process this material to make meaning and create change, updating old relational patterns. Both traumatized and thriving right-brain processes can be mirrored.

The Trauma Problem: Increased Relational Dysregulation and Insecurity

When our therapist's right brain unconsciously mirrors our client's traumatized right brain, the emergent sensorimotor, affective, or cognitive countertransferences and enactments can limit or even hijack our self- and co-regulatory abilities. Trauma state resonance can result in enactments, like dissociative attunement, defined as an unintegrated, out-of-awareness synchronization between two individuals that leaves the therapist with a fragmented, elusive, inconsistent narrative as they attempt to integrate the relational experience in their own mind (Hopenwasser, 2008, 2016).

Supervision is often needed to reveal dissociative attunements because of the complicated and exhausting relational dynamics that arise, accompanied by a lack of mindful awareness and disembodiments. These relational dynamics cause the healing process to get stuck. As a result, cycles of implicit relational trauma memories (sometimes both the client's and therapist's) loop, preventing meaning-making of the trauma. This causes therapists to feel out of sync with clients and their clients may feel unreachable. Since right brain-to-right brain resonance is the basis of attachment (Schore & Schore, 2008), relational misattunements and ruptures prevent the earning of a secure attachment (Marriott & Kelly interview with Sroufe, February 15, 2021)—a necessary component of the healing relationship. Affective co-dysregulation combined with enacted toxic countertransferences and projective identifications can subvert our best efforts to stay present, connected, and wisely facilitate change.

Reciprocally, clients may feel out of sync with us, their therapist. When feeling deeply misattuned, clients may experience us as unable to see, feel, or know them which triggers relational trauma themes of victimization. Clients may act as if the dangerous relational past is happening now, shifting from left- to right-hemisphere dominance (see Chapter 2) and disconnect-and-protect mode (DV states). This may plunge them into new cycles of hopelessness and doubt that any relationship can be safe. As healing professionals, we can appreciate how courageous trauma survivors are to enter therapy in the first place.

To complicate matters, the therapist's personal trauma memories may interfere with co-regulating affect and helping the client earn security. Therapists may also experience vicarious traumatization and burnout. Bearing witness to left brain–narrated trauma facts and stories wears us down. What's more, we are co-experiencing trauma with our clients as we live together in a post-pandemic world filled with cultural, national, socioeconomic, political, religious, and global divisiveness, war, and climate change. Understandably, therapists can feel beleaguered as we play whack-a-mole, resolving traumas as quickly as they pop up again for our clients and ourselves. Affective co-regulation and secure, earned attachment formation are deeply challenged, slowing or even stalling our client's healing.

The Play Solution: Increased Relational Co-Regulation and Security

Relational ruptures and enactments are unavoidable, yet what can minimize the therapist's tendency to get hijacked by right brain-to-right brain mirroring of the client's trauma states? You may have guessed it: intentional, attuned, appropriately timed playful, relational engagement.

Adding an attuned playful spirit to relational trauma work may be enjoyable and lessen intense affect by bringing a lightness, distance—and therefore containment—to difficult affect, sensation, and cognition. Playfulness helps engage our own and our clients' social engagement system (VV) and activates their PLAY circuits and related CARE and SEEKING explorative ones. In tandem,

ANS arousal is self- and co-regulated, keeping clients in their WOT or at its regulatory edges. Playfulness helps clients gain distance and contain their level of affect and arousal (covered in greater depth in Chapter 10). We can personify sensations or parts of mind and use objects, crafts, or other creative media to foster objectivity and affect management and tolerance. For example, we can guide our clients to create a miniature version of their perpetrator with Play-Doh and then smash it, facilitating affect regulation and emotional expression. Vagal brake tone can be strengthened as clients repeat this exercise. Both client and therapist may benefit from this type of containment and catharsis, which further enhances self- and co-regulation of affect.

Engaging playfully with our clients also fosters right brain-to-right brain neural resonance, synchrony, and rhythm (Feldman, 2007; Siegel, 2020b; Stevens, 2018), which can help us connect with states of withdrawal or dissociation (Kestly, 2016). In relational play states, we share strong emotions, social proximity, interactions, and synchronized and mirrored behaviors using multiple sensorimotor channels and modalities (e.g., art, music, dance) (Vaisvaser, 2021). Together, these shared relational play experiences foster attunement and bring us into harmony with the other—homing in on the heart of therapeutic change which is feeling felt by another and not alone (Stevens, 2018). As a consequence, empathy, mentalization, and intersubjectivity grow out of these play-based right brain-to-right brain experiences, as does an earned secure attachment. Through relational, playful co-regulation, our insecurely attached clients can earn security by being and feeling safe, seen, and soothed (Marriott & Kelley interview Sroufe, February 15, 2021; Siegel & Payne Bryson, 2020).

Brain integrative functioning emerges out of secure relationships, fostering the brain's ability to change and grow neural networks across the lifespan known as neuroplasticity. Therapy fosters neuroplasticity as the implicit and unconscious right brain-to-right brain exchanges between therapist and client affect procedural knowledge—how to act, feel, and think with others (implicit relational knowing) (Stern et al., 1998). Playfulness facilitates this growth and change in the healing relationship.

Playfully using objects (e.g., dolls, figurines, arts and crafts, music), movement (e.g., dance, yoga), or symbols and metaphors (e.g., storytelling) can support our clients to make meaning of their trauma. The right-brain language of play helps make implicit right-brain encoded trauma memories explicit, letting them "speak." After making the implicit explicit, we can further unfold the trauma memories relationally and experientially, allowing us to update and transform old meaning into new (Korn, 2012). Play states help make meaning playful and enjoyable and may connect clients to a higher and deeper spirituality (McCarthy, 2007).

Regulating attention, mood, emotion, the narrative making-sense process, thought, behavior, morality, and relationality (Siegel & Payne Bryson, 2020) support our brain to act in flexible, adaptive, coherent, energized, and stable ways (Siegel, 2020b). The most adaptive brains are characterized by maximum integration. Play is a superpower that supports earned security. Its connection to self- and co-regulation of affect and neural integration scaffolds the brain's natural push toward wholeness (Siegel, 2020a, 2020b).

Superpower #3 Case Example: Forty-one-year-old Luenell (whom we'll visit again in Chapters 10 and 11) struggled chronically with vacillating states of extreme agitation leading to paralysis and collapse, or rage resulting in storming out or emotionally and physically harming others. She frequently attended sessions with her 62-year-old mother Gloria. Over years of treatment, I misattuned many times. For example, early in treatment when Luenell became disturbingly agitated at her mother's misattunements, I'd ask her to breathe to calm. This further agitated Luenell, causing her to leave the room. Unconsciously, I was enacting a parallel process: just like her mother had (since Luenell's colicky infancy), I leaned on Luenell to calm herself and others who felt disturbed by Luenell's distress. Instead, I needed to identify and soothe Luenell's unmet needs. Once aware, I changed my approach.

After confirming this fit Luenell's experience, we explained to Gloria that Luenell's agitation reflected not feeling or being safe or seen. Leaving the room was Luenell's wise attempt to prevent herself from hitting Gloria (which she had done in the past). It also helped Luenell calm. Yet, Luenell and Gloria needed more practice before they could effectively and appropriately express their feelings, and be heard and soothed. So, we got playful.

Going forward we created playful, safe ways to objectively "see" each other's dysregulation and respectfully support self-soothing efforts. When triggered by her mother, Luenell was encouraged to physically move to a different place in the room or erect boundaries with pillows. Meanwhile, when triggered by Luenell's dysregulation, Gloria was supported to use a time-out signal to alert herself to calm and visually remind Luenell it's not her responsibility. I too would model playful ways to feel and be safe, seen, and soothed while facilitating the repair of ruptures.

Across sessions, Luenell playfully used the pillows to build high protective walls or cover her eyes and ears. Once, Luenell angrily tossed a pillow at her mother, who spontaneously and angrily tossed it back. An impromptu pillow-toss game ensued in which they shifted their anger into a laugh-filled experience. I narrated and applauded their regulatory accomplishment. Meanwhile, Gloria practiced using her time-out signal and pacing around the room to regulate. Through playfulness, I guided Luenell and Gloria to name and express their feelings, see and empathize with each other's experience, take responsibility to regulate (alone or with appropriate help), and earn longed-for relational security.

Superpower #4: Promoting Mindfulness and Embodiment

Mindfulness means paying attention with intention and acceptance. When we are mindful, we are present in the here-and-now in mind, body, emotion, and spirit. Mindfulness allows us to cultivate the relational connections that heal (Kestly, 2016, p. 22). Mindfulness promotes neuronal connection and integration because "where attention goes, neural firing flows, and neural connection grows" (Siegel, 2020a, p. 19). The end product of mindfulness is likely connected human relationships and balanced caregiving abilities (Forner, 2019) to self and others, including greater openness, curiosity, self-acceptance, and compassion (Heller & Kammer, 2022, p. 253).

The Trauma Problem: Hijacked Mindfulness and Embodiment

Trauma states trigger a shift from left- to right-hemisphere dominance (van der Kolk, 2014), causing us to have the experience of trauma time (Wesselmann, 2014). Instead of being in the here-and-now, we feel as if we are there-and-then (Fisher, 2017). Clients hijacked by trauma time lack presence, mindful awareness, objectivity, and perspective. Sometimes highly dissociative clients are disoriented to time, place, and person, experience depersonalization, derealization, and flashbacks, and may engage in post-traumatic play. Clients can be mindless and disembodied.

Maladaptive mind-wandering correlates with trauma states and interferes with healing. We get lost in our self-generated inner world, lose attention and focus, and disengage from perceiving the outside world and others (Chan & Siegel, 2018, p. 45). Our brain shifts from processing the stimuli in our external world to an internal processing mode, which is called "perceptual decoupling" (Cohen et al., 2022). In this state, we lack cognitive control and awareness, experience rigid thinking, disconnect from an internal experience of flow between mind, body, and emotions, and experience impaired problem-solving and mood regulation (Chan & Siegel, 2018, p. 45).

The Play Solution: Supported Mindfulness and Embodiment

Play is a superpower of mindfulness for trauma states as it fosters a here-and-now presence (Malchiodi, 2023), a focused and relaxed attention with a state of acceptance and receptivity (Chan & Siegel, 2018, p. 47). This may seem ironic because we can get lost in play, like when we are alone playing video games or daydreaming. Our mind wanders, taking us away from external demands as we abandon a task or goal-focused mindset. Yet, these same facets of play are excavated in therapy to grow mindfulness in relationship to oneself and others (e.g., the therapist).

Therapists must stay personally mindful to guide our clients to do the same. In the role of not-client, therapists consciously ground ourselves so we can re-anchor clients if they get lost in play, particularly looping, toxic, post-traumatic play. Therapists work relationally and intentionally to make the mind-wandering aspects of play adaptive (Chan & Siegel, 2018, p. 45). Mind-wandering might be linked to the exploratory SEEKING circuitry, activated with PLAY. As we facilitate clients to transition between internal and external worlds (activated by our default mode network) to become self-aware, we support the thriving, rather than the survival functions, of the SEEKING circuit.

As a client toggles to notice internal and external experience, they grow affect regulation, their WOT, and neural integration. Therapists can support a client's mindfulness to grow by exploring pretend and fantasy play like daydreaming, or sensorimotor play like dance, yoga, sand, clay, or finger paints. Clients learn to notice and be with their inner experience of sensations, emotions, and thoughts. They become embodied, having in-the-moment, mindful awareness of bodily sensations, emotions, and movements (Schwartz & Maiberger, 2018). Being aware of and connected with our body helps us get to know ourselves and others (Merleau-Ponty, 1962) and informs the scripts and meaning we develop.

The therapist helps anchor mind-wandering to harness its adaptive qualities (like receptivity and acceptance) and focus with relaxed and nonjudgmental attention (Chan & Siegel, 2018, p. 48). Mind-wandering's other benefits are delayed gratification, creativity, finding meaning in personal experiences, fostering well-being and health, reducing undesirable mood states, and preparing for potential stressors. Play's superpower abilities to promote mindfulness and embodiment are far-reaching.

Superpower #4 Case Example: Gretchen, a 15-year-old war and interpersonal violence survivor, often apologized in session saying, "Sorry Dr. Monica, my ADHD or something distracted me. What did you say?" I often responded sincerely and playfully, "Oooh, that's great! Where did you go?" and followed up with questions like, "Can you bring me there with you?" or "What were you feeling and noticing inside before you got distracted? And now that you're back?"

Gretchen had learned in our work that losing her present orientation could be a protector part (like flight) trying to distract from a trauma-related disturbance: an unconscious spontaneous association to important and relevant information, or even instinctual solutions. Learning to playfully embrace the "symptom" (see Chapter 6) became a repeated practice in promoting presence. I playfully encouraged Gretchen to "Thank that part of your mind for getting your attention. Ask it, 'Were you trying to pull me away from something or lead me somewhere?'" When Gretchen felt discomfort in sessions I'd request, "Hey Gretchen, can you ask your distractor to come help you out now?" By playfully growing a cooperative relationship with her distractibility and embracing its helpfulness, Gretchen grew appreciative of her mind's resourcefulness and increased her mindful awareness and sense of embodiment.

Superpower #5: Broadening and Building Positivity and Neuroplasticity

The Trauma Problem: Increased Negativity, Decreased Neuroplasticity, and Adaptability

Trauma states limit and hijack positive affect, replacing it with negative affect. This may reflect our brains' negativity bias that helps us protect against danger (Vaish et al., 2008)—especially important for chronic trauma victims. Negative emotions correspond with vagal braking problems, resulting in high arousal. In the face of life threats, this is a good thing—mobilizing us to escape or defend against the danger. However, ongoing states of high SNS activation (e.g., high heart and breathing rates, high energy expenditures) may shift us into DV states where thoughts and action tendencies are survival focused, causing shutdown, dissociation, or collapse. Staying in survival mode stunts our ability to experience joy and thrive. Also, states of chronic negative affect have been linked to decreased neuroplasticity seen at molecular/cellular, neural network, cognitive functioning, and affective information processing levels (Price & Duman, 2020). Put simply, chronic negative affect impairs integrative brain functioning and our cognitive ability to flexibly adapt to whatever life presents.

The Play Solution: Increased Positivity, Neuroplasticity, and Resiliency

We know play is fun and feels good, and we want to do more of it. The broaden-and-build theory of positive emotions (Fredrickson, 2001) explains why. Experiencing positive emotions (e.g., joy, fun, contentment, love) broadens our inventory of novel thoughts and actions, which builds our resources/skills, reflecting a change in the old and growth of new, adaptive neural networks. Positive emotions create an upward spiral of more positive emotions (Fosha, 2007; Fredrickson & Joiner, 2002).

The positive emotions of play states correlate with feeling safe and connected, as well as modulate vagal braking, affect, and arousal. They also decrease overall SNS activation (e.g., heart rate), conserve energy, increase oxygen supply to the brain, and promote self-soothing and the ability to reflect upon, savor, and thrive (Yeung, 2021). Positive emotions activate the brain's orbitofrontal cortex, which supports neurobiological integration while regulating affect and stress (Yeung, 2021, p. 356). Play's broaden-and-build powers of positive emotions also grow resilience, adaptability, and support flourishing. Who wouldn't want to bring the superpower of play's positive emotions to their clients?

However, the relationship between play and positive emotions is a bit complex. Too much of a good thing can cause a downturn in the positive upward spiral (Fredrickson, 2013) as when children have no limits set on their gaming time, rough and tumble play escalates in intensity and someone gets hurt, or two people are joking and one goes too far and hurts the other's feelings. Flourishing or thriving in play is best supported when we find an optimal ratio or balance between positive and negative emotions (Fredrickson, 2013, p. 818). As we learned, play is a neural exercise that helps us find the right balance. For example, a father who tosses his baby girl in the air may excite and delight her the first eight times, but as she starts to tire or get disoriented she'll start to cry. Or the woman who jams with her band until 4 a.m. is too tired to drive her kids' carpool to the championship game at 6:00 a.m. Through play, we navigate the highs and lows of positive and negative emotions and the corresponding regulatory edges of what feels safe and exciting or crosses the line. This process builds enduring skills, knowledge, and resiliency.

We would imagine most clients would prefer positive, light states of play compared with the negative, heavy ones of trauma. However, for healing and deep change to happen, clients need receptive positive affective capacity—the ability to viscerally experience and take in what the therapist offers them (Piliero, 2021, p. 277). The barriers limiting a client's receptive capacity can sometimes be softened by attuned playfulness. Playfulness, especially when spontaneous and unpredictable, can effectively disarm protector parts, lowering clients' walls. Clients more safely and freely take in compliments, plus feel seen and good.

Superpower #5 Case Example: My adult client, Reena, raised with a disorganized style of parenting, explained this challenge beautifully: "It is too hard and painful to feel safe, seen, good, and excited (VV engagement) and then be treated as invisible, unlovable, and be left alone (DV states)." To Reena, each positive followed by negative emotional cycle was a reenactment in which hope would be found then lost and grieved. Her narrow WOT protected her from having to navigate these dramatic ANS shifts.

To interrupt this cycle and grow her positive affect tolerance, I encouraged Reena to draw using charcoals, which she loved. During and between sessions, Reena creatively expressed herself through this medium which helped her practice feeling skilled, proud, and competent. We expanded Reena's tolerance of positive affect in therapy: she grew to safely take in and feel good, positive, and seen. She broadened and built positive affect tolerance, receptive capacity, and her WOT bandwidth. Reena brilliantly figured how to "lift the lows so when they follow times I feel good, the roller coaster dip doesn't feel as big and dysregulating." She had fewer depressive episodes and pulled herself out of them more quickly. As Reena shows us, engaging playfulness in therapy naturally derives benefit from the broadening and building superpowers of positive emotions, which can be transformative, foster personal growth (i.e., enhanced health and well-being), and promote thriving (Fredrickson & Losada, 2005).

Superpower #6: Connecting with Authenticity

The Trauma Problem: Disconnecting from Self

When life threat occurs in chronic and complex relational trauma and there is ANS dysregulation, brain disintegrative functioning, and disconnection, we prioritize our physical and intrapsychic (i.e., our vitality, essence, or soul) survival at all costs. To manage these disturbances, we disconnect and protect: our "realness goes underground," and we show up with a False Self (Tuber, 2020, p. 27, discussing Winnicott). This enables us to continue with daily tasks and responsibilities. Defenses that prevent trauma-related disturbances from overtaking us are protectors like the Apparently Normal Part of the personality in Structural Dissociation terms (van der Hart et al., 2006) or managers and firefighters in Internal Family Systems terms (Schwartz & Sweezy, 2020) (see Chapter 2 for more details). The intrapsychic protection systems form the template of how we relate to self, others, and the world (Bowlby, 1969) further disconnecting us from our authenticity.

The Play Solution: Increasing Connection with Self

Being real or authentic in a relationship with others supports our essence, core, or true Self. We feel safe, seen, and accepted for who we are. According to Winnicott (discussed in Tuber, 2020), children's play enables developmental achievements including the capacity to be alone, create intermediate space between inner fantasy and external reality, sustain a True Self, use objects, and expand and process reality. Even in adulthood, we express our authenticity, vitality, spontaneity, and creativity reflected in our core being through play. Using playfulness in therapy for children and adults facilitates communication of one's truth. Moreover, play is the medium that allows safe communication for all parts of one's being.

Superpower #6 Case Example: Fifty-year-old Mitch had often been shamed and shunned by his church community, similar to how his abusive mother and wife had treated him. Mitch was full of contradictions. Despite becoming a deacon and holding deep faith, he spoke bluntly to his fellow parishioners, used profanity unabashedly, and made double entendres frequently. And yet, he was very respectful of physical boundaries, selfless and devoted to his friends, children, and the needy, served responsibly on the Church council, acted as a volunteer Emergency Medical Technician, and was generous with his time and money. One day he brought me a personalized hat that said: "Team Mitch." He gave one to each person who supported his painful divorce process. I was deeply touched.

Midway through a subsequent session, I put on the hat and boldly declared, "Mitch, I am so proud of your growth and how fiercely you fought for liberation from your ex and full custody of your children. You are free of panic attacks, heart medication, and can now climb 90 flights on the stepper." I picked up a glittery wand off my bookshelf, walked over to him, and motioned the wand over his head. I said in an affected British accent, "You are officially dubbed a *mensch*—the Yiddish word deeming you a wholly decent person, and then some. Or a fucking amazing man!"

I knew Mitch appreciated my deep faith and enjoyed related Jewish references. He started to laugh and then tear up. He said, "You get me. You really see who I am. I can't tell you how much it means to be seen, liked, much less respected! And it sure as hell helps that you're as crazy as I am!" Mitch experienced me as a True Other—someone who with great relational attunement, helped him feel meaningfully felt, known, understood, seen, and helped (Fosha, 2005). He felt appreciative, enlivened, and experienced connection with his authenticity and true Self—who he believed he was and was meant to be (Fosha, 2005).

Being playful with our traumatized clients as I was with Mitch harnesses the superpower of tapping into our clients' truth, which strengthens and reaffirms who they implicitly know themselves to be at their core—their Self. Reflecting back and relationally metaprocessing (Fosha, 2000; Yeung, 2021 see Chapter 9) our clients' personal rightness and truth deepens their connection to their authenticity. Change experienced at this level—emotionally, cognitively, and spiritually—is affirming, life-enhancing, and transformative.

Summarizing the Six Superpowers

The six superpowers of play are scientifically supported in how they exert an extensive and profound impact on healing trauma and supporting change. The superpowers of play include mechanisms of action related to engaging our PLAY circuitry to be safe and connected, exercising ANS flexibility through vagal braking, affect self- and co-regulation, relational attunement and security, the power of broadening and building positivity, and facilitating connection to our true Self. See Figure 5.1 for a summary.

Because playfulness can take many forms of verbal and nonverbal creativity (e.g., imagination, dance/movement, music, storytelling/humor, drama, or art) in multisensory ways, it engages clients holistically on emotional, somatic, cognitive, and spiritual levels. Play's superpowers also promote a mindful and embodied relational presence, neuroplasticity, and connection to our authenticity. In closing, let's now integrate how these superpowers of play are suited to promote change in trauma for all clients.

Combining Play and Trauma States: A Perfect Mismatch for Change

The basis for play being a superpower of relational healing rests in the incompatibility of and mutual exclusivity between play and trauma states at the level of our ANS and brain circuitry. While both play and trauma states are co-residents of the right hemisphere, they activate different pathways. Practically, we know we can't truly have fun and experience joy while feeling unsafe or under threat of life. For example, when a transgendered youth explains the distress of how

	The TRAUMA STATE **PROBLEM**	The PLAY STATE **SOLUTION** SUPERPOWER Mechanism of Action	SUPPORTIVE THEORIES
#1	- Fear/Danger/Life Threat - Disconnection - Immobilization	- Safety/Exploration/Thriving - Connection - Mobilization	• Affective neuroscience • Polyvagal theory
#2	- Weakened ANS - Rigid vagal braking - Constricted affect tolerance	- Exercised/Strengthened ANS - Modulated vagal breaking - Expanded affect tolerance	• Polyvagal theory • Affective neuroscience/ Window of tolerance
#3	- Relationally dysregulated ANS and affect - Insecurity	- Co-regulated ANS and affect - (Earned) Security	• Interpersonal neurobiology • Relational/Attachment theories
#4	- Hijacked mindfulness and presence - Increased disembodiment	- Strengthened mindfulness and presence - Supported embodiment	• Neuroscience on mindfulness
#5	- Increasednegativity affect/ cognitive inflexibility - Decreased neuroplasticity, adaptability, and resilience	- Increased positive affect/ cognitive flexibility - Increased neuroplasticity and resilience	• Broaden-and-build theory • Polyvagal theory • Affective neuroscience
#6	- Decreased connection from Others - Increased disconnection from Self (personal truth, rightness, essence) - Maintained connection to unsafe others	- Increased Connection to Safe Others - Increased intrapsychic integration/connection with Self - Decreased connection to unsafe others	• Structural dissociation of the personality • Internal family systems • Accelerated experiential dynamic psychotherapy

Figure 5.1 Summary of play's superpowers in treating trauma.

their physical body belies their true identity, they verbally and bodily lack feeling light and free.

Ultimately, healing professionals can use this inherent incompatibility between the right-hemisphere neighbors of play and trauma to shift our clients' experience and effects of trauma. This incompatibility holds the key to promoting memory reconsolidation, the essential and necessary mechanism underlying "decisive, lasting, therapeutic change" (Ecker, 2018; Ecker et al., 2015). Memory reconsolidation requires us to: (1) Activate the implicitly encoded (e.g., trauma) memory network and its related schema—embodied anticipations (Badenoch, 2017) or expectations about how life will unfold for us. (2) Create a "mismatch" or "juxtaposition" experience by making something novel or discrepant from expectation happen. The disconfirmed expectation unlocks old neural linkages. (3) Consolidate new memories by linking old memories with new expectations.

When we bring together play and trauma states, we create a mismatch or juxtaposition experience: a simultaneous holding of contradictory or mismatched, neurally linked patterns of play and trauma, which challenge the personally experienced and debilitating effects of trauma. An example of a mismatch might be if a client spills their coffee on the rug in the therapy room. Based on their past, they expect to be yelled at, shamed, or beaten. But the therapist instead laughs and says, "Thank you. You've finally given me reason to buy the new rug I've had in my Amazon shopping cart for months. I've hated this one for years!" This sincere statement deconsolidates or unlocks the old neural network, allowing for and fueling change. Play states give clients reprieve, even if momentarily, from their heavy mental, emotional, physical, and spiritual trauma burdens while providing them with the key to promoting change for the better.

We've seen through theory and practice how play states bring juxtaposition experiences to trauma treatment by their very fun, light, and enlivening nature, thereby supporting memory reconsolidation. We may inject appropriately attuned and timed humor, spontaneously toss a ball, or break out into dance, catching clients off guard. We thereby challenge their expectations about the therapy process itself and explicitly work through the specific contradiction and disconfirmation of their old belief.

Embodying our playful spirit with traumatized clients of all ages allows us to safely target and undo the six UNs experienced in response to trauma (see Chapter 1). Through the mechanisms of action or six superpowers of play combined with the mismatch experience they offer, clients learn to:

- Safely activate ANS pathways and brain circuitry;
- Exercise their ANS and grow affect tolerance and receptive affective capacity;
- Build relational co-regulation and earn security;
- Grow mindfulness and embodiment;
- Broaden and build positive emotions, neuroplasticity, and resiliency; and
- Connect authentically with others and Self.

Combined with supporting our clients to feel safe and connected with us, playfulness offers them a new expectation that trauma work doesn't have to be only painful, anxiety-provoking, or something to be avoided. We help them release the once-fixed stranglehold of fear and negativity related to trauma through relational playfulness. They grow to associate the healing relationship with a trust that change is possible in ways that include smiles and laughter along with hard work. The positive reinforcement of healing with playfulness leads to recursive, upward spirals of motivation to change and consistent treatment attendance. In the following chapters, we'll learn exactly how to apply these playful superpowers, reconsolidate old memories, and create new ones of thriving.

References

Badenoch, B. (2017). *The heart of trauma: Healing the embodied brain in the context of relationships.* New York: Norton.

Blum, M. C. (2015). Embodied mirroring: A relational, body-to-body technique promoting movement in therapy. *Journal of Psychotherapy Integration, 25*(2), 115–127.

Bowlby, J. (1969). *Attachment and Loss: Attachment* (Vol. 1). New York: Basic Books.

Brown, S. & Eberle, M. (2018). A closer look at play. In T. Marks-Tarlow, M. Solomon, & D. Siegel (Eds.), *Play and creativity in psychotherapy* (pp. 21–38). New York: Norton.

Chan, A. & Siegel, D. J. (2018). Play and the default mode network: Interpersonal neurobiology, self, and creativity. In T. Marks-Tarlow, M. Solomon, & D. Siegel (Eds.), *Play and creativity in psychotherapy* (pp. 39–63). New York: Norton.

Cohen, D., Nakai, T., & Nishimoto, S. (2022). Brain networks are decoupled from external stimuli during internal cognition. *NeuroImage 256* Article 119230. https://doi.org/10.1016/j.neuroimage.2022.119230

Dana, D. (2018). *The polyvagal theory in therapy: Engaging the rhythm of regulation.* New York: Norton.

Ecker, B. (2018). Clinical translation of memory reconsolidation research: Therapeutic methodology for transformational change by erasing implicit emotional learnings driving symptom production. *International Journal of Neuropsychotherapy, 6*(1), 1–92. https://doi.org/10.12744/ijnpt.2018.0001-0092

Ecker, B., Hulley, L., & Ticic, R. (2015). Minding the findings: Let's not miss the message of memory reconsolidation research for psychotherapy. *Behavioral and Brain Sciences, 38.* https://doi.org/10.1017/S0140525X14000168

Feldman, R. (2007). Parent-infant synchrony: Biological foundations and developmental outcomes. *Current Directions in Psychological Science, 16*(6), 340–345.

Feldman, R. (2020). What is resilience: An affiliative neuroscience approach. *World Psychiatry, 19*(2), 132–150.

Fisher, J. (2017). *Healing the fragmented selves of trauma survivors: Overcoming self-alienation.* New York: Routledge.

Forner, C. (2019). What mindfulness can learn about dissociation and what dissociation can learn from mindfulness. *Journal of Trauma & Dissociation, 20*(1), 1–15. https://doi.org/10.1080/15299732.2018.1502568

Fosha, D. (2000). *The transforming power of affect: A model for accelerated change.* New York: Basic Books.

Fosha, D. (2005). Emotion, true self, true other, core state: Toward a clinical theory of affective change process. *Psychoanalytic Review, 92*(4), 513–551.

Fosha, D. (2007 Summer). "Good spiraling:" The phenomenology of healing and the engendering of secure attachment in AEDP. *Connections & Reflections, the GAINS Quarterly,* 3–13.

Fosha, D. (Ed.) (2021). *Undoing aloneness & the transformation of suffering into flourishing: AEDP 2.0.* Washington, DC: American Psychological Association.

Fredrickson, B. L. (2001). The role of positive emotions in positive psychology: The broaden-and-build theory of positive emotions. *American Psychologist, 56,* 218–226.

Fredrickson, B. L. (2013). Updated thinking on positivity ratios. *American Psychologist, 68*(9), 814–822.

Fredrickson, B. L. & Joiner, T. (2002). Positive emotions trigger upward spirals toward emotional well-being. *Psychological Science, 13*(2), 172–175.

Fredrickson, B. L. & Losada, M. F. (2005). Positive affect and the complex dynamics of human flourishing. *American Psychologist, 60*(7), 678–686. https://doi.org/10.1037/0003-066X.60.7.678

Gallese, V. (2009). Mirror neurons, embodied simulation, and the neural basis of social identification. *Psychoanalytic Dialogues, 19*, 519–536.

Gallese, V. (2010). Embodied simulation and its role in intersubjectivity. In T. Fuchs, H. C. Sattel, & P. Henningsen (Eds.), *The embodied self: Dimensions, coherence and disorders* (pp. 78–92). Stuttgart: Schattauer.

Gendlin, E. T. (1981). *Focusing*. New York: Bantam Books.

Gil, E. (2010). *Working with children to heal interpersonal trauma: The power of play*. New York: Guilford.

Heller, L. & Kammer, B. J. (2022). *The practical guide for healing developmental trauma: Using the NeuroAffective Relational Model to address adverse childhood experiences and resolve complex trauma*. Berkeley, CA: North Atlantic Books.

Hesse, E. & Main, M. (2006). Frightened, threatening, and dissociative parental behavior in low-risk samples: Description, discussion, and interpretations. *Development and Psychopathology, 18*(2), 309–343. https://doi.org/10.1017/S0954579406060172

Homeyer, L. E. & Morrison, M. O. (2008). Play therapy: Practice, issues and trends. *American Journal of Play, 1*(2), 210–228.

Hopenwasser, K. (2008). Being in rhythm: Dissociative attunement in therapeutic process. *Journal of Trauma & Dissociation, 9*(3), 349–367. https://doi.org/10.1080/15299730802139212

Hopenwasser, K. (2016). Dissociative attunement in a resonant world. In E. F. Howell & S. Iltzkowitz (Eds.), *The dissociative mind in psychoanalysis: Understanding and working with trauma* (pp. 175–186). New York: Routledge.

Iacoboni, M. (2007). The quiet revolution of existential neuroscience. In E. Harmon-Jones & P. Winkielman (Eds.), *Social neuroscience: Integrating biological and psychological explanations of social behavior* (pp. 439–453). New York: Guilford.

Kestly, T. A. (2014). *The interpersonal neurobiology of play: Brain-building interventions for emotional well-being*. New York: Norton.

Kestly, T. A. (2016). Presence and play: Why mindfulness matters. *International Journal of Play Therapy, 25*(1), 14–23. https://doi.org/10.1037/pla0000019

Korn, D. (2012, July 14–15). *EMDR the next generation: Finding your way in the dark*. [EMDR Master Class presented in Iselin, NJ].

Lenzi, D., Trentini, C., Pantano, P., Macaluso, E., Iacoboni, M., Lenzi, G. L., & Ammaniti, M. (2009). Neural basis of maternal communication and emotional expression processing during infant preverbal stage. *Cerebral Cortex, 19*(5), 1124–1133.

Malchiodi, C. A. (Ed.) (2023). *Handbook of expressive arts therapy*. New York: Guilford.

Marks-Tarlow, T., Solomon, M., & Siegel, D. (Eds.) (2018). *Play and creativity in psychotherapy*. New York: Norton.

Maroda, K. (1998). Enactments: When the patient's and analyst's pasts converge. *Psychoanalytic Psychology, 15*(4), 517–535.

Marriott, S. & Kelley, A. (Executive Producers) (2021, February 15). How we become the person's we are, with Dr. Alan Sroufe. Attachment through the lifespan. (No. 141). [Audio podcast episode]. In *Therapist Uncensored*. https://therapistuncensored.com/episodes/attachment-through-the-lifespan-alan-sroufe/

McCarthy, D. (2007). *"If you turned into a monster": Transformation through play: A body-centered approach to play therapy*. London: Jessica Kingsley.

Merleau-Ponty, M. (1962). *Phenomenology of perception*. London: Routledge & Kegan Paul.

Ogden, P. (2019). Acts of triumph: An interpretation of Pierre Janet and the role of the body in trauma treatment. In G. Craparo, F. Ortu, & O. van der Hart (Eds.), *Rediscovering Pierre Jane: Trauma, dissociation, and a new context for psychoanalysis* (pp. 200–209). New York: Routledge.

Ogden, P., Minton, K., & Pain, C. (2006). *Trauma and the body: A sensorimotor approach to psychotherapy.* New York: Norton.

Ogden, T. (1994). The analytic third: Working with intersubjective clinical facts. *International Journal of Psychoanalysis, 75,* 3–20.

Olson-Morrison, D. (2017). Integrative play therapy with adults with complex trauma: A developmentally-informed approach. *International Journal of Play Therapy, 26*(3), 172–183.

Panksepp, J. (1998). *Affective neuroscience: The foundation of human and animal emotions.* New York: Oxford University Press.

Panksepp, J. (2011a). Child development and the emotional circuits of mammalian brains. In R. E. Tremblay, M. Boivin, R. DeV Peters (Eds.), M. Lewis (topic ed.), *Encyclopedia on early childhood development* (pp. 1–5). child-encyclopedia.com.

Panksepp, J. (2011b). The basic emotional circuits of mammalian brains: Do animals have affective lives? *Neuroscience and Biobehavioral Reviews, 35*(9), 1791–1804.

Pargament, K. I. (2007). *Spiritually integrated psychotherapy: Understanding and addressing the sacred.* New York: Guilford.

Perry, B. D. (2014). The Neurosequential Model of Therapeutics: Application of a developmentally sensitive and neurobiology-informed approach to clinical problem solving in maltreated children. In K. Brandt, B. D. Perry, S. Seligman, & E. Tronick (Eds.), *Infant and early childhood mental health: Core concepts and clinical practice* (pp. 21–53). Washington, DC: American Psychiatric Publishing.

Piliero, S. (2021). Fierce love: Championing the core self to transform trauma and pathogenic states. In D. Fosha (Ed.), *Undoing aloneness & the transformation of suffering into flourishing: AEDP 2.0* (pp. 269–291). Washington, DC: American Psychological Association.

Porges, S. W. (2009). Reciprocal influences between body and brain in the perception and expression of affect. A polyvagal perspective. In D. Fosha, D. J. Siegel, & M. F. Solomon (Eds.), *The healing power of emotion: Affective neuroscience, development and clinical practice* (pp. 27–54). New York: Norton.

Porges, S. W. (2011). *The polyvagal theory: Neurophysiological foundations of emotions, attachment, communication, and self-regulation.* New York: Norton.

Porges, S. W. (2015). Play as neural exercise: Insights from the polyvagal theory. In D. Pearce-McCall (Ed.), *The power of play for mind brain health* (pp. 3–7). mindgains. org.

Prenn, N. (2011). Mind the gap: AEDP interventions translating attachment theory into clinical practice. *Journal of Psychotherapy Integration, 21*(3), 308–329.

Price, R. B. & Duman, R. (2020). Neuroplasticity in cognitive and psychological mechanisms of depression: An integrative model. *Molecular Psychiatry, 25,* 530–543. https://doi.org/10.1038/s41380-019-0615-x

Rothschild, B. (2021). *Revolutionizing trauma treatment: Stabilization, safety and nervous system balance.* New York: Norton.

Schore, A. N. (2010). The right brain implicit self: A central mechanism of the psychotherapy change process. In J. Petrucelli (Ed.), *Knowing, not-knowing and sort-of-knowing: Psychoanalysis and the experience of uncertainty* (pp. 177–202). London: Karnac Books.

Schore, A. N. (2011). The right brain implicit self lies at the core of psychoanalysis. *Psychoanalytic Dialogues: The International Journal of Relational Perspectives, 21,* 75–100.

Schore, A. N. (2022). Right-brain-to-right-brain psychotherapy: Recent scientific and clinical advances. *Annals of General Psychiatry, 21*(46). https://doi.org/10.1186/s12991-022-00420-3

Schore, J. R. & Schore, A. N. (2008). Modern attachment theory: The central role of affect regulation in development and treatment. *Clinical Social Work Journal, 36,* 9–20.

Schwartz, A. & Maiberger, B. (2018). *EMDR therapy and somatic psychology: Interventions to enhance embodiment in trauma treatment.* New York: Norton.

Schwartz, R. C. & Sweezy, M. (2020). *Internal Family Systems* (2nd ed.). New York: Guilford.

Siegel, D. J. (2020a). *Aware: The science and practice of presence.* New York: Penguin Random House.

Siegel, D. J. (2020b). *The developing mind: How relationships and the brain interact to shape who we are* (3rd ed.). New York: Guilford.

Siegel, D. J. & Payne Bryson, T. (2020). *The power of showing up: How parental presence shapes who our kids become and how their brains get wired.* New York: Ballantine Books.

Stanley, S. (2016). *Relational and body-centered practices for healing trauma: Lifting the burdens of the past.* New York: Routledge.

Stern, D. N., Bruschweiler-Stern, N., Harrison, A. M., Lyons-Ruth, K., Morgan, A. C., Nahum, J. P., Sander, L., & Tronick, E. Z. (1998). The process of therapeutic change involving implicit knowledge: Some implications of developmental observations for adult psychotherapy. *Infant Mental Health Journal, 19*(3), 200–308.

Stevens, V. (2018). Resonance, synchrony, and empathic attunement: Musical dimensions of psychotherapy. In T. Marks-Tarlow, M. Solomon, & D. J. Siegel (Eds.), *Play and creativity in psychotherapy* (pp. 191–216). New York: Norton.

Tuber, S. (2020). *Attachment, play, and authenticity: Winnicott in a clinical context* (2nd ed.). Lanham, MD: Rowman & Littlefield.

Vaish, A., Grossmann, T., & Woodward, A. (2008). Not all emotions are created equal: The negativity bias in social-emotional development. *Psychological Bulletin, 134*(3), 383–403. https://doi.org/10.1037/0033-2909.134.3.383

Vaisvaser, S. (2021). The embodied-enactive-interactive brain: Bridging neuroscience and creative arts therapies. *Frontiers in Psychology, 12* April, Article 634079.

Valentine, L. & Gabbard, G. O. (2014). Can the use of humor in psychotherapy be taught? *Academic Psychiatry, 38*(1), 75–81.

Van der Hart, O., Nijenhuis, E. R. S., & Steele, K. (2006). *The haunted self: Structural dissociation and the treatment of chronic traumatization.* New York: Norton.

Van der Kolk, B. A. (2014). *The body keeps the score: Brain, mind and body in the healing of trauma.* New York: Penguin.

Warner, E., Westcott, A, Cook, A., & Finn, H. (2020). *Transforming trauma in children and adolescents: An embodied approach to somatic regulation, trauma processing, and attachment-building.* Berkeley, CA: North Atlantic Books.

Wesselmann, D. (2014, April 4). *Trauma Time.* https://debrawesselmann.com/2014/trauma-time/

Winnicott, D. W. (1971). *Playing and reality.* London: Tavistock.

Yeung, D. (2021). What went right?: What happens in the brain during AEDP's meta-therapeutic processing. In D. Fosha (Ed.), *Undoing aloneness & the transformation of suffering* (pp. 349–376). Washington, DC: American Psychological Association.

Chapter 6

How Trauma Symptoms Welcome Playfulness

From Enemies to Allies

Approaching Trauma Symptoms Playfully

Imagine a puppy, a kitten, or a newborn baby. Now, notice what comes up inside you when you do. For most of us, these images tend to evoke a tender "ooh" or "ahh." These tiny beings evoke words like "adorable," "innocent," "tiny," "helpless," "lovable," and "sweet." Most of us are drawn to such small beings; we love looking at them, and we want to approach, embrace, and even play with them. They spontaneously raise our empathy, compassion, and protectiveness. When we see hurting puppies, kittens, and babies on TV commercials soliciting donations, we feel an extra strong tug in our hearts—which is what the marketers bank on, of course. We want to help these innocent ones heal from all their wounds and delight in their explorations and discoveries.

But this powerful inclination is often challenged in us when we meet with hurt people's trauma symptoms: self-mutilation, drug or substance abuse, debilitating depression, crippling anxiety, dissociation, depersonalization, derealization, flashbacks, voices, and dysregulated affect like rage or complete submission. Whether we are therapists in training or seasoned, it is natural to feel frightened or overwhelmed in the face of such symptoms and even hope the client gets assigned to or goes to a different therapist.

Over the years, I have heard many colleagues state, "I'm not a trauma therapist," hoping to avoid working with very dysregulated and dysregulating traumatized clients. Yet when we remember the six UNs of trauma (from Chapter 1)—a person feeling UNsafe, UNseen, and UNconnected (and alone) and their appraisals of the trauma as UNbearable (and intolerable), UNwilled (and unwanted), and UNresolved—we realize that all therapists, at some level are, and need to be, trauma therapists. We all treat people who experience overwhelming hurt.

Wouldn't it be nice to be unafraid of trauma work and related symptoms? And wouldn't it be even better to invite, welcome, embrace, and play with trauma symptoms and the people they're connected to—just like we would welcome an injured puppy, kitten, or baby? Let's explore how.

DOI: 10.4324/9781003509493-10

Symptoms: Allies in Trauma Treatment

Symptoms Signal That Something Is Wrong—Come See What It Is

To start, let's appreciate that a symptom is a brilliant, most often intuitive, construction of the mind and body. *Symptoms signal that something is not right, something is out of balance, or we are not functioning at our very best.* A symptom is like a gauge in our car that lets us know it's time for servicing, perhaps before our car becomes undriveable. In this way, a symptom is a wonderful ally that gives us a signal that repair is needed to restore balance.

More specifically, symptoms in the form of distressing thoughts, feelings, and body responses are "communications from trauma-related parts" (Fisher, 2017, p. 11). Symptoms wave yellow and red flags saying, "Hey, look at me, there's something amiss here. Can you please come, check me out, and help?" Symptoms invite us to explore two questions. First, what's going on, in the here-and-now, that triggered this response? Second, how is this action pattern related to something from the past that needs resolution and possible transformation?

Let's return to the Model of Structural Dissociation of the Personality (SD) (van der Hart et al., 2006, discussed in Chapter 2) to better understand symptoms. The five EPs, or emotional parts of the personality, are fight, flight, freeze/fear, shame/submit, and attach/separation distress. These are the emotional action systems with which we respond to triggers of stress, danger, or life threat. In this way, we can think of each EP as a protector system that lives along a continuum. As a person's experience of threat increases, so does their autonomic nervous system (ANS) dysregulation, which causes the EP to react in an unmodulated way. Symptoms signal us as to which EP protection system has been triggered and hijacks the person. When EPs kick into gear and a person reacts in a calm and regulated way (without symptoms), we know the EPs are working in unison with each other and wise Self (see Chapter 2).

For example, 42-year-old Todd was painfully bullied by a co-worker who repeatedly pointed out his mistakes. Each time, Todd successfully soothed his triggered feelings of inadequacy and self-doubt (shame EP), used choice words (fight EP) to shut the bully up, and walked away (flight EP). By contrast, in his synagogue's baseball league, Todd's fight reaction overtook him when dealing with the team's coach who won more votes than Todd to become chairman of the men's group. During a game, the coach replaced Todd with another pitcher (triggering the shame/submit EP). Todd lost his cool and started cursing and yelling at his coach (fight EP), which caused him to be expelled from the game (increasing shame EP).

Depending on the situation, our EPs can act in modulated or hijacking ways. I remind clients that our EPs are wired-in emotional action systems that we can learn to dial up or down through our intentional, here-and-now presence. When

EPs hijack our wise, resourced presence, they cause the very thing they tried to soothe. Todd's fight reaction to his coach increased rather than decreased his shame. Our symptoms signal which EP is working too hard and needs help from the other EPs and Self. I use Janina Fisher's flip chart (Fisher, 2022) to help clients identify which EPs are activated, assess how well they are working in tandem with their wise Self, and figure out how familiar this action pattern is. This curiosity often leads to a recognition that the response is familiar and in fact is a procedurally learned (sensorimotor) memory. The playing out of the memory is an enactment—a present expression of how the client showed up then in response to threat. We explicitly appreciate how a client's EPs helped them survive their trauma and explore related scripts further. Like using a knob, we help clients dial up or down the EP's activation. In this way, we are updating, not eliminating, the EP so it can fit the present need as a here-and-now adaptation.

Symptoms Then: Trauma-Time Adaptations That Were Protective

Symptoms are snapshots of the action patterns that were used as adaptations at the time of the trauma. These present-time snapshots are both *remnants of* and *windows into* what a person did to survive their trauma. These vestiges of trauma memories that show up in the present act like "living memories" (Fisher, 2017). Trauma memories are stored in the right hemisphere in implicit, fragmented ways without a coherent narrative. They present as body memories, primary process symptoms (i.e., sensations, images), and may include feelings of deep depression, fear/panic, stuckness, dissociation, separation anxiety, rage, intense control or micromanagement, substance abuse or other addictions, physical, emotional, mental, or sexual abuse of others, fleeing, or hiding. These symptoms can be reframed as present-time signals to client and therapist that something is wrong and direct us to see how they might have acted then in response to a similar threat.

How each of us adapts to life threat or danger is unique. We each spontaneously and intuitively react in ways that increase our chances of survival. These trauma-based adaptations are unconscious, tailor-made action patterns consisting of what is most relevant to the threat, best-suited to the person's developmental and cognitive levels, relationship dynamics, and life context at that time. In other words, everyone really does the best they can with the resources they have at that time in their lives. Adaptations are specific to that person, for that trauma, at that time, as are the related symptoms that emerge to signal something is out of whack.

One way that a therapist can reframe a symptom is by understanding that a behavior that "may appear to be an irrational 'disorder' is actually full of personal meaning and deep sense when viewed from the underlying emotional context from which it arises" (Ecker, 2003, p. 39). This is called *symptom coherence*, "a well-defined, cogent set of personal themes and purposes that necessitate the symptom and its production" (Ecker, 2003, pp. 39–40). Symptom coherence explains why cutting behaviors in two 13-year-old girls might hold vastly different meanings to each. While Treena used cutting to increase her sense of control over pain—both how much and whether she or others induced it—Ally cut to intentionally scar herself to never forget or forgive the harm her perpetrator caused.

Our ability to adapt so creatively and uniquely is truly incredible. Thus, calling all symptoms "maladaptive coping mechanisms" dilutes the rich wealth of functions they served in the past and their current relevance. Our responsibility as trauma therapists is to discover and unfold the unique emotional truths, themes, constructs, belief systems, sensorimotor patterns, and spiritual energies relevant to each person to reveal their specific resources, creativity, and resilience.

The signaling of distress with current symptoms beckons us to investigate why this particular symptom has appeared and how it was used adaptively in trauma time and became a protector part (Fisher, 2017; Schwartz & Sweezy, 2020; van der Hart et al., 2006). While this perspective is widely accepted, Western medicine–influenced approaches tend to focus on symptom reduction or elimination, per se. Eastern-influenced approaches like mindfulness or Focusing (Gendlin, 1981) make space for the symptom's presence and notice what unfolds. Such bottom-up trauma treatment approaches and creative arts and play therapies are more inclined to invite, welcome, and work with symptoms because they appreciate and lean into the brilliance of symptoms' functions and uniqueness.

Symptoms Now: Trauma-Time Protectors That Hurt Us

At the time of trauma, a person's survival-based coping response was "compellingly necessary and purposeful to avoid suffering" (Ecker et al., 2012, p. 68). It was protective and adaptive, allowing the preservation of the person's essence and integrity of their Self, body, mind, or spirit. As we learned in Chapter 2, ANS disturbance and affect dysregulation, disintegration of brain functioning, and disconnection from others and Self ironically function to help us survive.

However, when there is a lack of attuned fit between the current threat and the coping response, a "symptom" emerges. A symptom can appear as an over or underreaction to the trigger and does not resolve the issue. Symptoms indicate that a person is reacting to the *here-and-now* stressor as if they are in the *then-and-there*. If the response fits the current stressor or threat and the issue is resolved, there is no issue. A current maladaptive symptom or action pattern was adaptive to another time, place, and interpersonal context (Russell, 2015, p. 27) when it was comforting and/or life-saving. Used in non-threatening situations, these responses become life-limiting and often hijack a person, causing the very thing they wish to prevent (i.e., self-sabotage).

For example, going into a fetal position, rocking, and putting his hands over his ears might have been comforting when gunfire surrounded Pat's home at age 8, but not when 16-year-old Pat tries to enjoy celebratory fireworks. These once adaptive, protective responses are no longer sufficiently effective at resolving the distress. In fact, using outdated or ill-fitting protectors can hurt us and leave us more symptomatic.

Internal Family Systems (see Chapter 2 and Schwartz, 1995; Schwartz & Sweezy, 2020) provides a map of how our minds adapt to trauma by developing an internal system with manager and firefighter parts to protect the trauma-burdened exiles stuck in trauma time. Even when the traumatic event ends, the complex and clever internal system of protection remains intact. Managers are constantly at work in the background to proactively prevent exiles from breaking through and hijacking us by dysregulating our ANS and leaving us unable to function. Managers help us go on with normal life *as if* everything is peachy keen: "Nothing's wrong here. We're good."

However, events in current life have a way of breaking through this *as if* all-is-fine experience (maintained by our "Going on With Normal Life" [Fisher, 2017] or Apparently Normal Part in SD, [van der Hart et al., 2006]). When the proactive actions of the managers fail to protect the exiles, the firefighter parts enter the scene, reactively shutting down the triggered exiles who threaten to upend the entire system with intolerable trauma memories and related affects, behaviors, feelings, sensations, etc. The exiles send SOS signals, or symptoms, to the person and the world that say, "See us and rescue us from the burdens of our unresolved traumatic past." The firefighter-driven behaviors show up as the big, in-your-face symptoms such as cutting that requires an emergency room visit or sexual addiction that results in a gang rape. Ultimately, destructive symptoms signal the need to update the once-effective protective internal system through the leadership provided by the present-day wise Self and the therapist.

Protectors in Disguise—Good Intentions, Poor Execution

We can appreciate that protector parts like disturbing emotional parts (EPs) or firefighters don't look or feel like "protectors" when they cause more harm than good. Used in non-threatening situations, these trauma-produced protectors can feel life-limiting and often hijack a person, causing the very thing they wish to prevent (i.e., self-sabotage). So perhaps we can think instead of these stuck-in-trauma-time protective symptoms as protectors *in disguise*.

No matter how well-intentioned our defenses and protective functions are, they will be limited if stuck in the time of trauma. For example, just like we'd never ask our 5-year-old parts to complete a geometry test, nor would we expect a 40-year-old to rely on her 4-year-old trauma-time protectors that coped with paternal incest to adequately handle sexual advances by the senior partner at her law firm. Trauma-time protectors only benefit from the skills and resources available at that time, at that age, in that context of relationships and life.

When constructs, beliefs, emotions, sensorimotor expressions, and action patterns are formed in trauma time, the coping repertoires or scripts they yield tend to be binary and inflexible and represent the dialectic of victim-victimizer, perpetrated-perpetrator, or death-survival. The symptoms that emerge cohere with and reflect this trauma-related protection system.

When clients' protector parts identify with sadistic abusers, this process can become more fraught. Clients who behave aggressively, masochistically (i.e., self-mutilate or repeatedly put themselves in harm's way), treat their "loved ones" abusively, or sabotage all treatment efforts test their therapist's ability to connect with compassion and empathy. These darker sides of our clients need to be remembered as protectors in disguise. The bolder, scarier, and uglier the symptoms, the more vulnerable, horror-filled, and burdensome the experience of trauma being guarded is. We must go through repeated cycles of teaching these symptomatic clients about their trauma-time protectors' attempts to pre-serve attachment at all costs to enable survival. Attachment to sadistic abusers sometimes entails internalizing and identifying with them to survive. We may need extra supervision or consultation to find ways to connect with these clients because of the fear and vicarious traumatization pulled up in us.

It follows and is not surprising that a vast number of my clients have looked at me askance when I've framed their dysregulating symptoms as protectors. They've said, "Protectors? You call my overeating to the point of becoming obese *protective*?" Or, "Who's the one who belongs on the couch? How can my staying in bed and binge-watching Netflix for days and not going to work be protective?" Or, "I see that my anger was defensive, but not the part when I threw the chair and got expelled. Now my college acceptance is jeopardized!"

These are all opportunities to help clients identify and appreciate that the *intention* behind the behavior was protective, but the execution was misattuned, misaligned, or went off the rails completely. Many clients can relate to the expe-rience that even when people have the best of intentions, they can fail miserably. As the saying goes, the road to hell is paved with good intentions. When clients understand the limitations of their trauma-time protectors' efforts, they may gain compassion for how they tried valiantly yet insufficiently to soothe their internal distress. When grounded and connected to their Self, clients grow appreciative that symptoms or dysregulation results from actions of misguided protectors in disguise. We support our clients to grow compassion for these parts which opens up space to update their protectors to their current developmental-relational con-text. We help clients integrate their updated protectors to become well-resourced to collaboratively and effectively work with all parts of mind.

Other clients are less receptive to compassion for their protectors in dis-guise, which may reflect a blend between present and trauma-time orientation and parts. For example, Robin, an 84-year-old client who had a childhood and marital history of dismissive and hurtful attachments, consistently challenged me on the point that behind every symptom lies a protective, good intention. She'd call it "pitcher-stone" (a term she picked up from *Man of La Mancha*). She'd say, "Yes, I hear you Monica, but whether the stone hits the pitcher, or the pitcher hits the stone, the glass pitcher lies there in shattered pieces."

When Robin's adult daughter, Zeena, made minimal to no contact with her for weeks on end, Robin's stuck in trauma-time, attachment-driven protectors were triggered: she felt abandoned, ignored, dismissed, and irrelevant. In an effort to reconnect with, be seen, and appreciated by her daughter, Robin's very young (ages 3–13) attach EPs took over the reins. She'd push connection on Zeena, offering financial help, treating her to go shopping and out for meals together, or volunteering to "help" lessen Zeena's stress by physically and financially caring for her four children.

These protectors in disguise inadvertently enabled Zeena to stay distanced from Robin; whether or not Zeena reciprocated Robin's efforts to connect, Robin would do all the work to maintain connection. In addition, Zeena unconsciously learned that her states of distress triggered her mother's rescuer parts. Robin's attachment-motivated and good-girl rescuer protectors left her feeling disabled—exhausted by twisting herself to accommodate her daughter's schedule, used "like a sucker," and unseen. "Zeena wouldn't care if I dropped dead as long as there was money for her in my will!" Robin would invoke "pitcher-stone," explaining that while understanding (in her left brain) that her protectors were trying to help her, her symptoms of feeling dismissed, abandoned, and exhausted left her heart shattered in pieces like the broken pitcher. Whether her protectors intended this or not, the result was the same.

At this point, I reminded Robin that *her protectors were only trying to protect that which is worthy* and were reacting to the need to maintain connection, at all costs, with her daughter. This reflection of worthiness and good intentions did not land. Robin beat herself up even further: "I'm such a shmuck. What's wrong with me?" Helping Robin access self-compassion was ineffective. Her wise Self was blended (see Fisher, 2017; Schwartz & Sweezy, 2020) with her critical (Fight EP) and shaming (Shame/Submit EP) protectors.

Also, Robin could not objectively appreciate that her protectors in disguise were well-intentioned because they caused her to feel terrible. Robin needed me to acknowledge her "pitcher-stone" experience. However, my caring intentions to relieve her pain (my countertransference) caused me to focus on the positive intentions of her protectors. This was a misattunement, leaving Robin feeling dismissed as had her parents, daughter, and husband. Once I admitted how I missed what she needed, and acknowledged and empathically processed her anguish, Robin could deeply, securely, and finally experience and grieve her anger and pain at feeling misunderstood and invisible. Together we repaired the enactment of relational misattunement and invalidation. We also co-created a new, transformative experience of me reflecting and sitting with Robin's emotions, allowing her to be and feel safe, seen, and soothed in a secure and steady way with her protector-induced pain (see Siegel & Payne Bryson, 2020). This repair paved the way for Robin to mirror the same attunement intrapsychically and with others.

Robin's "pitcher-stone" challenge highlights the importance of acknowledging the pain inflicted by the misattuned internal protectors and the resulting destructive symptoms left in their wake. Through the earned, secure attachment with our clients, we pave a path for clients to approach their misattuned protectors more caringly, as Robin and I did. This helped Robin grow to appreciate and validate her own pain and ways her stuck-in-trauma-time defenses hurt her. She repaired her internal ruptures by creating more integrated, cooperative, and attuned protection and soothing. Robin recognized that while it was her very nature to be charitable and giving, she noticed imbalance in how she didn't give enough emotional nurturance to herself and gave too much to others when her attach-seeking protector parts detected abandonment or rejection. For example, Robin tried to give me lavish gifts of gratitude and appreciation, which, as her therapist, left me uncomfortable. Robin worried she was getting more from me than I was getting from her and that this would cause me to resent her. This was Robin's "pitcher-stone" in reverse, which we explored quite intimately, with many shared tears of mutual love.

Eventually, Robin learned to modulate her gift-giving to be appropriate and comfortable for me and others. She developed more attuned ways of giving to herself, too. Rather than allowing her 3–13-year-old protectors to take charge of threats to or imbalances in her attachments, she learned to thank them for their efforts, telling them they were no longer alone and didn't need to lead the way in protecting her. Robin brought her additional 70–80 years of lived experience to update her attach, fear, shame/submit, and fight protectors. Over time, Robin smiled and relaxed as her trauma-time protectors felt increasingly heard, seen, and soothed by her adult, compassionate wise Self. Her protectors softened and became cooperative, more readily stepping to the side as they felt more trust in letting her wise, current-day Self lead the way. The lessons learned from history remained accessible but now lacked the heavy, burdensome pain.

With practice, Robin increasingly connected with and genuinely appreciated the following points, which are relevant to our work with all trauma clients:

1. Symptoms signal that historic, stuck-in-trauma-time protectors have been triggered.
2. Protectors' or defenses' resourcefulness is bound to the time of the trauma when they emerged. We did the best we could with what we had access to back then.
3. Protectors are well-intentioned at their root—that's why they're called protectors!
4. Defenses and protector parts emerge out of a given truth that our core essence is worthy of protection and care.

THEN

Trauma

TRAUMA TIME Survival Response/Adaptation
• Life-saving and life-preserving
• Protective and comforting
• Perfect-fit for the D-R-C

NOW

Trigger

TRAUMA TIME Survival Response/Adaptation
• Life-limiting
• Can be destructive and distressing
• Poor fit to here-and-now (D-R-C)
• Blocks needs from getting met
• Causes symptoms that cause the effect they tried to avoid

D-R-C = Developmental Relational Context

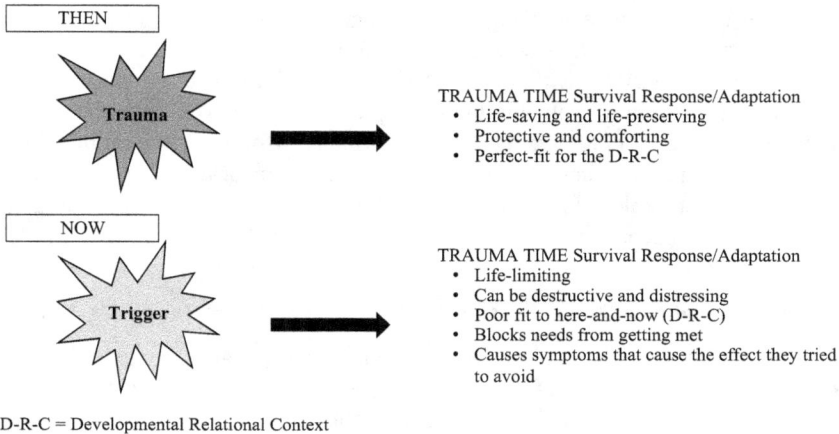

Figure 6.1 Trauma-time protectors—then and now.

5. Protectors function dynamically within ourselves, with others, and in the world, mirroring the blueprint of our earlier attachment dynamics.
6. When trauma-time protectors take us over or hijack us, they act as protectors in disguise, causing harm not help.
7. By revealing the wisdom of our once life-preserving, survival-promoting protector systems through exploring our intrapsychic system, we can facilitate the repair of attachments internally and with others to better show up in our current life.
8. Trauma-based symptoms can be transformed in the present, from life-limiting to safe, relevant, contingent, life-enhancing, and affirming protectors.

Figure 6.1 summarizes how trauma symptoms function differently at the time of the trauma compared with the present when the trauma has passed.

In summary, symptoms are true allies of trauma treatment. They are visible and available to lead us to their right-hemispheric origins and related circumstances. However, when symptoms show up as protectors in disguise, they belie—to client and therapist—the gifts and golden treasures they contain to promote tailored-made healing. As trauma therapists, we must hold in mind the true nature and worth of symptoms, no matter how disturbing and dark they appear.

How to Invite, Welcome, and Embrace Symptoms Playfully: Learning from Children's Intuitive Wisdom

When we reframe symptoms as protectors in disguise, we feel more comfortable and curious to approach and work with them: we encourage clients to do the same. Yet this can be challenging for adults. First, how can someone learn to trust the very symptom that causes them distress or harm? Also, some cultures, particularly industrialized nations, intentionally prioritize comfort and ease, discouraging people to welcome their symptoms. People go to great lengths to avoid, demonize, or eradicate their uncomfortable, off-putting symptoms. Pharmaceutical companies and Western medicine have historically leaned into an elimination-not-exploration mindset with physical expressions of psychological and emotional discomfort.

Symptoms Embody Deep, Personal Wisdom—Let Them Teach Us

Instead, McCarthy (2007), based on Carl Jung's work, beautifully explains how symptoms are expressions of our shadow sides. We tend to relate to our shadow sides as "not me" or the "anti-me" because of their unacceptable, disturbing, and even uncivilized qualities which do not fit into our family systems and larger community, culture, or world. The shadow holds energy related to loss, pain, grief, fear, or rage and can feel like a "monster" within us (McCarthy, 2007, p. 13). In cultures where we downplay or outright deny our dark, scary, and threatening monster sides, we cut ourselves off from our associated vitality—our life-affirming energies. By contrast, some cultures (e.g., the West African Dagara tribe, see Somé, 1997) teach us not only to embrace but intentionally connect with the shadow sides, revealing their evolutionary and ancestral powers.

But consider that we don't have to look far to see this wisdom enacted. Children, who welcome their monster or shadow sides, are our everyday shamans. Through play, children model and teach us to approach, welcome, and embrace all symptoms, regardless of the level of discomfort they trigger. All day long, children play out dark and scary themes as well as light and beautiful ones. For example, children may play out aggression or destruction themes when they build and destroy block towers or sandcastles, pour red and black paint all over their carefully drawn city scene, or make dolls fight each other. Kids draw or become monsters and scare anyone in their midst with loud roars or a surprise "attack."

Symptoms are interwoven through children's play, driving its purpose and meaning. Kids just go for it; it's as if their play says to the onlooker, "Now that I've got your attention, look at what's going on in my life. Here's what's right— let's enjoy it. Here's what's wrong—let's fix it and enjoy what emerges!" Children seem to connect with their evolutionary wisdom, intuitive "knowing," and trust that the symptom holds the solution. The energy behind a symptom provides the push toward wholeness and exactly what we need to instigate healing, growth, and development (Bakur Weiner & Simmons, 2009, p. xi) and achieve regulation. In play, children demonstrate that "the sense of what is wrong carries with it, inseparably, a sense of the direction toward what is right" (Gendlin, 1981, p. 86).

When children are supported wisely and safely to playfully follow and explore their process, possibilities for change and transformation appear. "The child's fiery passion and life force must be tolerated and even encouraged . . . [because] the energy needed to change is embedded in the symptom itself" (McCarthy, 2007, p. 112). For example, when 5-year-old Molly kicked her doll hard and broke off its head, I explored rather than reprimanded her. "Wow, your foot had so much power when kicking the doll!" (I made the language experience-distant to minimize Molly's shame of having done something wrong.) "What did your foot say to dolly when kicking it? How did your foot feel when it moved that way? What did dolly say to your foot?" The dialogue that emerged revealed Molly's anger at her aunt who gave her the doll. Molly said, "She promised she would play dolly with me when she had her sleepover (during a weekend visit). But she left because of a 'mergency.' She didn't say good-bye." Molly was mad and sad that her aunt left suddenly and unpredictably. This raised early abandonment memories which now could be further explored.

Molly's example represents the premise of play and creative therapies. Therapists need to embrace the safe expression of our client's intuition and creativity, which reflects all facets of their being. This support encourages the emergence and strengthening of the client's drives toward growth and change for the better. This is seen poignantly in play therapy with traumatized children. The way children express and use symptoms in play shows they got the memo: symptoms are valuable signals from trauma-time protector parts asking for attention and repair. Paraphrasing McCarthy (2007, p. 15), the experience of being with the symptom (that appears like a monster) is like entering a doorway to a labyrinth which leads us deeper and deeper to the treasure that lies within. We can embrace symptoms as a portal for healing with clients of all ages.

Along these lines, somatic-based therapies used with adults (e.g., Dance Movement Therapy, Sensorimotor Psychotherapy, Somatic Experiencing, and Body-Mind Therapy) similarly and intentionally mine the body symptoms, follow them, and allow them to unfold to reveal trauma-transforming movements and affects. Even for those of us not schooled in creative, play, or somatic therapies, we can embrace trauma symptoms to affect change by embodying a playful mindset with an open, curious, and supportive stance.

Symptoms Hold Treasured Solutions—Let Them Lead Us

Through play, children show us how embracing and unfolding symptoms leads to solutions and releases transformational energy. Even post-traumatic play can be unfolded with clinical acumen to reveal the wisdom held within the symptoms (Gil, 2017). Since symptoms hold the solutions, we must follow them, whether they manifest as a collapsed depression and submission, paralysis or stuckness, panic, separation anxiety, rage, dissociation, disintegration, annihilation, fear of death, etc. Welcoming and embracing symptoms is relevant to clients of all ages.

When playing follow the leader, trust in the leader is assumed. By mirroring and copying what the leader does, we trust we will not be led down a path of harm. This same trust is implied when we as therapists follow the lead of the client's scary and monstrous symptoms. We do so by mirroring and reflecting the symptoms' sensorimotor expressions of what is wrong. By dropping into the body to join with and explore symptoms, fears may arise in us. *Where will the symptom-leader bring us? Will the client handle what emerges? Will I be able to handle it?* When these anxious questions arise, I lean into my experience that no symptom has ever failed me in finding answers and bringing more clarity to me and my client, as long I surrender with faith to the symptom's wisdom. I also hold these words as truth:

> By heading straight into the core meaning at the heart of the symptom, therapy becomes a place where a deeper sense of order replaces the apparent senselessness of presenting complaints, and clients awaken to areas of self that have control over what previously seemed utterly out of control. The emotional truth of the symptom is always there, waiting to be discovered and embraced.
>
> (Ecker, 2003, p. 48)

When we ask adult clients to welcome, invite, embrace, play with, or magnify the very disturbance they wish to eliminate, it may cause pause and curious laughter. The irony of embracing and following otherwise disavowed or shame-filled parts can feel disarming, confusing, or even playful. Our nervous system relaxes as we move from a phobic response to a calm, welcoming one, activating safety and connection. In moving toward a symptom with curiosity, we are adopting a tend-and-befriend (Taylor, 2021) approach rather than a fight-or-flight one. This approach creates a juxtaposition experience (discussed in Chapter 5) which enables memory reconsolidation.

When we follow the symptom-leader and explore its emotional and somatic expression, we are led to the right hemisphere, which houses the original trauma memory and its affects, sensations, and procedurally learned action patterns. Related left hemisphere–held belief systems and scripts will emerge. When therapists follow the symptom-leader, we are led to the disturbing trauma fragments in need of transformation. By releasing the need to control the course of treatment and surrendering to the lead of our client and their symptoms, therapists discover sometimes unimaginable treasures. Trusting our client's symptoms' wisdom sets an example for clients to do the same. It also grows our own, our client's, and our mutual trust in the therapeutic relationship and process, while increasing hope that deeply reparative experiences are possible. We can metaprocess (see Chapter 9) these moments of change, which further fuels healing and transformation.

As a novice trauma therapist in the 1980s, I learned that following trauma symptoms would lead me directly to the right hemisphere's golden treasure, the motherlode of the original trauma memory/memories, and facilitate trauma resolution and symptom soothing. So, I strived to find the motherlode. This goal was relatively straightforward when I worked with single-incident traumas, whether big T or little t. However, the bulk of my caseload consisted of clients with chronic and complex trauma, and I failed to discover the golden treasure. In part, this was because chronic trauma results in the development of extensive neural networks of associations (Shapiro, 2018), which means there may not be one huge golden nugget, no motherlode, no single, original trauma memory that can be quickly processed to bring lasting relief. When unsuccessful at discovering the motherlode, I relied more heavily on techniques and protocols than the relationship, which often moved the therapy astray of my intention.

Fortunately, with supervision, further training, and commiserating with colleagues, I learned that the golden nuggets were right before my eyes in the here-and-now relationship with my clients. This made so much sense to me; many of my clients had attachment trauma histories combined with situational traumas. While true for all clients, it is especially true for our clients with chronic complex trauma: the healing journey requires a secure, attuned relational foundation that can then scaffold all that unfolds. Each symptom, along with its associated neural networks of emotional, affective, sensorimotor, and cognitive protector systems, needs repeated experiences and cycles of attuned, safe connection to allow healing.

The relational journey is scattered with tiny specks, chips, and dust of gold. Following many different symptom-leaders helps us accumulate the golden flecks or dust of attachment repair. A ton of gold is a ton of gold—whether comprised of thousands of golden glimmers or one golden boulder. Through practice and experience, I learned that above all else, when working with trauma, especially attachment trauma, therapists need to have deep patience, attunement, care, respect, and trust. With trust, we follow the numerous, if not seemingly endless, symptom-leaders on many different paths and sometimes repetitive-feeling cycles toward healing.

Being and Playing with Symptoms—A Mantra to Guide Trauma Work

When we view symptoms as our right brain–based, trauma treatment allies, we can feel more comfortable and curious about them. I'd like to share a mantra inspired by AEDP (Accelerated Experiential Dynamic Psychotherapy, Fosha, 2000, 2021) which I adapted (from Halliday, 2022—the bold is AEDP language, the italics are my addition) to remind me to hold a playful and welcoming mindset toward trauma-related symptoms: **come (and stay) here (with me)** *now, so we can explore and play safely*. This stance communicates: I want to meet and learn about you, and I want to hang out in this space together and creatively explore whatever comes up.

Embedded in this playfully welcoming attitude are Tibetan Buddhist, mindfulness, attachment, and play-inspired themes. Through this mantra, we convey implicitly and explicitly that we: (1) welcome what was formerly unwelcomed (Chödron, 2019); (2) offer a mindful, nonjudgmental, open, and curious holding environment for all parts of you; (3) genuinely want to be with you in relationship; (4) are focused just on the now, this present moment, to help you ground, feel contained and safe with me, a caring other; and (5) can go anywhere together, and it can even be fun.

This mindset helps us embody a playful spirit. A playful attitude with symptoms enables work with our clients to feel good, pleasurable, and satisfying. Ironically, playfulness with trauma may even encourage us to even feel drawn to the work—and maybe even want to do more of it. Who would ever imagine describing trauma work this way? Clients who can use playfulness to heal and transform trauma would and do. It doesn't mean trauma work isn't hard, it means that, with a playful spirit, we work smarter, not harder, and decrease, if not eliminate, the fear of doing it. Emboldened with this playful mindset, we now move forward to Part IV of this book, which guides us on how to practically infuse our playful spirit into the therapy setting and relationship to promote healing.

References

Bakur Weiner, M. & Simmons, M. B. (2009). *The problem is the solution: A Jungian approach to a meaningful life*. New York: Jason Aronson.

Chödron, P. (2019). *Welcoming the unwelcome: Wholehearted living in a brokenhearted world.* Boulder, CO: Shambhala.

Ecker, B. (2003). The hidden logic of anxiety: Look for the emotional truth behind the symptom. *Psychotherapy Networker, 27*(6), 38–43.

Ecker, B., Ticic, R., & Hulley, L. (2012) *Unlocking the emotional brain: Eliminating symptoms at their roots using memory reconsolidating*. New York: Routledge.

Fisher, J. (2017). *Healing the fragmented selves of trauma survivors: Overcoming self-alienation*. New York: Routledge.

Fisher, J. (2022). *The living legacy of trauma flip chart: A psychoeducational in-session tool for clients and therapists*. Eau Claire, WI: PESI.

Fosha, D. (2000). *The transforming power of affect: A model for accelerated change.* New York: Basic Books.

Fosha, D. (Ed.) (2021). *Undoing aloneness & the transformation of suffering into flourishing: AEDP 2.0.* Washington, DC: American Psychological Association.

Gendlin, E. T. (1981). *Focusing*. New York: Bantam Books.

Gil, E. (2017). *Posttraumatic play in children: What clinicians need to know.* New York: Guilford.

Halliday, K. (2022, March, 13). Experiences Teaches Meeting #3. AEDP Experiential Learning Online Course.

McCarthy, D. (2007). *"If you turned into a monster": Transformation through play: A body-centered approach to play therapy.* London: Jessica Kingsley.

Russell, E. (2015). *Restoring resilience: Discovering your clients' capacity for healing.* New York: Norton.

Schwartz, R. (1995). *Internal family systems therapy.* New York: Guilford.

Schwartz, R. C. & Sweezy, M. (2020). *Internal Family Systems* (2nd ed.). New York: Guilford.

Shapiro, F. (2018). *Eye Movement Desensitization and Reprocessing (EMDR) third edition: Basic principles, protocols and procedures.* New York: Guilford.

Siegel, D. J. & Payne Bryson, T. (2020). *The power of showing up: How parental presence shapes who our kids become and how their brains get wired.* New York: Ballantine Books.

Somé, P. M. (1997). *Ritual: Power, healing, and community: The African teachings of the Dagara.* New York: Penguin Books.

Taylor, J. B. (2021). Whole brain living: The anatomy of choice and the four characters that drive our life. Carlsbad, CA: Hay House.

van der Hart, O., Nijenhuis, E. R. S., & Steele, K. (2006). *The haunted self: Structural dissociation and the treatment of chronic traumatization.* New York: Norton.

Part IV

Infusing a Playful Spirit into Trauma Treatment

Chapter 7

Creating a Playful Therapy Setting

A Safe, Sensorimotor-Sensitive Space for Exploration and Healing

In this chapter, we will explore how to infuse a playful vibe into the treatment setting that promotes safety and healing opportunities for traumatized clients of all ages. The therapy space literally and figuratively helps us create a holding environment for our clients. We will examine how to capitalize on using the office space, online and in-person, to fully welcome clients—including their important others and all parts of mind. With sensitivity to our clients' trauma histories, we will explore how to use our senses—with sensorimotor and object play—to decorate and relationally play with the therapy milieu to support healing. Illustrative examples from my office space and practice will be shared.

Creating a Physical and Playful Holding Environment for Our Traumatized Clients

Clients seek therapy to get relief and heal. However, they reach for help to an unfamiliar person who practices in an unknown setting. This would be triggering for any of us, especially trauma survivors. From this perspective, we can appreciate how brave and bold starting therapy is.

Therefore, from the first client contact through the last—whether by email, phone, online, or in-person—we need to intentionally create a space that allows our traumatized client's autonomic nervous system (ANS) to detect safety. The therapy environment first must support somatic regulation before attachment-building and trauma processing can occur (Warner et al., 2020). Loosely borrowing from the concept of the holding environment (Winnicott, 1960), trauma therapists aim to create a physical space that can metaphorically and literally help clients feel safely held and secure for their best self to emerge. Making this therapy space playful makes clients want to return.

Let's keep in mind that our physical office space (in-person or online) represents the therapist's emotional and relational holding abilities, too. Therefore, as if speaking for us, we want our therapy setting to convey to our clients that you are "welcomed here" and can feel "at home with safety." We imbue our office

DOI: 10.4324/9781003509493-12

space with a sense of *mi casa es su casa*—my safe holding space is your safe holding space, let's share it.

We strengthen this implicit message with explicit statements that the space contained by the office walls secures confidentiality, keeps out what is unwanted and in what is wanted. We establish rules to further support these messages. For example, when clients accidentally curse, I might say, "I am okay with you cursing *in here*." For young children, I ask permission from caregivers about their swearing rules to align with their values. For teens or religious adults, I might remind them that we are sitting in a "no-judgment zone" and if they're ok, I'm ok. They know the regular rules of life turn back on when leaving the space.

In addition to conveying welcoming, safety, and holding, we can decorate our therapy space to communicate that "playfulness is encouraged here." We arrange objects around our offices that are easily accessible and promote playful or creative interaction. We may place fidget toys, puzzle gadgets, or objects of tactile interest (e.g., that are squooshy, flexible, soft) in easily accessible places. Arts and craft materials can inspire exploration and creativity. After decades of practicing with adults, a colleague placed a basket of colorful yarn, pipe cleaners, and markers next to the couch where her clients sit. She shared how this small addition put a smile on her face, helped her younger, more creative parts of mind emerge to help out in session, and stimulated long-standing clients to become playful and creative like never before. We can arrange pictures, books, and artwork throughout the setting to promote visual curiosity, lightness, and fun. We can remove objects that might be triggering to clients (e.g., artwork of nudes). We can encourage clients of all ages to feel free to use the objects contained in our holding environment and bring in their own. Tweaking our holding environment with playful touches may help us and our clients become more engaged.

Let's now explore how we can make the holding environment even more attuned, welcoming, and playful by recruiting our traumatized clients' sensory and movement channels.

Engaging Sensorimotor Sensitivity and Safety in the Therapy Setting with Our Traumatized Clients

To promote our client's engagement in the therapy space and subsequently the therapy relationship, we can use sensorimotor sensitivity that is trauma-informed and individually oriented—thereby synthesizing left- and right-brain facets, respectively. Let's see how.

Our Five+1 Senses during Times of Trauma and Safety

Let's remember (from Chapter 2) that when a life threat occurs, all available brain resources attend to and remember the traumatic situation with all of its sensory information—sights, sounds, smells, taste, touch/pressure/pain/injury, movement, temperature, position, balance, etc. The right brain holds these sensorimotor fragments which create a brain trauma imprint—a sensorimotor map of trauma associations—that helps us better predict, identify, mitigate, and avoid trauma's recurrence. Throughout life, nerves on the inside and outside of our bodies detect signals that might trigger danger and the sensorimotor map of trauma associations, signaling our ANS (via the central nervous system) to up or downregulate—become more alert or collapse.

It follows that trauma therapy will activate trauma imprints. So, we need to engage sensorimotor sensitivity with clients of all ages in the therapy milieu (online or in-person) to signal safety, welcoming, connection, and exploration. Sensorimotor refers to our five+1 senses: smell, sound, sight, taste, and touch plus movement. Included in the "+1" of movement is kinesthesia—the awareness of body and how to move it—and proprioception—the sense of our body parts' position, location, and orientation, the effort needed for movement, and sense of balance. Movement is integral to all five senses, especially touch, and will be discussed in examples of touch interventions.

In particular, growing client awareness of and attunement to their movements in the therapy space opens up an important and useful channel in trauma processing. Relational and environmental trauma correspond with boundary violations and the inability to move freely or complete movements (Levine, 1997; Ogden et al., 2006). Therefore, therapists want to explicitly highlight client movements that are self-driven (not reactive), uninhibited, and comfortably and appropriately use the space around them.

When trauma therapists hold sensorimotor sensitivity, we can better notice and discern when our clients' five+1 senses are getting triggered by the therapy space (and relationship). Then we can work together to calm their dysregulation. Adding playfulness to our sensorimotor sensitivity further supports this intention. Successfully co-regulating disturbance in the therapy environment grows success for clients to do the same outside of therapy's four walls.

Sensorimotor Uniqueness: What's Safe to One Is Triggering to Another

We can all agree that each person has preferences—some like it hot, some cold, some love the taste of chocolate, while others hate it, some love listening to the Beatles, while others find their sound annoying. Sensorimotor likes and dislikes are personal and therapists must honor this. Similarly, each client will take in and interpret sensorimotor signals in unique ways owing to their wiring—especially neurodivergent clients—and developmental-relational-contextual (D-R-C) lens (see Chapter 1). It is impossible to create a perfectly safe and comfortable environment for all clients at all times. Depending on which part of mind shows up, the same client can feel soothed one day and triggered the next by the therapy setting. As attuned healing professionals, we make adjustments, whether physical or emotional, to support sensorimotor sensitivity. Let's look at two examples of how what feels safe to one can be triggering to another.

I used to have a "fresh spring" scented deodorizer in my waiting room. The smell soothed me when I entered. Some clients also commented about enjoying the scent that greeted them. However, one client fortunately shared with me that the specific scent conjured disturbing olfactory memories. She explained that, when she was a child, her father would reek of beer as he drank himself into a stupor in his recliner chair. She recalled how during episodes when her father passed out, her mother tried to bring stability and control to her and her siblings by plunging herself into a disinfecting and cleaning frenzy. My waiting room deodorizer triggered these scent memories. While we worked to separate past from present and calmed her ANS to not respond in the same way upon entering my waiting room, I wanted her to know I heard her. So, I found another calming and soothing scent which we both enjoyed. Most importantly, she felt seen, heard, and comforted.

Of course, it may not always be possible to change the physical therapy space. In my waiting room, I have three framed pictures of ocean scenes, which many clients find relaxing. However, this wasn't the case for one client who had memories of nearly drowning at the beach. Changing the pictures was not an option, so we used a different approach. I validated their experience of discomfort, processed the disturbance, and reframed their ability to now sit surrounded by waves and feel stable, safe, and calm. I reiterated this new skill a couple of times in future sessions and playfully joked, "Now that you find these ocean scenes so calming, you'll probably want me to change out all the pictures in my office to ocean scenes!"

When the therapy setting triggers our clients' five+1 senses, we can playfully co-regulate while we convey professionalism, appropriate boundaries, privacy, and a welcoming of all parts. After, clients can experience that trauma work is not just a serious, somber, and hard endeavor.

Playful Engagement of Our Five+1 Senses

Together with our clients, we can co-create safety, soothing, attunement to self and others in fun, healing ways through metaphorical and explicit communication. One client shared how the overhead fluorescent lights were like harsh "death rays." I reflected, "I agree they're harsh. Clearly, though, your resilience to destructive forces is incredible!" Another client commented how hard and scratchy her seat felt, to which I replied, "I hear you." Later in the session, this client soothed herself with a tranquil, warm beach scene at which point I commented, "Wow, you're a texture shifter. In less than 20 minutes you transformed hard and scratchy to peaceful and warm!"

We can co-create sensorimotor safety in telehealth sessions as we actively guide our clients to engage their five+1 senses in their natural setting (e.g., their home, car, dorm room, office). During COVID, one client only found privacy for her online sessions in her bathroom, sitting on the lid-down toilet. I reflected, "While not ideal, you're exuding regal vibes. Talk about being on your throne! Next time bring your scepter and crown!" By transforming the therapy setting to something calming and fun, we help our clients know wherever they find themselves can be imperfectly perfect. Also, we help them associate the less-than-ideal setting with safety and connection, making self-regulation generalizable or more readily re-created outside of the therapy session.

What's more, as telehealth therapists, we are brought into our client's personal space which can increase our intimate knowing and experience of them. In real time, we can see how our client and those around them use and respect their boundaries for separateness and connection. With curiosity, we can find out about their surroundings by looking at photos on the wall, toys or objects they show us, or how they have decorated. We can have coffee or a snack together or enjoy an impromptu group or family session. In one group I run online, Mike the dog often joins and settles down on the floor next to his human mother. Our group has observed how Mike is his human's and the group's ANS dysregulation barometer: when uncomfortable affect rises, he starts moving, goes to comfort his human, or leaves the room entirely. These windows into a client's personal space provide invaluable information.

Clients' and therapists' use of a virtual background can reflect creative self-expression (i.e., use of photographs of themselves and important people and places to them), a need for privacy (i.e., using the blurring feature), change (i.e., different sessions take place in different spaces), or stability. Online therapy also presents a great exercise in mentalizing (see Chapter 8): does our client or do we have any idea what the other sees? How aware are we of how the other feels when the camera is angled, for example, at the ceiling, our neck, or the floor? What is it like for the viewer when the camera bounces up and down or moves unpredictably? We can use these moments to playfully direct clients and ourselves to re-attune and re-establish connection. When we accompany a client on a walk, online or in-person, we share a co-regulating experience of moving together. The right-left walking movement activates both hemispheres—a form of bilateral stimulation (BLS) (see Shapiro, 2018)—which assists the processing and integration of healing.

Let's now look at ways to use sensorimotor sensitivity to make our office settings more playful for the five+1 senses of clients of all ages. The examples shared are intended to spark each therapist's individual creativity to bring their playful spirit into their online and in-person office spaces while supporting clients to feel safe and connected from the outset of treatment.

Smell

Unlike the other senses, smell is most strongly linked to emotion. Odor cues bypass the brain's relay station and directly link to memory and endocrine function (Fung et al., 2021; Gomez, 2013; Zhou et al., 2021). Therefore, odors can rapidly signal the flight response (see Iravani et al., 2021; Lanius et al., 2014) as when "we smell trouble" or soothing when we inhale essential oils to affect mood (i.e., aromatherapy).

Using scents in our office space or inviting clients to do so online can have rapid calming and orienting effects to the present (Gomez, 2013, p. 160). In addition to the deodorizer in my waiting room, I have a fragrant hand lotion, a tube of Bain de Soleil suntan lotion/gelée, and scented markers. I tell clients how the Bain de Soleil scent reminds me of going to the beach during high school, a memory that is relaxing and enjoyable and then offer them to try it. While they smell it, I invite them to focus on the oily smoothness of the gelée on their skin and its appealing orange color: the more senses we link to these calming effects, the more brain regions are activated and the stronger the association to this safe and connected state will be. Clients may or may not like the scents I offer, but are invited to find their own (in therapy or at home) whether in lotion, aftershave, deodorant, perfume, etc. I remind clients that *self-soothing with a sniff* is a very resourceful tool and explain the brain basics of why. Anna Gomez (2013) creatively uses aromatherapy with child clients, offering them different scents they can mix together to create their own lotion to take home. This is a beautiful and personalized exercise of creativity, self-soothing, empowerment, and generalizability that can be used with clients of all ages.

We can support clients to *self-soothe with a sniff* during teletherapy sessions, too. I've encouraged clients to sniff whatever calms them at the start of or during a session. Clients have sniffed and applied moisturizers, smelled and put on their partner's shirt, or inhaled their freshly shampooed dog and started petting them. As clients self-soothe with different scents (touch and movement), we can use BLS to deepen that safe state and strengthen associations to positive feelings and beliefs about themselves and connections with others. We can metaprocess (Fosha & Thoma, 2020 and Chapter 9) mastery affects related to self-soothing. We can encourage clients to make these scents portable and even share them with us.

Sound

I have a white noise machine in the waiting room and an audibly ticking clock in the consultation room. The first helps promote confidentiality, drowning out any sounds coming from inside the office. The second, like a metronome, is loud enough to offer a consistent rhythm that, when focused on, helps clients slow down their breathing, heart rate, rate of speaking, or movement. In office or online, I invite clients to bring music to play in the background to help them regulate their ANS. Binaural beats embedded in sounds like the ocean, a rainstorm, etc., can be used alone or accompany Eye Movement Desensitization and Reprocessing (Grand, 1999; Shapiro, 2018).

Clients can use movement with sound to soothe. They can create beats by drumming on their lap, tapping the couch or a tabletop with a soothing rhythmic movement. We can encourage synchrony and connection with clients, by asking permission to join them in this practice. We always support clients to find the type of sound soothing that best fits them.

Sight

My office is set up to visually appeal to all developmental ages. One corner is inviting to children and young parts of mind. There is a brightly colored, child-size table and chair sitting on top of a blue rug of a hopscotch board, a large wicker basket filled with stuffed animals, and affixed to the walls, four framed cards of brightly colored cartoonish animals, four wooden flowers, and two pillows with outstretched arms—one of a red heart and the other a yellow sun. A double bookshelf sits next to this area with shelves organized developmentally from the ground up. Toddlers and young children can reach the bottom two shelves, which hold age-appropriate toys, games, cars, balls, and sandplay miniatures. The next shelf up holds crafts (markers, finger paints and paints, colored pencils for older children and adolescents) and young children's board and easy-to-read books. The next shelf holds clinical/adult reading level books, and on the very top of the bookshelf sits a stuffed six-foot-long green snake, a gumball machine, and a carved wooden robin. Therapists can place small wooden, glass, or ceramic figures, stuffed animals, and colorful and inviting crafts (like pipe cleaners, markers, clay, and kinetic sand) all around the consultation room to evoke playfulness and creativity. The objects we choose can symbolize themes we'd like to convey to our clients.

On my waiting room side table is a little wooden zebra sticking its face into an attached, round shallow bowl. I filled the bowl with turquoise glass stones to make it look like the zebra was drinking. It symbolically communicates to all who enter that they can drink-in their fill of nurturance in this space. I tell little kids that the zebra is thirsty and has lots of water to drink. Ironically, PJ, an 11-year-old boy on the autism spectrum, blew me away with how he used this wooden figure. An adult client, whose session followed PJ's asked me, "Monica, did you do this?" PJ had taken the blue glass stones and spelled out, "Hello?" I told him I hadn't. Although this adult was a keep-to-himself kind of guy, after our session he rearranged the stones to spell out, "Hi 2 U."

It amazed and touched my heart how a boy who struggled to connect with others was the first person in 20 years to use these glass stones to connect with other clients, anonymously. What's more, the quiet adult client became eager to see what messages were left "for him." He always replied. Ironically, other clients who were very social would look at the glass stone messages, smile, and leave them untouched. Through the playful anonymity afforded by these accessible glass stones, two socially isolated clients found a delightful way of connecting and scanning for opportunities to practice.

Finally, playing with different Zoom or Doxy backgrounds can be fun. Child and teenage clients have taught me how to change and share different background scenes. Sometimes theirs are quite kooky, which helps them be seen for their creativity. When I share the whiteboard option on Zoom with clients, we can draw and modify each other's creations, create stories, and play cooperatively. A number of adults shared their creative sides as budding photographers by selecting background photos from trips and family events. Exploring their choice, the story behind the photo, their felt sense of taking the photo, and their experience of my reactions to it opens up avenues for exploration.

For example, one adult client shared photos of her wheelchair-bound nephew across the first few years of his development. Through this show-and-share experience, this client chronicled her initial grief and anger at God for her nephew's and family's suffering. Eventually, her photos reflected the joy and blessings she felt when taking pictures of him and celebrating his life. I cherished how my client included me in her visually creative and expressive journey from pain to celebration.

Taste

I offer water and tea to my clients, accessible while they wait for our session. Some colleagues offer k-cups, candies, and granola bars. Depending upon personal preference and the types of clients we work with, this choice can vary. My decision reflects a wish to provide some nurturance and implicitly let the youngest parts of all clients know they can drink from my well. Online and in-person, I invite clients to eat snacks or meals while in session. Since many clients come to therapy right after work, school, or extracurricular activities, I emphasize the importance of refueling to reenergize mind and body. When our basic needs are met, our ANS and affect calm.

For child, teenage, and some young adult clients, I will offer to take them for a milkshake, ice cream, or donut next door to celebrate their birthday. I get parental or guardian permission first. Or we might plan a birthday celebration where I promise to buy the pizza and they will bring their favorite dessert.

Sometimes I invite clients with eating issues to bring their "forbidden" foods to the office. Together we engage in mindful slowing down to notice their smells, textures, flavors, and temperatures, how the food moves, and its consistency in the bowl or on their tongue. We use the five+1 senses to realign their relationship with food. In sessions with adult clients, I've played with foods—just like toddlers do—making taffy out of York Peppermint Patties, watch and sniff ice cream as it melts, or aggressively and loudly crunch pretzels or potato chips in our mouths while savoring the flavors. Therefore, inviting playful engagement with taste in a safe holding environment may both soothe and expand our client's tolerance for sensorimotor activation.

Touch and Movement

With guidance, clients can use their sense of touch to ground in endless ways in the office or online. We can comment on how clients touch themselves to soothe—stroke or twirl their hair, pat one hand with the other, and many other actions. We can also focus on ways clients use their physical environment to ground. For example, we can ask them to slow down to notice the calm they feel with the firmness or mushiness of the seat cushions, the soft texture and warmth of the throw blanket across their legs, or the solidity of the floor under their feet. When combined with proprioception, we can explore how calm, strong, coordinated, or embodied they feel when they use force to pull open the heavy door or play catch with us.

Therapists can reflect wise, self-attuned sensorimotor recruitment in statements like, "You seem so at ease when you twirl your hair. Can I try that with my hair, too?" or "You know the just-right way to cuddle yourself up in that snuggly blanket. How does your body feel now?"

We can help clients notice how their sense of touch with movement promotes balance, comfort, and mastery. I encourage children and teens with sensory integration difficulties to practice gaining proprioceptive awareness through dancing, playing hopscotch, and tracking how their bodies move in space and near another person—me. We can help clients of all ages learn to assert and protect their physical boundaries by having a "safe" in-office pillow fight—a behavior not always possible at home. Movement offers countless opportunities for clients of all ages to practice empathy and mentalization by noticing their physical impact on others and their physical surroundings. We can guide clients to notice the strength in their muscles and the force used to protect their personal space. During a safe pillow fight, we can reflect, "Wow, you are so strong" or "You are so good at protecting yourself."

We help clients gain awareness of their micro and macro movements that help them calm. These might include tracing their fingers over the decorative rivets on the couch; moving their legs from the footrest to the floor; stretching or shifting positions (to relieve pain and discomfort); or shielding vulnerable parts of themselves by placing a pillow, blanket, or jacket on their lap. When we direct clients to focus on what their movements do for their senses and nervous system, they often express surprise. We can help clients appreciate that when they connect to their body's intuitive, spontaneous wisdom, they feel more grounded, strong, and embodied.

Online and in-person, we can invite clients to check in with their body and move to adjust their posture, and breath, and use their space and objects in their environment. One adult client was wiggling uncomfortably in her seat. I asked her, "How would your body like to move right now?"

She laughed and said, "If I could, I'd do one of my yoga poses—a downward dog and sun salutation."

I replied, "If I could? Of course you can! Be my yoga instructor for just a moment." She laughed, and jumped off the couch. I mirrored her yoga posture and breathing, her slow rounding up, one vertebra at a time, and then reached my arms as she did toward the sky. She got a kick out of me following her. I explained, "How good that felt after sitting on my butt for hours!" We laughed. I reminded her how attuned she is to her body, just like to her feelings.

She smiled, acknowledging, "I guess I am!"

Teaching our clients to convert a therapy office into a yoga studio is one example of how we can help clients engage their imaginative playfulness in any environment to promote self-attuned calming.

It's Not the Space, But How We Engage It with Our Traumatized Clients

Just like helpful therapy techniques lose their impact or may be triggering if the therapy relationship isn't attuned, safe, and secure, the same is true when offering a playful therapy space. It's *how* we use our space and co-create the experience of it *with* our clients that is more important than how the space is appointed, per se. We don't need an interior designer or elaborate budget to create a safe and playful space. Many of us work in generic, impersonal offices with harsh fluorescent lighting, industrial furniture, and bland carpeting, yet we can still convey a playfulness, warmth, and homeyness to soothe and regulate our traumatized client's ANS and affect.

Playing with the Therapy Setting

We strive to put our clients centerstage in the playfully, co-created therapy space that is attuned in sensorimotor ways and relationally. We can make the therapy setting about them by using purposeful language that is explicit or verbal, implicit or nonverbal (e.g., primary process, see Chapters 3 and 4), or hypnotic and metaphorical (see Corydon Hammond, 1990). Let's explore some play-inspired examples of how to intentionally use the physical space as opportunities to transmit therapeutic messages of sensorimotor safety and welcoming.

We can act on this intention when we first meet our client. How we open the door and welcome our client into the office is important. We want to attune in developmentally and culturally appropriate ways and use sincere enthusiasm—to their level of tolerance. Saying with an accompanying sweeping arm gesture, "C'mon in. Feel free to look around and get comfy," conveys welcoming and extends a playful invitation to be explorative and at ease. Clients may wonder unconsciously or consciously, "Is this the place where we do deep

painful trauma work? Why is this therapist so enthusiastic?" From the beginning, we challenge our clients' expectations of uncomfortable trauma work with
an ease-filled space and welcoming; creating a juxtaposition experience to promote change.

We can use objects in the therapy space to earn secure attachments. When I
see clients hesitating to get a drink from the water cooler, after huffing and puff-
ing to get to the session on time, I will ask, "Would you like some water? I'm
happy to get it for you. Just sit and catch your breath. And thanks for allowing
me to practice my waitressing skills, which I never had the chance to do and
always wanted to." Clients have responded, "Oh, I'm glad I could be of help
with your unrealized career!"

Other times, I have said, "Let me get some water for you. Enjoy the service, there's no extra charge!" reassuring clients that they will not have to pay a
price for receiving extra attention and care. Other times, this gesture might feel
intolerable to those who have not learned to receive or receive without strings
attached. Also, encouraging the client to get their own water can communicate,
"I trust you know how to take care of yourself."

Depending upon the client's readiness and the trust we have co-created, I
might make the implicit explicit and metaprocess it relationally (see more in
Chapter 9): "What's it like for you to let me do this for you?" Or I might reflect
and explore the change in the client's capacity to receive, "Do you remember
when we first started meeting, you were so uncomfortable letting me get you
water? Now look at you, not only are you accepting my offer, you asked me
if it would be okay if I got you some. Wow! Notice that change. What's it feel
like?" This exchange around water illustrates how we can use many different
objects related to the five+1 senses in our therapy space to address important
attachment-related themes like giving and receiving nurturance.

At each moment, we can seize opportunities to engage the holding environment to attune with emotional and sensorimotor sensitivity. As we settle into our
seats to begin the session, I remind each client that I want them to feel comfortable at every level—which hypnotically suggests all parts of mind. I offer ways
to feel comfortable in sensorimotor ways. "Please let me know if it feels too hot,
too cold, or just right, because I can change the thermostat." I might say, "Isn't it
great that we have the power to fix things with the flick of a switch or by pressing a button?" This metaphorical message lets clients know they have control to
address any physical discomfort, and I am supporting them to use their agency.
With chronic, complex trauma clients, we can look for opportunities to *find and
mine* the tiniest examples of self and other attunement to soothe discomfort.
With little kids, I sometimes invite them to come with me to change the thermostat setting. This action metaphorically communicates how they have some
control over their space, which is especially empowering as this is not frequently
the case for a young child.

With open-minded curiosity, therapists can playfully support our clients in countless ways to use the therapy setting metaphorically and playfully to increase their self-attunement, choice, control, agency, and mastery. For example, asking, "I see the sun is on you, would you like me to adjust the blinds?" allows a client to feel the warmth of the sun's energy and to leverage choice and control over their body temperature, their vision being obstructed or not, etc. We can play with puns, "Wow, you seem *enlightened* today." "Talk about shining a light on this issue!" "Don't you love being in the limelight?" Asking, "Would you like another pillow? Would you like to use a blanket?" helps the client become sensorily self-attuned, connected to their body's needs, and gives themself permission to adjust things to promote feeling "just right." Across sessions, we can remind and reinforce our clients to better self-attune and soothe by changing things about the therapy setting.

Similarly, we can use ordinary objects in our office to hypnotically and metaphorically communicate messages to our clients. For example, offering the garbage can to clients before they ask for it is especially helpful for those who have struggled to reach for support or lived with others misattuned in meeting their needs. It communicates, "I see you have stuff you want to get rid of. Here, let me help you with that." For clients who have been overly attended to or had things done for them, limiting their agency and independence, I wait until they ask for the garbage can. To promote competence, I might bring out the garbage can and invite the client to make a three-point shot or announce "swoosh" when their trash lands in it. If they miss the can, I've communicated sincere statements that they are not alone, like, "Oh my gosh, I missed the can three times this week when it was right under my hand!" Playing with how we use and communicate about the therapy space and the objects in it offers endless ways to address themes related to safety, attachment, boundaries, competence, empathy, mentalizing, reciprocity, and more.

Reframing Unpredictable Changes to the Therapy Setting

One of the most fun and creative ways to bring sensorimotor sensitivity and safety to our clients using the therapy environment, in-person or online, is when the unpredictable happens. Unexpected scenarios I've encountered include loss of electricity, erratic internet connection, the landlord walking into the office without permission, children screaming or crying nearby, a bus backfiring outside the window, and smells coming through the window or ventilation system.

We narrate these uncontrollable occurrences and reframe them as imperfectly perfect events related to the work we are doing with our clients. Nothing is random or coincidental. This reframe keeps our clients centerstage and, in a lighthearted way, makes the world revolve around them. In essence, we are appealing to the young child parts who believe, "The sun rises because it's time for me to get up, and the moon appears because I'm ready to go to sleep"; such interventions reflect their developmentally egocentric innocent side. While therapists need to insure reframes are developmentally attuned, they playfully help clients feel truly important.

Let's look at some examples of how to reframe unpredictable changes in the therapy setting using the five+1 senses. These reframes support regulation and strengthen our clients' belief that "I can tolerate change and discomfort and work with it effectively." The snippets shared reflect how I have reworked the unpredictable and uncontrollable occurrences and hopefully will spur you to creatively discover ways to promote sensorimotor re-grounding using the five+1 senses.

Smell

In-person. The ventilation system in my office blows all kinds of odors into my room from the entire floor. The chemicals used to clean the bathrooms sometimes send overpowering ammonia and Lysol scents into my office. I've said, "Isn't nice to know we are in a really well disinfected building? Any germ will be killed on contact!"

The musky scents used by the down-the-hall acupuncturist for moxibustion sessions have been soothing for some clients and triggering for others. One client happily recalled when inhaling the scent, "That was the scent my acupuncturist used to help turn my breech baby around in my womb. Ahhh, I love it." I grabbed this moment and said, "Yes, the acupuncturist and I coordinated before your session to remind you to use this smell and your intention to turn the upside-down things in your world right-side up!"

Another client expressed worry, "Is someone smoking pot? Will I get a contact high?" First, I reassured her this was a form of Eastern medicine therapy meant to aid healing. Then I asked, "Since this scent doesn't do it for you, which scent does?" She identified how the Lady Emma Hamilton Rose scent calmed her. Then we practiced ways she could recall its fruitiness in her imagination. She settled herself. I joked, "Maybe we can convince the acupuncturist to send oils from the Lady Emma Hamilton Rose through the vent for our next session."

Online. I have commented on how I wish computer monitors had a scratch-and-sniff option or how one day computers could transmit scent the same way they do sound, like in 4D theaters. When clients eat during online sessions or comment how they are cooking or baking something, I might breathe in and say, "Mmmm, that roast smells good" or "My mouth is watering as your chocolate chip cookies are baking." These light statements let my clients know I am imagining savoring their creation and am trying to be there with them in all ways possible.

Sound

In-person. It is not uncommon to hear emergency vehicle sirens outside my office window. If clients don't seem distracted, I might let the sound pass. But if the client seems shaken, I might first give a reality-based understanding of what might be happening. "Wow! Loud sirens! They must be helping put out the car fire on 1st Ave." Otherwise, I might say playfully, "This truly is an urgent topic!" or "The rescue team is here to help!" or "Your boss has clearly called 911 hearing your plans to expose his behavior!" Similarly, when banging or construction noises interrupt a session, I might say, "Sounds like somebody's knocking to join us. I guess this is the place to be!" or "I hope they are constructing my rooftop office with chaise lounges and a pool!" With children in particular, I might engage their imagination, "What do you imagine the people are building?" "Wouldn't it be cool if they could build us the fortress you wanted? But since they probably aren't, shall we?"

Online. Erratic internet connection can cause all kinds of sensory interruptions. When mouth movements are out of sync with the spoken word, I sometimes imitate the problem to make it less annoying or might joke, "I didn't realize you were a ventriloquist—your mouth didn't move, yet you said so much!" Online I've had instances where wind-like sounds get loud, making it hard to hear the person. Saying things like, "Oooh, it sounds like you're at the seashore on a windy day. Ahhh, shall we go there together for a moment? Okay, how did that feel? Now let's mute and unmute as we come back to my office and your kitchen."

Sight

In-person. I have had power outages during sessions on a number of occasions. I've joked, "Whoops, I guess the landlord forgot to pay the utility bill." Once during an evening session, I had to move the session to areas with emergency lighting. For one client who had fears of the dark, we sat in the dark together during a thunderstorm. While helping them calm with breathwork and the sound of my voice, I joked, "Don't you think I'm the coolest therapist ever—arranging a power outage during a storm to help you practice your grounding skills?"

Clients often comment sarcastically or with a sigh implying, "Monica, you're so ridiculous!"

I acknowledge and validate, "Okay, that was stretching it," and highlight, "You seem grounded again. I no longer have go to extreme measures for you to practice these skills!"

Online. This is a fun one. Sometimes when clients start their telehealth session on their phone or tablet, the orientation is off so they appear to be on their side or upside down. I'll joke about how flexible or acrobatic they are. I might mirror their orientation by moving my camera angle. I might say, "What a talent—spinning upside down without leaving our seats! Even better, we know how to right ourselves." These implicit, metaphorical comments remind clients they have the ability to settle when unsettled or orient when disoriented. When clients disappear into the Zoom background, we play around with themes like which part of them wants to show up. I may intentionally encourage the client to leave out parts of themselves (e.g., their head) from view and joke around about integration, feeling split off, or dissociation. This neutralizes dissociative experiences and helps us talk about them playfully.

Taste

In-person and online. Ruptures in taste (by mouth or figurative) may occur when a client shares something they made or bought with the therapist, yet don't get the acceptance or acknowledgment they want. I remember a home visit to an 89-year-old woman who said, "I don't care that you have dietary restrictions, you are insulting me that you won't eat what I bought for you!" She felt personally rejected. Because the wounds cut so deeply and her ability to empathize or mentalize was so limited, no intervention that was gracious, much less playful, landed well for her. All I could do was return for subsequent home visits to show her *even if I don't accept what you bought me, I want to be with you.*

In-person or online, we can explore how tasting the same food and having different preferences is welcomed. One teenager offered me a piece of bittersweet dark chocolate, which I declined because I only eat and love milk chocolate. She was incredulous, believing only dark chocolate was worthy of consumption— milk chocolate was "totally gross" to her. I remarked, "We need to be thankful to each other, because if all people only liked dark or milk chocolate, we might not have enough for everyone!" I made the metaphor explicit, addressing the importance of accepting differences and how this helps create balance in the world.

Touch and Movement

In-person. One time, a client sat on the couch in a big wet spot; my previous client's water bottle had leaked without anyone's awareness. I used paper towels to absorb the water and my client moved the couch cushion to the side. Then we joked about this strange way to cool off. I celebrated her ability to "go with the flow"—yup, this kind of humor is what my clients have to endure—and show resiliency in the face of all types of emotional and physical discomfort.

As much as therapists try to make the therapy space developmentally appropriate, fun, and safe for little children, the ways kids explore and interact with their environments can lead to injuries or safety ruptures more frequently than those who are sedentary in session. Once, a 6-year-old client playing with the dollhouse took off the removable roof and one of the pieces that secures the roof broke off so it couldn't be reattached securely. I reflected, "Wow, that stinks! Maybe we can come up with a way to make that roof better?" Together we physically adjusted the roof and glued on the broken piece. I announced, "What a great fixer you are!" and gave her a high five. Therapists can use these touch and movement ruptures as opportunities to metaphorically and hypnotically communicate clients' creative, spontaneous, and unique abilities to repair.

Online. In virtual sessions, a client or therapist might tap their laptop close to the microphone, disturbing what we can hear. We need to know our client's receptivity to direct feedback, puns, and metaphors, to guide how we address issues. We can ask them directly if they would be careful not to tap on the microphone, or playfully ask, "Was part of you sending me a hidden message in morse code?" Interesting themes might emerge.

Ruptures through touch—possibly linked to problems with depth perception, mentalizing, or proprioception—may raise shame. For example, when virtually "high fiving," clients and therapists have accidentally knocked over their laptops or cameras. We can lighten the shame through levity *and* stay with the theme that needs to be addressed. For example, "Whoa, your high five is powerful! What did you notice inside when that happened?" or "When you high-fived me with such force, I felt you wanted to connect with me, which felt good to me. What was it like to connect with me in a way that nearly broke your camera?" Different metaphors and themes for healing can emerge, as in connecting isn't safe or coming on too strong pushes others away.

In therapy, we always improvise, learning to work with what we've got, even if it sometimes means flying by the seat of our pants. Opportunities for healing and transformation abound, just waiting for us to discover what may be hiding in plain sight. We can seize the possibilities for learning and growth in random or spontaneous occurrences by asking, "How might this be important here and now?" "How might this fit with the theme we are working on?" "What might the universe be telling you/us?" It might be a reach or a stretch, it might not fit, but go for it anyway. When we infuse relational playfulness in the holding environment, we grow our personal and client's openness and explorative capacities to repair ruptures.

Inviting Our Clients' Worlds into the Therapy Setting

When we invite clients to bring in their important beings and things into therapy, different purposes are served. Who and what our client brings into the therapy setting is a form of Show and Tell—it helps us learn about our client and their values, gain insights into what brings them joy, and see how they interact in different relationships—to people and things. The more our client literally and figuratively fills the therapy space with their world, the more it will feel like their own which supports therapy engagement.

Welcoming Important Others and Objects

Let's explore how we can welcome people, pets, spiritual presence and objects, or transitional and comfort objects from our clients' lives into the therapy space.

People

Clients of all ages have asked me whether they could invite relatives to sessions. Teenagers have asked if their friends or significant others could join them. Adults have wanted to include family members or partners. After reviewing the purpose and agreeing about whether or not the presence of this person will further treatment goals, the client and I discuss confidentiality, boundaries, and how their important other will handle what happens during and after the sessions. With little kids, I might joke about the private nature of therapy and even ask, "Can your dog JoJo keep what happens here private and not bark about it to other dogs in the neighborhood?"

When clients bring their important others to therapy, an incredible opportunity presents itself to see how they show up with others. For example, we can find out if the relationship promotes each person to feel safe, seen, soothed, and secure (Siegel & Payne Bryson, 2020)? Are communication and boundaries healthy and balanced? Is there mutual respect? The dynamics that unfold provide rich information to inform treatment, especially when addressing attachment issues.

Sometimes clients have invited friends to therapy in an effort to sidestep uncomfortable treatment topics. Therapists can carefully and creatively play with this type of defense, as long as they have a deep trust with their client and a good sense of how things will land. For example, after about six months of therapy, 17-year-old Darby and I had established a rhythm. She was highly dissociative and avoidant, having established multiple levels of protection against the sequelae of her extensive history of sexual abuse, severe learning disabilities, and multiple abandonments since birth. I had developed a sense of how much Darby could tolerate me pushing her boundaries and defenses, while Darby had figured out how much of her high-risk behavior I could tolerate without over or underreacting.

One day after bringing her cat to therapy, she hypothetically asked if I ever worked with clients' friends or significant others in sessions. While we had had many family sessions—which I requested and Darby had agreed to—Darby's request for friend sessions was completely self-initiated and therefore might increase her investment in making positive changes. We navigated many tricky layers of confidentiality (for all parties involved), gained her parents' permission, and mapped out her intentions. Darby explained having her friends in session could help me see how good her friendships were and would help me support her to deal with conflicts with them. We both agreed to welcome her friends, yet I had not explicitly asked Darby to give me a head's up when this would be.

Weeks later without forewarning, Darby showed up to a session with not one but two of her close friends. While initially surprised and thrown by this unexpected "visit," I saw great opportunity. I slowed down Darby's and her friends' eagerness and asked them to hang out in the waiting room while Darby and

I briefly checked in. I asked if their parents had consented for them to join. Darby giggled saying, "Yeah, my parents spoke with theirs. Mom said that their parents hoped it would light a fire under my friends' asses to get into therapy too!"

Also, I confronted Darby about pushing my comfort, asking, "Darby can you appreciate that I would have preferred a head's up to be prepared?" She smiled slyly and agreed that that would have been best. I then took responsibility for not making this need clearer when I agreed to a friend session.

Then I welcomed her friends into the consultation room. First, we reviewed confidentiality. Next, we established how lucky Darby was to have them in her life and vice versa. After about five minutes of rapid bantering about how they have been there for each other, one friend commented on how "dumb" Darby is. "I tell her all the time how that guy is an absolute dick and T-R-O-U-B-L-E (she spelled it out), but she won't listen."

Darby laughed uncomfortably, told her friend to "shut the fuck up or you can leave," and changed the subject.

This was my cue to directly address what was unfolding in real time. "Have the two of you noticed that Darby's cool having you guys in session with her as long as things remain comfortable and easy, yet she's ready to rip you a new asshole and kick you out when triggering topics and emotions emerge?"

Her friends chimed in, "Yeah, that's Darby. We give her shit for this all the time!" Her friends felt validated when I called out Darby, while Darby felt safe to own her avoidance and minimization because of her friends' loving support mixed with some chops-busting. Darby and I had developed a similar relationship, which enabled us to explore and reshape this dynamic more fully in that and future sessions. By supporting our clients to welcome safe and important others into the therapy space, we may quickly uncover concerning relational dynamics and facilitate their repair with the assistance of their trusted others.

Pets

Other important beings that clients have brought to session include pets—I've seen dogs, cats, bearded dragons, snakes, ducks, gerbils, hamsters, and ant farms. The relationships people have with their pets can be incredible—filled with unconditional love, attention, playfulness, and safe connection. When we notice and track how these attuned and loving relationships unfold in the therapy setting, we can explicitly comment on their dynamics. We can reflect on unconditional attunement, love, soothing, and synchrony. For example, when pets function as emotional supports, we can say, "Oh, Jojo knows you so well. He jumped into your lap to warm and soothe you. Jojo, you're so smart. What does it feel like that Jojo is so tuned into you? What do you imagine it feels like to Jojo that you're so tuned into him?" We can explain how they are each other's neurobiological regulators (Fisher, 2017, p. 55) or nervous system soothers. We can explicitly narrate how our clients intuitively know how and when to cuddle, pet, groom, or play with their pets to calm their pets or themselves. We can verbalize how well-attuned the client is when they know their pet's sweet spot and make them purr or roll with delight.

The presence of pets can also reveal how our client handles their relationship with their pet (and others) when things go wrong or they act unpredictably. Even in this cherished attachment, clients might scream at, humiliate, hit, or antagonize their pet, reflecting other "loving" attachments in their life. How passively or aggressively do they go after their cat who refuses to come out from under the couch? How do they set limits on their bearded dragon who starts nibbling on a nerf ball or a doll's hair?

The way clients use their pets to communicate messages can be very telling, too. For example, an 8-year-old client brought in his very old dog. My client noticeably grimaced after his dog dropped a massive poop and hesitated to clean it up with his mother. His dog communicated directly what my client couldn't— *I don't like coming to therapy: it makes me feel like poop!* After he and his mom cleaned the mess, we explored and processed the discomfort of being in a place you don't want to be. In a different case, discussed briefly in Chapter 3, 1½-year-old Tanya spontaneously started "playing" with her dog Scooby, while her mother and I were discussing the visitation schedule with the father—who had been accused of incesting this toddler. Tanya's "playing" meant inserting her pointer into Scooby's anus and pulling him closer and laughing each time he resisted. Through her actions with Scooby, Tanya re-enacted what had happened to her with her father. Scooby's presence helped Tanya express important themes of violated touch which she could not yet articulate with words. We see that including important, trusted others in the therapy space can uncover essential information to healing.

Spiritual Presence and Objects

Finally, welcoming our clients' important beings into the therapy setting may involve their spirituality, which for many can be a very central part of their lives. This welcoming may take a metaphysical form. We need to nonjudgmentally and openly encourage clients to feel safe to discuss and even invoke their spiritual connections to God, higher powers, spiritual beings, Mother Earth, etc. into the therapy space. Therapists don't have to believe what our clients do, but support them to share whatever is important, stabilizing, and supportive of their resiliency. For example, I have asked clients to take a moment to pray or make contact with their higher power. Even when my belief system differs from theirs, clients feel sincerely supported to welcome and infuse their grounding higher power's presence into the therapy space, making the setting more personally comforting and supportive. Spiritual connections can be some of the most intimate, grounding, and transformative for people.

Welcoming a client's spirituality into the therapy space may also take physical form. Clients may want to share religious or spiritual amulets, photos, music, etc. with us. We can even encourage them to leave their item/s in the therapy room in a safe space (e.g., a drawer, a cabinet) to help them feel anchored and understood. This sends a number of powerful messages: I will safely hold something precious to you; we are co-creating a space that helps you feel held; and you know how to hold and soothe your dysregulated parts and I see that. Clients may also talk about comforting objects or signs of reassurance ranging from visions of Jesus, God, and Allah, to a blue avatar; protective messages from the deceased coming in dreams or visitations; or "random" and "coincidental" events that feel like universal signs of hope (i.e., seeing a double rainbow reminding them that beauty can exist even in dark times). When we safely and nonjudgmentally welcome our clients to bring in their beloved spiritual symbols/objects, we are giving them permission to freely share important aspects of their true and full Self.

Transitional Objects

Young children may spontaneously bring transitional objects, like dolls, toys, or blankets, to therapy to help them feel comfortable with an unfamiliar person or space. A child's transitional object can serve as a wonderful helper to the therapist. Therapists can speak directly to the object (to get to know its role for the child) or speak through the object (to facilitate connection with the child). Transitional objects can help a child speak to the therapist for them and safely hold disavowed parts of themselves—their "not me" parts.

For example, when 6-year-old Timmy brought in his Ant-Man action figure, I introduced myself, saying, "Hi, Ant-Man. I'm so glad Timmy brought you in so I could meet you. Did he tell you who I am?" Timmy made him shake his head no. I explained, "I am a feelings doctor. I play and talk to people about all their feelings, and help them be the best they can be. How does that sound to you?"

Timmy in the deepest voice he could muster said, "Good. Do you have superhero powers like me?"

I answered, "I wish I did. Maybe you can show me your superhero powers and together we can help Timmy grow his powers. How does that sound?" Timmy moved Ant-Man's hand to motion a thumbs up.

"Awesome," I said. I added, "Ant-Man, Timmy told me he doesn't think he's very good or have any powers at all. Can you let him know we all feel that way sometimes?" Timmy brought Ant-Man up to his ear and nodded. "Ant-Man, I don't know if you ever feel that way because you're a superhero," Timmy nodded Ant-Man's head. I ended, "I feel happy to know that all of us can feel weak and strong at times and we still can have awesome powers!"

Comfort Objects

Preteens, teens, and adults also bring objects into sessions, which function similarly to transitional objects because they can be soothing and grounding. These objects offer an opportunity for the therapist to playfully explore important aspects of the client, including their interests, talents, and creative expressions connected to their life force, spirituality, and joy. Teens often share music, videos, games, texts, and things they may have purchased (like jewelry, tattoos, or clothing), created (like drawings), or gifts received as a way of bringing parts of themselves into the therapy space and relationship. Adults may bring healing crystals, pictures of famous sculpture or artwork, their photography, or something they baked and feel proud of. One man brought in a beautiful stained-glass window that took him months to create. When clients bring these objects into the therapeutic space and relationship, they are co-creating safety and connection while opening up an opportunity for us to get to know them more deeply on their terms.

Now let's see how to welcome all parts of mind into the therapy space to further encourage a safe and welcoming holding environment.

Welcoming Internal Parts of Mind

Each client enters our virtual or in-person waiting and consultation room with their full positive and traumatic history in tow. Traumatized clients arrive accompanied by their intrapsychic protector parts. Depending upon a client's age, they can simultaneously experience us and the therapeutic milieu through their current and historic D-R-C lenses of their lived experiences—traumatic or not—as an infant/baby, toddler, child, adolescent, and/or younger or current adult self.

Holding this in mind, we can appreciate how Levaya, a 57-year-old female client, may simultaneously see the therapy room through multiple visual lenses. That of her: (1) current, wise adult Self; (2) 26-year-old part who attended therapy with a misattuned employee assistance counselor; (3) 15-year-old part who was forced to meet a student assistance counselor for alcohol use; (4) 10-year-old part who was brought to family therapy during her parents' toxic divorce; and (5) 4-year-old playful, well-adjusted part. Current-day adult Levaya and her 4-year-old part may really like the wall photo of the therapist's family, which brings up warm feelings of her current family and early, loving memories of her nuclear family. In contrast, Levaya's 10- and 15-year-old parts may feel envy and grief because they did not have the family togetherness they perceive in the picture. Those parts of her mind may not trust that this therapist can understand them. Similarly, while Levaya's 4- and 10-year-old parts feel at ease to see a stuffed bear on the couch, her 26-year-old part might feel infantilized, believing this therapist will undoubtedly be misattuned to the needs of an adult.

Clients who can verbalize these discomforts enable exploration and repair. Those who can't may keep their discomfort hidden and their ANS and defensive parts remain on high alert. Levaya reminds us that to help each traumatized client feel safe and connected we need to be sensitive to the competing needs of and triggers to their multiplicity of parts (informed by their D-R-C). Without attuning to and exploring how the therapy setting can dysregulate or alienate some parts of mind but engage others, we may inadvertently trigger more internal discord which can block client engagement and the healing process. Therefore, to welcome all parts of mind, we must remember to purposefully check to see how the different things clients notice in the therapy space may elicit different reactions. By inviting clients' feedback and validating related feelings, we ensure each part of mind feels and is safe and seen. By making reasonable adjustments to the therapy setting or how we engage it, we can empower our clients and enhance their sense of soothing and security with the physical setting (and with us). Their positive associations to and engagement with the therapy space help make it a truly safe holding environment.

Playing with and in Our Holding Environments

In this chapter, we've explored how the therapy setting in-person or online serves as our auxiliary medium for healing: a literal and figurative holding and reparative environment that supports our traumatized clients to experience welcoming, a playful spirit, safety, and sensorimotor sensitivity. We learned that it's not just about setting up the physical space, per se, but how we use it that safely engages and regulates our traumatized clients' five+1 senses to promote connection and a healing experience. We gained awareness about how to playfully and metaphorically communicate implicit and explicit healing messages through the therapy space. We saw the importance of openly welcoming our clients' important others and all parts of mind into the therapy milieu. When we include our clients' worlds into the therapy space, we increase their treatment investment and engagement, and freedom to be fully themselves. With the know-how we've gained, we can intentionally develop and engage a playful, sensorimotor-sensitive holding environment that aligns with trauma-informed practice.

Having explored how to use the physical holding environment for playfully spirited trauma treatment, we can now move into Chapter 8 in which we'll explore how to relationally and playfully hold and attune with our clients to further promote their change and healing.

References

Corydon Hammond, D. (Ed.) (1990). *Handbook of hypnotic suggestions and metaphors.* New York: Norton.
Fisher, J. (2017). *Healing the fragmented selves of trauma survivors: Overcoming self-alienation.* New York: Routledge.

Fosha, D. & Thoma, N. (2020). Metatherapeutic processing supports the emergence of flourishing in psychotherapy. *Psychotherapy*, *57*(3), 323–339.

Fung, T., Lau, B., Ngai, S., & Tsang, H. (2021). Therapeutic effect and mechanisms of essential oils in mood disorders: Interaction between the nervous and respiratory systems. *International Journal of Molecular Sciences*, *22*(9), 4844. https://doi.org/10.3390/ijms22094844

Gomez, A. (2013). *EMDR therapy and adjunct approaches with children: Complex trauma, attachment, and dissociation.* New York: Springer.

Grand, D. (1999). Inner Mirror CD#2. BioLateral Sound Recordings. www.biolateral.com.

Iravani, B., Schaefer, M., Wilson, D. A., Arshamian, A., & Lundström, J. N. (2021). The human olfactory bulb processes odor valence representation and cues motor avoidance behavior. *Proceedings of the National Academy of Sciences*, 118(42), e2101209118. https://doi.org/10.1073/pnas.2101209118

Lanius, U. F., Paulsen, S. L., & Corrigan, F. M. (Eds.) (2014). *Neurobiology and treatment of traumatic dissociation: Towards an embodied self.* New York: Springer.

Levine, P. (1997). *Waking the tiger: Healing trauma.* Berkeley, CA: North Atlantic Books.

Ogden, P., Minton, K., & Pain, C. (2006). *Trauma and the body: A sensorimotor approach to psychotherapy.* New York: Norton.

Shapiro, F. (2018). *Eye Movement Desensitization and Reprocessing (EMDR) basic principles, protocols and procedures* (3rd ed.). New York: Guilford.

Siegel, D. J. & Payne Bryson, T. (2020). *The power of showing up: How parental presence shape who our kids become and how their brains get wired.* New York: Ballantine Books.

Warner, E., Westcott, A, Cook, A., & Finn, H. (2020). *Transforming trauma in children and adolescents: An embodied approach to somatic regulation, trauma processing, and attachment-building.* Berkeley, CA: North Atlantic Books.

Winnicott, D. (1960). The theory of the parent-child relationship. *International Journal of Psychoanalysis*, *41*, 585–595.

Zhou, G., Olofsson, J. K., Koubeissi, M. Z., Menelaou, G., Rosenow, J., Schuele, S. U., Xu, P., Voss, J. L., Lane, G., & Zelano, C. (2021). Human hippocampal connectivity is stronger in olfaction than other sensory systems. *Progress in Neurobiology*, *201*, 102027. https://doi.org/10.1016/j.pneurobio.2021.102027

Chapter 8

Growing Our Playfully Spirited Therapist Self

In this chapter, we will focus on how therapists can nurture their playful spirit and infuse it into their work with traumatized clients. We will explore how play's superpowers (discussed in Chapter 5) boost the healing qualities in the therapeutic relationship, catalyzing and deepening healing and change. This chapter will also look at how therapists fueled by their playful attitude can *attune on steroids* and learn how it magnifies and accelerates the earning of security and change for the better. Once embodied, we will see how our playful spirit is a true facilitator of trauma healing and change.

Cultivating a Playful Mindset and Attitude

When we as therapists cultivate our unique and personal playful spirit, we strive to embody play's qualities of feeling good, wanting to do more of what we're doing, immersing ourselves in the experience with a go-with-the-flow attitude, exploring with curiosity, and connecting with our personal truth (see Chapter 3 for more details). Our playful spirit can't be taught but must be discovered and practiced through lived experiences. To aid this discovery, we need to intentionally explore our worlds—inside and outside of the therapy milieu—with curiosity to identify what makes us laugh and smile, encourages our creativity, motivates us, lightens our mood, and supports us to thrive.

Nurturing our playful spirit makes navigating the hard work of trauma treatment easier and the process itself more enjoyable and fulfilling. It more importantly helps us impart positivity and hope to our clients. We communicate a powerful implicit and explicit message: although we work with the most painful and dehumanizing aspects of victimization and victimizing, our ability to laugh, feel joy, and believe that healing is possible are very much alive in us. We are proof that life-enlivening energies and affects can exist in the face of bearing witness to and healing the worst that life presents.

When therapists share a playful mindset with clients, we infuse the therapy relationship with an essential ingredient of change—positive affects. In fact, positive affects are "the raw materials of transformational work" and signal that

DOI: 10.4324/9781003509493-13

healthy change is occurring, can be the result of it, and can generate recursive spirals of more positivity and transformational change (Fosha, 2021, p. 378). And of course, positivity feels good to us and our clients.

The therapist's very embodiment of a playful attitude in the context of trauma work creates mismatch experiences for clients (see Chapter 5 and Ecker et al., 2013) about the therapy process and content. Instead of anticipating that the trauma treatment process will mainly evoke fear, overwhelm, and pain, clients notice (consciously and unconsciously) that it can be associated with safety, positivity, and even enjoyment. Clients also notice that when they share distressing narratives and symptoms, therapists with a curated playful attitude stay mindful, grounded, curious, and welcoming about all things dysregulating. The therapist's attuned, appropriate, and playful attitude disarms and confuses clients about what they may have expected trauma treatment to be and feel like. Their mismatched expectations prime memory reconsolidation, thereby accelerating trauma healing and change. In short, therapists and our clients benefit tremendously when we cultivate a playful spirit.

Boosting the "Healing" of the Healing Relationship with Play's Superpowers

A therapist's cultivated playful spirit naturally infuses itself into the relational work with our clients. Because our playful spirit derives from and harnesses play's superpowers—the mechanisms of action that promote change (see Chapter 5)—we, in effect, boost the healing aspects of the healing relationship. Let's briefly review what these are.

When therapists engage a playful attitude, clients witness and experience how we use playful positivity in action to self- and co-regulate affect. Returning to calm and connected (ventral vagal) autonomic states is the prerequisite for and hallmark of a safe and effective healing relationship. When therapists invite clients to be playful with them, clients learn to mobilize (sympathetic nervous system engagement) to promote a sense of mastery, confidence, accomplishment, and positivity. Clients watch and learn how to prevent and handle getting hijacked as play states are incompatible with (dorsal vagal) states of shutdown and immobilization with fear. In fact, through the superpowers of playful engagement, clients gain experience with the healthy autonomic (dorsal vagal) state of rest and restore which corresponds with a mindful and embodied presence. Playful interactions with therapists support clients to experience co-regulation, going with the flow (with increased affect tolerance and modulated vagal braking), and the earning of security to feel and know they are safe, seen, and soothed in relationship to others and themselves (intrapsychically).

When we as therapists engage with genuine playful spiritedness, we bathe ourselves, clients, and the therapy milieu with positivity which supports neuroplasticity and resilience. Also, when therapists and clients interact with genuine playfulness, authentic connection to personal truths and core Self grows. Playful authenticity enhances qualities of compassion, creativity, curiosity, connectedness, courage, confidence, calm, clarity (nonjudgmental objectivity), patience, perspective, persistence, presence, and, of course, more playfulness (see 8 C's and 5 P's of Self in Internal Family Systems, Schwartz and Sweezy, 2020).

Finally, when we juxtapose the superpowers of playful healing relationality with trauma-based relational expectations, we prime our clients for deep healing and lasting change. Infusing the positivity of our playful spirit into the healing relationship truly boosts healing for traumatized clients of all ages. Yet, as the next section reminds us, our playful spirit needs to be attuned to be effective.

Accelerating Healing and Change through Attunement on Steroids

While the therapist's playful mindset can boost and accelerate healing, we must make sure it fits each client's style and needs. More specifically, it's not that we are playfully spirited but *how* we are that facilitates healing and transformation. We can't force or impose playfulness into the therapy relationship, it needs to unfold organically and spontaneously. For example, my client Marcy once told me how her former therapist—who had fine arts training—pulled out a color wheel and asked her to identify the color of her feelings. When she couldn't decide, the therapist tried selecting the colors for her. Marcy described, "I don't feel in colors. My therapist's persistence left me feeling unseen and kind of invalidated." Marcy explained that, over time, her therapist's adherence on using creative arts over what felt right to her, triggered Marcy to leave the misattuned relationship.

Fortunately, we can facilitate trauma healing by attuning in just-right or right-enough ways with clients that are attachment-focused, playful, and person-tailored. In keeping with our playful spiritedness, I call this process and stance *attunement on steroids*—an enhanced way of tuning into and being with our clients that accelerates healing and change in therapy. Attunement on steroids is transtheoretical, can be used with clients of all ages, and is particularly helpful with traumatized clients because it derives from healthy and playful attunement behaviors found in caregiver-infant relationships that promote growth and repair. It relationally supercharges the emotionally corrective experiences of therapy while enrobed in wisdom, compassion, and sincerity.

The professionally imposed bounds and dynamics of the therapy milieu and relationship make attunement on steroids possible. These include clients paying for a safe, healing relationship; having their needs focused on and met consistently, contingently, and confidentially; being vulnerable with and relying on a stranger; and having boundaried meetings with agreed time limits and frequency. How beautifully ironic: the unique-to-therapy boundaries and dynamics that clients deem artificial and contrived, are the very same ones therapists intentionally capitalize on to catalyze healing when we attune on steroids. In other words, we take what's unnatural about therapy and magnify it to unlock and harness our clients' natural healing abilities. Attunement on steroids is a form of playing with and befriending the monsters (see McCarthy Chapter 6) of therapy, if you will. Therapists embrace the very qualities of therapy that clients disparage and mine their beauty, positivity, and reparative qualities.

As we've come to appreciate all things playful in trauma treatment, when we attune on steroids, we create a mismatched expectation. Clients consciously and unconsciously must contend with the contradiction between what happens in therapy versus everyday life or traumatic experiences. In effect, we metaphorically provoke clients to scratch their heads and ask, "What's going on here?" "Is this for real?" Or they might notice, "This feels different, unfamiliar, or weird." Their trauma-related neural linkages unlock, priming clients for positive change to be encoded.

While different from everyday life and trauma, therapy still is a microcosm of and metaphor for our client's relational and experiential history, which are experienced in magnified ways through enactments, transferences, etc. Therapists, in parallel, need to hold a magnified awareness of how to make the experience healing through being attuned on steroids. Similar to playing with symptoms, we can playfully and relationally embrace what is unique to therapy to strengthen our clients' commitment to the hard work of positive change.

The Purpose of Attunement on Steroids for Clients

Since "the therapist is the intervention" (Piliero quoted by Frederick, 2021, p. 197), when therapists attune on steroids, we magnify our interventional efficacy. The attunement-on-steroids motto is as follows: everything therapists do and all that unfolds in the therapy relationship and environment can be used in the service of helping our client to: (1) tolerate, trust, and integrate authentic care, protection, and positivity; (2) earn relational security; and (3) support the embodiment of their wise, self-at-best (Fosha, 2021) to emerge and blossom. First, let's define these client goals before digging into what we do when attuning on steroids.

Tolerating, Trusting, and Integrating Authentic Care,
Protection, and Positivity

The attuned-on-steroids relational stance challenges the foundational wiring of clients with complex and chronic relational trauma. They may ask, "How could, and why, would this stranger, who has no genetic or personal investment in my well-being, care for and protect me?" It's a great question that therapists must welcome. We can remind clients to keep their skeptical protectors close by to wisely assess if we are truly trustworthy allies, yet not stand in the way of positive change and healing.

Years of experience reminds me that trauma therapists make mistakes and misattune, which can further "prove" to clients that healing is hopeless. While our misattunements or relational ruptures offer us rich and complex opportunities for repair (Hopenwasser, 2008, 2016), some clients will not stay in therapy long enough to allow repair. Paying for therapy just to experience more hurt can feel masochistic. Bringing attunement on steroids and playfulness to our work may sometimes soften the blows of our ruptures and mistakes, while other times magnify misattunements for which we need great sensitivity and awareness to repair.

We need to hold in mind and heart that feeling safe, attuned with, and securely connected may feel destabilizing and therefore unsafe to some clients. Clients with relational trauma histories may find it hard to tolerate and trust feeling genuinely close, valued, cared about, and joyful. Skeptical of genuine care and safety, clients may focus on how *therapists get paid to care*, believing any connection and protection is transactional and inauthentic. They may minimize the value of the therapy relationship, saying things like, "That's your job. I pay you (or you get paid) to listen, show me care, or treat me nicely." They are right. And they're not.

Even when we engage our wisest, most compassionate, and attuned selves to help clients be safe, seen, and soothed, they may not *feel* it due to their limited receptive affective capacity or ability to "take in and experience" (Frederick, 2021, p. 191) positive, protective, or reparative messages, actions, emotions, or sensations. Difficulty letting and taking in these types of positivity and care might reflect our client's preverbal adaptations stemming from early complex and chronic relational trauma. For example, infants use dissociative shutdown to protect their tiny selves against the deep, unbearable, and life-threatening pain of unseen and unmet vulnerabilities and needs. Connecting with these seemingly unreachable clients takes patient perseverance, requiring us to be "transformance detectives" (Fosha & Frederick, 2014)—tracking then finding and mining the tiniest glimmers of positive change. We attune on steroids to help clients accept and viscerally take in all the positives we have to give. We can always begin this process by acknowledging that our client has made it into our office—whether self- or other-motivated.

Skepticism and minimizing therapy's and the therapist's value (literally and figuratively) may also reflect a deep, underlying fear and conflict about trusting and hoping positive change is possible. Healing work challenges the client's internal working model (IWM) (see Bowlby, 1969 in Chapter 2) and their evolutionarily driven negativity bias (Vaish et al., 2008), which promoted their survival. Clients may feel it's easier to resign themselves to the familiar "devil they know" rather than risk the upheaval of changing all that they've ever known to trust and hope for better.

Attunement on steroids helps therapists tap into our compassion, sensitivity, and empathy to remember that negative (e.g., life-threatening or traumatic) compared with positive (e.g., supportive and loving) experiences are learned faster; require greater attention and processing time; form more complex cognitive representations; weigh more heavily in our judgment, decision-making, and forming impressions; and correspond with greater brain activation (Vaish et al., 2008, p. 383). Negativity is more resistant to extinction. Therefore, therapists need sincere and magnified patience and consistency to earn our clients' tolerance of and trust in our authentic care and protection.

Earning Relational Security

Unlike biological caregivers who start attached to their infant to ensure survival and through attunement promote thrival (Fosha, 2010), therapists first attune to each new client to grow an attachment. When we show up attuned on steroids, we intentionally and genuinely give care in healthy, balanced, stable, predictable, consistent, and loving ways. Clients earn security with us as they internalize that we are available and contingently responsive to their needs. Then, we can guide them to internally mirror the same with all parts of mind and externally with others. This practice helps clients rewire their insecure attachment-related schema or IWM into one of an earned security (Marriott & Kelley interview with Sroufe, 2021).

Attuned on steroids, we earn security by letting go of a strict agenda or expectations about and for our client, which might prevent us from really grasping our client's feelings and experience. We act with a playfully-inspired nonjudgmental, open, gracious, creative, and go-with-the-flow mindset and welcome whatever and however things show up. We prioritize our clients' need to be and feel safe, seen, and soothed to promote security (Siegel & Payne Bryson, 2020). We appreciate misattunements will happen and work to repair them and take appropriate responsibility.

While a therapist's attuned-on-steroids stance and behaviors are intentional and conscious, the right brain-to-right brain process of earning security is unconscious (Lyons-Ruth, 1999)—which integrates right brain-to-right brain implicit, unconscious, and nonverbal connection between therapist and client. As Interpersonal (Siegel, 2020) and Affective (Schore, 2022) Neurobiology highlight, right brain-to-right brain connections enable us to move in sync with others and follow their rhythms. Meanwhile, left brain–based thinking and communicating help us integrate the experience. Attunement on steroids capitalizes on brain-to-brain mirroring of synchronous (Feldman, 2007; Fosha & Lanius, 2019; Stern et al., 1998) and dissociative (Hopenwasser, 2008, 2016) rhythms at cognitive, affective, somatic, or spiritual levels. In other words, attunement on steroids helps us move in sync with our clients at every level as our brains mirror each other's as we co-earn relational security.

Establishing Healthy Boundaries

Attunement on steroids helps therapists support clients of all ages to establish and implement healthy boundaries through our magnified attention to their needs for, and comfort with, physical proximity. We help our clients define: "Where do I begin and end in physical space?" "Where do you begin and end?" "What are my sensory and movement preferences?" "How do we share space in safe and respectful ways?" "How do our boundaries stay safe, effective, and intact?" "In what circumstances do we need to shift our boundaries?" and "How do we reestablish healthy boundaries?" Thus, therapists can play with sensorimotor boundaries to support a client's individuality, separateness, their sense of Self, and sensorimotor safety (discussed in Chapter 7).

Through our all-about-the-client stance, we intentionally ask clients, "Do you feel more comfortable with me sitting this close or further away?" or "Do you prefer the room be cooler or warmer? Darker or lighter?" These simple questions implicitly communicate a profound message that our client's comfort is important, is separate and different from ours, and deserves to be tuned into and respected. Attuned on steroids to our client's sensorimotor comfort, we support their increased self-awareness, self-attunement, and self-soothing. Our heightened sensorimotor attunement helps clients value their personal comfort. We can further help them assert their needs to grow their embodied agency so they can spontaneously ask us to close the blinds or make the room warmer or cooler.

On occasion, a client spontaneously makes changes (e.g., turns off the light or lowers the temperature) in the office without asking me. For example, early in their therapy, a 5-year-old client frequently took figurines off the top of my desk or opened the desk drawers without asking my permission. One 62-year-old client, without checking with me, went to my desk and removed pens from the pen holder which had confidential files next to it. We can explore these boundary-violating behaviors and themes of regard and respect for someone else's space or property, privacy, or sensorimotor comfort.

Engaging our attunement on steroids helps us ground, slow down, and create spaciousness to explore and see what unfolds. For example, we can neutrally narrate the behavior to prevent or minimize shame. "Oh, you shut off the light" or "I see you took the pen out of my pen holder." We can pause to see whether they spontaneously mentalize and share how their behavior might affect us. Then we can say, "I wonder what you imagined I might feel when you did that?" giving them an opportunity to reflect on how we might feel different than them. We can distinguish our needs, comfort levels, etc. and make clear the importance of checking in with us. We can say, "If it is something that belongs to me or my space, please check in with me first before you use (or change) it because I want both of us to feel comfortable sharing this space together." Then, we take responsibility to make clear boundaries we may not have previously.

Our attuned-on-steroids stance is intended to leave room for growth and learning for both us and our clients. We welcome a sensorimotor dance or back-and-forth experimenting and playing with boundaries. For example, when either we or our client changes physical proximity or emotional presence, the other is affected. We interactively adjust to reestablish safe and comfortable boundaries. While attuned on steroids, we more effectively engage this sensori-motor dance to support clients to earn relational security and seek our physical and emotional closeness for comfort when in distress, and distance to autonomously explore when calm.

Supporting Connection with Self

Through attuning on steroids, we engage relational healing at its finest, helping clients feel seen and known for their authentic being and Self (Schwartz & Sweezy, 2020). As we respond to our clients in deeply meaningful and contingently attuned ways, we facilitate their sense and embodiment of being real and alive (Winnicott, 1960, pp. 148–149) and connection with their genuine essence—who they have always known they were meant to be (also called a True Self relational experience [Fosha, 2005; Winnicott, 1960]). When recognizing their embodied, authentic Self, clients may say, "This is me," "That fits me," or "This feels right," which are often accompanied by smiles, tears, and a sense of ease and rightness. Engaging playfully further enlivens our clients and facilitates them to access and act from their Self. We purposefully attune in magnified, intentional, and authentic ways and act from our authentic Self, modeling ways for our client to discover and embody the same. Through this process, clients grow trust in us to safely integrate attuned care, protection, and connection.

What We Do to Attune on Steroids

When therapists attune on steroids, we amplify aspects of natural caregiver attunement practices to help us fully take in our clients with our minds, hearts, spirits, and bodies—with ethical constraints on touch. Reminiscent of early attunement play which flows from caregiver to infant, attunement on steroids has a unidirectional flow of care, connection, and safety from therapist to client. When attuned on steroids, therapists meet the client where they are, not the other way around. We show up in the service of our client, for our client, tuning in to meet their needs in ways to help them genuinely feel met and understood (van der Kolk, 2014) consciously and unconsciously. Attunement on steroids is not about perfectly attuning and meeting all of our client's needs: this is neither realistic nor healthy, just as with caregiving a child. Instead, when we attune on steroids, we genuinely and deliberately show up as the "good-enough mother" (Winnicott, 1971)—acting in ways that are just-right or right-enough to help our clients be and feel safe, seen, and soothed (Siegel & Payne Bryson, 2020), so they can ultimately learn to do the same for themselves and with others. As clients internalize our amplified attunement, they learn to self-attune, enabling them to attune with and securely attach to others and the multiplicity of their minds. The therapy dynamic then can become a bi-directional, interactive flow of attunement.

Let's see what we can do to intentionally cultivate aspects of our emotional-relational mindset and our behaviors to aid our magnified attuned practice.

Emotional-Relational Mindset

To start, we can amplify our attunement emotionally and relationally by using a developmental-relational-contextual lens (D-R-C discussed in Chapter 1), holding our clients metaphorically and sometimes literally, and delighting in them.

Seeing with our D-R-C lens. Therapists must get to know and experience our clients from scratch, which can feel daunting to us and them. Yet, we have the benefit of seeing clients with fresh eyes. To see them most fully, objectively without bias, and with curiosity we use the phenomenological D-R-C lens integral to the attuned-on-steroids stance. The D-R-C lens is fueled by mind and heart as it compassionately supports us to nonjudgmentally take in our clients for all that has contributed to their vulnerability and resiliency. How we take in our clients' being influences our understanding, perception, and the way we show up for and with them. It also affects how our clients feel seen and known. Different than many who give our clients care, while being attuned on steroids, we hold ourselves accountable to examine our positive or negative biases to prevent anything destructive to earning trust and relational security.

Holding: taking around. For therapists, communicating messages of holding our clients near and dear can be challenging, especially when physical touch is not appropriate. Still, we want to effectively communicate, "I see you." "I will soothe you." and "I am giving you concrete, physical, metaphorical, and emotional validation and care that will help you feel and be secure."

Robin, an 84-year-old, long-term client, shared how she searched for 50 years to find a therapist who would "take her around"—a phrase her grandmother would say before scooping her up, holding her firmly in her strong arms, and enveloping her with love and care. To Robin, a therapist who could "take her around" meant they would emotionally embrace and guide her through her struggles and reintroduce her to a life where she could be seen, understood, and supported to live more fully as her best Self. Clients of all ages, with all their parts of mind, hope for the same as Robin: they wish to be *taken around* by their therapist.

Taking our clients around is an essential relational attunement-on-steroid ingredient. It goes beyond a stance of welcoming that is open, curious, compassionate, and nonjudgmental. It communicates implicitly, explicitly, somatically, and verbally, "Let me fully hold you—allow me to safely take you in with my arms, my heart, and my mind." Taking our clients around conveys a warmth and loving holding that is deep, broad, and spacious. It gives the client the felt sense that we want to be with them and they are important to us.

Taking our clients around with attunement on steroids says more than "you are not alone." We convey, "Feel me with and near you as you move through life in your fullest truth. Together we will support you to become the very best version of yourself." This is especially important for relational trauma survivors as we seek to impart hope and possibility for change through relationship.

For example, we can take around our clients even in our initial meeting in sensorimotor, playful ways. We can greet them with a happy tone of voice or a smile, hold eye-to-eye gaze, make welcoming arm and hand gestures, call them their preferred name with a slightly melodic tone, or engage an open body stance. We take our clients around when we welcome every aspect of their being, inviting their angry or suicidal parts to show up in session or physically leaning in as they share a painful or joyful story. Through these forms of taking around, we convey, "I am with you," or "I want to take you in," and even, "You are a gift to me." One client said with confusion, "You actually seem excited to see me?" We slowed down and stretched out this reaction into a wonderful exploration of how shocking that felt because, while growing up, they always felt like an imposition and a nuisance.

Some clients, particularly children, literally want to be taken around—or even to take around the therapist. They may ask for hugs or even spontaneously give one to the therapist. While this is a natural way to behave with child clients, those whose physical boundaries have been violated (i.e., through sexual or physical abuse) pose challenges. Similarly, teenagers and adults make the act of taking around with physical connection more complicated. Still, we can take them around by hugging ourselves and saying, "Can you feel me hugging you?" We can put our hand over our heart and tilt our head to the side as we gently smile and say, "Hmmm. Can you sense how much I care for you?" The sensorimotor ways to take our clients around are limited only by our creativity. Fully holding our clients deepens their experience of being met (Stern, 2004) and holds vast reparative possibilities for relational healing.

Authentic delighting in. The attuned-on-steroids mindset also involves therapists freely allowing ourselves to appropriately and spontaneously express genuine delight in our clients which expands and deepens messages of authentic care and their importance to us. When I *kvell*—a Yiddish term meaning "burst with pride or excitement in and for someone"—about my client's accomplishments they tend to feel proud, important, seen, and celebrated for their strengths, abilities, and achievements. I explicitly share with clients that I am *kvelling* and explore what it feels like to them.

Our delight in clients can surprise and disarm those unaccustomed to this strong, positive reception. "Such a disconfirmation of expectations can rapidly soften defenses, yielding access to more viscerally felt, right-brain-mediated emotional experiences" (Fosha, 2010). The therapist's delight in the quintessential qualities of the client's Self is a powerful antidote to their shame (Hughes, 2006). Being delighted in amplifies the experience of being seen and increases positive affect tolerance. In turn, feeling positively impactful on others grows relational competence, pride, and efficacy.

Experimental attitude. When therapists are attuned on steroids, we intentionally engage an experimental attitude (Ogden et al., 2006). We bring curiosity, creativity, and out-of-the-box thinking to facilitate our client's exploration, growth, and change and their learning of how they effect and can be affected by people and experiences. To facilitate our clients' healing, we playfully experiment with their boundaries of affect tolerance and physical and emotional closeness/distance. We make our growth-encouraging intentions explicit and process them relationally and experientially. We encourage our clients' buy-in to change and improve what is not best serving them.

Our experimental attitude requires us to notice and grow openness and flexibility. Fortunately, when grounded and present the social engagement pathway of our ANS and both prefrontal cortices are online enabling us to access memories and life experiences, replete with their cognitive, emotional, and sensorimotor knowledge. With our whole brain online, we can combine left-brain objectivity, logic, and linear thinking with right-brain holistic, nonjudgmental, and flexible thinking.

When attuned on steroids, we act with an open mind and heart, flexible to our client and the dynamics that unfold in the therapy process. We can stay goal-oriented yet fluid and adaptable. We let go of assumptions that treatment and healing are linear (Rothschild, 2021), strictly adherent to phases and stages. This is especially relevant when treating chronic and complex trauma which occurs in a spontaneous, recursive, cyclical, and/or spiraling fashion (Badenoch, 2017; Fosha, 2021; Herman, 2022; Rothschild, 2021). Our flexibility supports our experimental attitude, too.

In essence, all intentional therapist self-attunement practices help us harness the best qualities of healthy and playfully attuned caregivers to benefit client attachment and healing needs.

Relational Behaviors

Therapists engage in different actions that facilitate our ability to attune on steroids including frequently checking for fit, tailoring the ways we communicate, and trusting our clients to lead the process.

Frequently checking for fit. We will inevitably misattune and cause ruptures in relationship with our clients. This is fortunate since the co-regulated relational repair not the rupture is important in developing/earning a secure attachment (Tronick & Gianino, 1986). In fact, when therapists avoid ruptures or conflicts, we implicitly send the message to clients that we can't handle it. This avoidance may also increase our anxiety as we avoid stepping on emotional landmines. Lastly, this prevents clients from engaging in conflict that could present opportunities for healing.

While attuned on steroids, we identify the rupture and guide its relational repair. We model ways to take responsibility for our mistakes with self-compassion and hold our clients accountable with love when they cause ruptures. Additionally, we try to identify misattunements and not good enough fit as *a matter of course*. This is not to avoid landmines, per se, but to potentially catch them from being as destructive. By consistently, explicitly checking in with our clients for fit, we also accomplish a number of things:

1. Establish the client as the ultimate authority on themselves. They know what's right for them.
2. Build the client's self-attunement and awareness (of body, mind, emotions, and spirit).
3. Support the client to articulate their personal needs.
4. Support the client to help/guide another person to attune to them.
5. Keep our therapist self humble: we don't know everything. We make mistakes.
6. Model self-awareness, empathy, mentalization skills, and responsibility-taking to repair mistakes.
7. Compassionately welcome and experience the reality of being human in relationship.

Tailoring Communication. When attuned on steroids we need to tailor how we speak to the multiplicity of our clients' minds and address the effects of trauma.

Speaking to all parts of mind. Attuning on steroids also includes mindfully shaping the content of our verbal, nonverbal, implicit, and explicit messages *and* the process of how we convey them. Our verbal and nonverbal communications are geared to be accessible and understandable to the youngest, preverbal parts of the client's mind. Therefore, when attuned on steroids, we are mindful of what we say and how we say it with our words and our body language. As best as possible, we convey that every facet of our client's being is important to us.

In addition, when we have well-practiced prompts or sayings that communicate our full client's importance to us, we can be more present, embodied, and facilitate the right brain-to-right brain experience of therapist with client (Halliday, 2022). Here are some prompts to use with clients to check whether they feel fully seen, heard, known, and felt:

- "Did I get it?"
- "How does that fit for you?"
- "What am I missing?"
- "Does that feel right (or right enough) to you?"
- "How would you direct me to get it so it's just right?"
- "'Sort of' is not good enough; I'd really like to get your experience better."
- "I think I'm hearing you, but I'm not sure. Will you help me?"
- "Thanks for your patience. It sometimes takes me a while to get it, and I hope you know and feel I really want to."

UNs of Trauma	Therapist Messages to Earn Security	Client's Feelings & Self-Beliefs
UNsafe	• I will protect you the best I can. How does my protection feel?	• I feel safe. • I am worthy of protection.
UNseen	• I see and feel your: - Distress/pain/discomfort - Full being - Growth/becoming	• I feel seen and accepted for all that I am, feel, and experience. • I am important and worthy (e.g., of being understood, validated, supported).
UNconnected (and alone)	• I am here with you. Do you feel me with you?	• I feel connected to you. • I am not alone. I belong.
UNbearable	• I see and sense your overwhelm/ fear/terror and am here to move through it with you. How does that feel?	• I feel calmer, soothed and seen. • I can handle the discomfort/pain.
UNwilled (and unwanted)	• I see and sense how you feel helpless/hopeless/out of control. Let's be with that together.	• I feel soothed handling this together. • I am agentic/have choice and control in how to cope.
UNresolved	• I see and sense how this is unending/has no closure. Let's make space to notice that together.	• I feel held and soothed. • I am able to handle the uncertainty/open-endedness.

Figure 8.1 Attuned-on-steroids messages to earn security and target repair of the six UNs of trauma.

Undoing the six UNs of trauma. When attuning on steroids and promoting relational security, we simultaneously target repairing the six UNs of trauma (see Chapter 1). Figure 8.1 shows some therapist messages that promote earned security to help clients feel and know they are safe, seen, and soothed. Emergent feelings and self-appraisals show how our messages correspond with helping undo the six UNs.

Sometimes conveying these messages to earn security through play and playfulness softens our clients' defenses, allowing them to be taken in more easily. Other times they may require further exploration. Owing to our clients' different affective receptive capacities, we need to check whether our client has felt or taken in our intended message. It is a win-win situation, whether or not the security-promoting message lands. If it does, the client takes it in and we can strengthen and deepen its integration with bilateral stimulation (see Eye Movement Desensitization and Reprocessing Shapiro, 2018) or metaprocessing (see Chapter 9 and Fosha, 2021; Fosha & Thoma, 2020). If it doesn't, we explore the block to integrating the felt-sense experience of being and feeling safe, seen, and soothed. Connecting with and learning from blocking beliefs and protector parts often leads to shifts in the internal system of parts, positive feelings and beliefs about Self, and to the dismantling of the six UNs of trauma.

Trusting our clients to lead. When therapists attune on steroids, clients grow intrapsychic and relational security, become more self-attuned, and expand their ANS's regulatory abilities and window of affect tolerance. As clients learn to repeatedly check-for-fit internally and relationally, they grow discernment about what they need and how to get it—increasing their coping and problem-solving flexibility. The attuned therapist needs to know when to hand over the reins and let the client lead because this process gives the client practice handling challenges, repairing ruptures, and savoring and deepening successes in the context of a supportive healing relationship.

Treena, a 17-year-old client, tried to protect me from what her borderline mother might do to me. After each session, Treena's mother would interrogate her and try to rupture her alliance with me, even though the mom had referred Treena for treatment. Treena's mother felt threatened by Treena's growing attachment to me and Treena's calm and reduced symptoms after sessions. Parts of her mother felt inadequate and shamed and perceived me as the enemy who was trying to show her up as a "better mother" figure. Treena feared her mother would physically harm me.

To reassure Treena, I shared bold messages about how, "Your mother does not intimidate me from doing the right thing for you" or "I can handle whatever she does." However, Treena knew her mother better than me and sensed a real threat to me. While some clients try to protect themselves or their therapists as they historically protected themselves from discomfort, this felt and was different. Treena explained her mother's long-standing history of erratic and violent behaviors. She could not feel safe working with me until she knew and felt that I was safe.

Once I took Treena's lead—based on her knowledge of her mother—our alliance grew stronger and Treena felt seen, respected, validated, and soothed by me. I agreed not to invite her mother into sessions to work on the mother-daughter relationship. I deferred to her wisdom to navigate feeling "better enough" from therapy, but not "too good," for fear of triggering her mother's inadequacy. Treena knew she had to play both sides. With me, she enjoyed and bubble-wrapped herself in the safe and honest earned security we co-created. With mom, Treena downplayed how much therapy was helping her. Treena said that her mother just wanted her to stop cutting and expressing her suicidal feelings at school because, each time, the school forced and inconvenienced her to take Treena for risk evaluations before she could return to school. If Treena sensed her mother was going to yank her out of treatment, she threatened to cut herself but reassured me it would be superficial. It amazed me how effective her strategy was. I expressed deep respect for Treena's conscious and complex adaptations to protect herself and me.

Treena's isolation in navigating her relational pain was somewhat lessened as I validated her insight and ability to successfully navigate different relationship styles—with me, her mom, dad, friends, teachers, and her boyfriend—all while connecting with her essence or Self. Increasingly, she felt seen by me and supported to become more wisely independent and more safely dependent and connected. Treena became more empowered, resourceful, embodied, and validated through our work. She managed to complete her school year, improve her connection to her boyfriend, distance from harmful friendships, and end treatment on her terms when she was ready enough.

Treena taught me that when we work with severe and complex relational trauma, staying attuned on steroids can reveal unpredictable and client-specific solutions that we never imagined nor were taught in graduate school or at conferences. Ironically, just being with our clients without fixing or changing anything can be one of the most reparative and challenging things we can do. Being curious and open to all possibilities, while trusting our clients' innate healing wisdom, can strengthen their sense of safety, being seen and soothed, and practically grow their interpersonal and intrarelational security, even if we accomplish this in somewhat unconventional ways. For example, creating real safety with Treena meant the client protected the therapist, not the other way around, per se. Just like our clients, trauma therapists dealing with clients who live in less-than-ideal relationships and contexts have to do the best we can with what we've got under the circumstances.

This case illustrates how being attuned on steroids can help us navigate complicated and challenging clinical relationships and situations. Through my magnified attunement, Treena grew trust in my authentic care, earned relational security, connected with her wisdom and authentic Self, and benefitted by living a better life. This was accomplished by the attunement-on-steroids process of repeatedly checking for fit, tailoring my communication and interventions, and trusting Treena to guide me through her relational world. Deep down, each client holds the solutions to their problems; discovering these is facilitated when we are attuned on steroids.

Therapist's Use of Self

Attunement on steroids means we use our full being–including body, personal feelings, and experiences–to best serve our clients. We mindfully connect to our life experience and the wisdom of Self (Schwartz & Sweezy, 2020), self-regulate (i.e., mind, body, emotions, and spirit), and ground ourselves in the here-and-now to be the most effective neurobiological regulator (Fisher, 2017, p. 55) for clients especially when they get activated by the there-and-then of trauma memories. This means that we cultivate an embodied mindful presence which allows us to go into the therapy process and, "release our own Being in order to Be-with our client in the moment," be open and touched by them, move to their rhythm, and welcome whatever becomes important at the moment (Finlay, 2016, p. 57). With our embodied mindful presence, we can ease and let go of our own and our clients' tendencies to be pulled into the past or future. "When we are present, we feel energized, balanced, effective, and less burdened by the difficult emotional work of psychotherapy" (Geller, 2017).

Attunement on steroids also assumes we intentionally and continuously scan our body to deepen our embodied presence; this heightens our interoceptive awareness to guide our use of somatic countertransferences in the service of relational work (Blum, 2015). The more tuned into our body we are, the better. When we monitor the experience of our inner sensory system, we more readily recognize optimal moments to respond—and to respond in ways that will offer the greatest impact while in precise resonance with what is emerging in the now (Finlay, 2016; Geller, 2020).

Using our body. Attunement on steroids includes the use of our bodies through the intentional verbal and nonverbal mirroring of our clients. While we unconsciously and spontaneously mirror our clients with some frequency (e.g., by crossing our legs in tandem or reciprocating a smile), bringing attention and intention to mirroring may feel somewhat contrived. Yet, it increases our synchronizing with clients and our ability to mentalize, empathize with, and have an interoceptive experience of our clients—and them of us (Blum, 2015). As opposed to just observing our clients, mindfully imitating them strengthens our felt sense of their bodily, emotional, and cognitive experiences (see Carr et al., 2003; Rizzolatti & Craighero, 2004). This augmented experiential felt-sense knowing can guide our interventions to be more empathic and compassionate. As the use of the embodied mirroring technique (Blum, 2015) demonstrates, intentional and attuned mirroring can help us relationally move more effectively and efficiently through our clients' stuck states, helping them feel less alone. Owing to the protective bounds of therapy, we can explicitly mirror and explore its reveals through slowing down, unfolding, delighting in, and deepening new and positive experiences.

While mirroring in general helps us better synchronize and move into rhythm with our clients, intentional mirroring when attuned on steroids logically magnifies these effects. It deepens our shared relational presence, resonance, synchrony, and rhythm with clients helping optimize therapeutic movement (Geller, 2017), resolve therapeutic impasses (Blum, 2015), support the earning of relational security (Lyons-Ruth, 1999), and promote change and relational healing (Schore, 2022).

We can also use our body with heightened attunement in sensorimotor practices with clients. For example, we can support our clients to gain mastery to meet their needs by following the sequential movements of the satisfaction cycle including yield, push, reach, grasp, and pull (see Body-Mind Psychotherapy, Aposhyan, 2004; Body-Mind Centering, Bainbridge Cohen, 2012; and somatic psychology, Schwartz, 2018). We encourage clients to experiment with changing their sensorimotor, procedurally learned action patterns they relied on to survive (Ogden et al., 2006) to now promote satisfying their needs and thriving. Having learned their old action patterns in traumatic relationships, clients need to learn new ones in the reparative relationship with us. This requires therapists to literally move with our clients.

For example, if a client needs to gain practice with assertiveness and pushing, we can provide the safe, resistant force with our hands or a pillow. If they struggle to reach outward (e.g., due to adapting to parents with dismissive attachment styles), we need to comfortably receive or reciprocate their reach. Since our historic adaptational action patterns may get triggered, we will need to engage our mindful embodied presence to unblend these dynamics from those of our client. In fact, being attuned on steroids can help us make the process explicit and model how we, like our client, can choose a different movement. Using our own body with an internally focused D-R-C lens can help us ground and then act in the best service of our client.

Self-disclosing/sharing. Using our therapist self in the service of our client involves sharing personal vulnerability and transparency *for the client's benefit*. We share personal experiences, feelings, sensations, and thoughts with the intention of meeting the client in a relationally authentic way to augment the earning of security. When using our therapist self in service of the client, we literally enact "the therapist is the intervention" credo: we self-disclose and share in grounded, sincere, discerning, and intentional ways meant, for example, to normalize, validate, and teach life lessons and support clients to feel less alone. Clients with relational trauma histories may be sensitive to narcissistic motivations or overtones; our attunement on steroids helps prevent our gratuitous sharing.

Similar to caregivers with their children, therapists with our clients can share stories about ourselves to deepen the relational bond. As a result, clients feel more meaningfully connected to us and grow to feel we are more human, approachable, and relatable. Self-sharing can also be powerful and fun. For example, clients really get a kick when I share that I, too, am actively engaged in the hard work of helping my best Self show up. "Yup, after all my therapy, I'm still working with my fight protectors to help them soften. If you don't believe me, ask my therapist, my husband, or my kids!"

Sometimes my clients sigh with relief, saying, "So, it's not just me!" or say, "At least I'm in good company," or joke, "And I'm paying *you* for help?" Each of these reactions can be explored. We can bond over our shared human struggle with vulnerability and connection. Ultimately, self-sharing and self-disclosing aim to soften defenses, earn relational security, and help our clients know they are not alone and feel "felt" (Frederick, 2021, pp. 196–197). For clients whose sense of agency, impact, and efficacy have been stripped interpersonally, they gain empowerment learning that they can positively and meaningfully affect the therapist, and not just the other way around.

In addition, therapists can share sincere messages about how a client is in their heart and mind between sessions. I tell clients I chose to wear a certain color or necklace because I knew they liked it or it reminded me of them. My clients feel touched when I tell them how I thought about them in between sessions. For example, I might share I heard a song they played in session with me, I prayed for their mother's recovery, or I watched the show they told me about. Through this sharing, clients learn they are always with me and our relationship is meaningful and real, not just a business transaction. It strengthens object constancy, too.

Attuned on steroids we can also share physical items—personal or purchased. I have shared objects like a book, a crystal, or a poem with clients to hold until I return from vacation as a way of staying connected to me—like a transitional object. I have also given objects to keep as anchors and regulatory reminders. For example, I gave one client a fake toy potato as a concrete, playful reminder she can hold whenever she gets triggered by her teenage daughter. We called her daughter's tendency to project or deflect onto my client "hot potatoing" personal shame and upset. My client used the potato to unblend from her tendency to take on her daughters' feelings as her own. The potato also would help her smile and calm.

Sometimes, in discerning and financially responsible ways, I purchase a small item—like stickers, certain types of crafts, extra soft tissues, or crystals—intended for a particular client's exclusive use in session. This type of client-specific sharing communicates that they and their preferences are important to me. One 10-year-old client was floored when I purchased poop stickers for her. Her eyes lit up in disbelief that I bought these solely for her use. Even after realizing she couldn't have them all at once (a practice in patience), but could choose one each time we met, she seemed to feel important to me like never before. Another client who taught me about crystals loved when I shared that I bought a crystal for us to use together in session. She shared that she felt I accepted her "weird, woo woo" beliefs and was deeply touched that I was open to learning from her.

Catalyzing Change with a Playful Spirit

This chapter detailed that a therapist's playful spirit facilitates trauma healing in the relationship with clients of all ages. It then introduced the concept of the therapist's attunement on steroids stance, its purpose, and how to engage it. When therapists cultivate both of these embodiments, we magnify and catalyze corrective emotional healing experiences for clients because we activate their mismatched expectations of relationships and therapy: memory reconsolidation—a necessary component of lasting healing and change—ensues. When engaging a playful spirit and being attuned on steroids, therapists access their fullest, truest, and best therapist self to act in full service of and for their traumatized clients. As a result, a co-created field of synchronized movements and psychodynamics emerges enabling clients to grow and deepen their self at best in resonant, creative, and life-enlivening ways. Trauma treatment becomes deeply experiential, dynamic, rewarding, and therefore self-reinforcing for both therapist and client as positive recursive cycles of healing and change emerge.

This readies us for Chapter 9 in which we will define what change is and how to deepen and expand it using playfulness, metaprocessing, and spirituality.

References

Aposhyan, S. (2004). *Body-mind psychotherapy: Principles, techniques, and practical applications.* New York: Norton.

Badenoch, B. (2017). *The heart of trauma: Healing the embodied brain in the context of relationships.* New York: Norton.

Bainbridge Cohen, B. (2012). *Sensing, feeling, and action: The experiential anatomy of Body-Mind Centering.* Middletown, CT: Wesleyan University Press.

Blum, M. C. (2015). Embodied mirroring: A relational, body-to-body technique promoting movement in therapy. *Journal of Psychotherapy Integration, 25*(2), 115–127.

Bowlby, J. (1969). *Attachment and Loss: Attachment* (Vol. 1). New York: Basic Books.

Carr, L., Iacoboni, M., Dubeau, M, Mazziotta, C., & Lenzi, G. L. (2003). Neural mechanisms of empathy in humans: A relay from neural systems for imitation to limbic areas. *Proceedings of the National Academy of Sciences of the United States of America, 100*(9), 5497–5502.

Ecker, B. (2003). The hidden logic of anxiety: Look for the emotional truth behind the symptom. *Psychotherapy Networker, 27*(6), 38–43.

Ecker, B., Ticic, R., & Hulley, L. (2013). A Primer on memory reconsolidation and its psychotherapeutic use as a core process of profound change. *The Neuropsychotherapist, 1,* 82–99. https://www.coherencetherapy.org/files/Ecker-etal-NPT2013April-Primer.pdf.

Feldman, R. (2007). Parent-infant synchrony: Biological foundations and developmental outcomes. *Current Directions in Psychological Science, 16*(6), 340–345.

Finlay, L. (2016). *Relational integrative psychotherapy: Engaging process and theory in practice.* Chichester: John Wiley.

Fisher, J. (2017). *Healing the fragmented selves of trauma survivors: Overcoming self-alienation.* New York: Routledge.

Fosha, D. (2005). Emotion, true self, true other, core state: Toward a clinical theory of affective change process. *Psychoanalytic Review, 92*(4), 513–551.

Fosha, D. (2010). Wired for healing: Thirteen ways of looking at AEDP. *Transformance: The AEDP Journal, 1.* https://aedpinstitute.org/journal/wired-for-healing/

Fosha, D. (Ed.) (2021). *Undoing aloneness & the transformation of suffering into flourishing: AEDP 2.0.* Washington, DC: American Psychological Association.

Fosha, D. & Frederick, R. (2014, October 9–10). *AEDP in clinical action: Becoming transformance detectives and facilitating healing change.* AEDP Institute workshop Stockholm, Sweden.

Fosha, D. & Lanius, R. (2019). *The neuroscience of trauma and its healing: The road back to the neurobiological core self.* AEDP Institute on Demand Seminar.

Fosha, D. & Thoma, N. (2020). Metatherapeutic processing supports the emergence of flourishing in psychotherapy. *Psychotherapy, 57*(3), 323–339.

Frederick, R. J. (2021). Neuroplasticity in action. In D. Fosha (Ed.), *Undoing aloneness & the transformation of suffering into flourishing: AEDP 2.0* (pp. 189–216). Washington, DC: American Psychological Association.

Fredrickson, B. L. (2001). The role of positive emotions in positive psychology: The broaden-and-build theory of positive emotions. *American Psychologist, 56,* 218–226.

Geller, S. (2020). Cultivating therapeutic presence: Strengthening your clinical, heart, mind, and practice. *Transformance: The AEDP Journal, 10*(1), 1–25. https://www.sharigeller.com/_images/pdfs/2_Journal-August_2020-Geller.pdf

Geller, S. M. (2017). *A practical guide to cultivating therapeutic presence.* Washington, DC: American Psychological Association.

Halliday, K (2022). Experiences Teaches Meeting #3 March, 13. AEDP Online Experiential Learning Course.

Herman, J. L. (2022). *Trauma and recovery: From domestic abuse to political terror.* London: Basic Books.

Hopenwasser, K. (2008). Being in rhythm: Dissociative attunement in therapeutic process. *Journal of Trauma & Dissociation, 9*(3), 349–367. https://doi.org/10.1080/15299730802139212

Hopenwasser, K. (2016). Dissociative attunement in a resonant world. In E. F. Howell & S. Iltzkowitz (Eds.), *The dissociative mind in psychoanalysis: Understanding and working with trauma* (pp. 175–186). New York: Routledge.

Hughes, D. (2006). *Building the bonds of attachment: Awakening love in deeply troubled children.* Lanham, MD: Jason Aronson.

Lyons-Ruth, K. (1999). The two-person unconscious: Intersubjective dialogue, enactive relational representation, and the emergence of new forms of relational organization. *Psychoanalytic Inquiry, 19*(4) (January), 576–617. https://doi.org/10.1080/07351699909534267.

Marriott, S. & Kelley, A. (Executive Producers) (2021, February 15). How we become the person's we are, with Dr. Alan Sroufe. Attachment through the lifespan. (No. 141). [Audio podcast episode]. In *Therapist Uncensored.* https://therapistuncensored.com/episodes/attachment-through-the-lifespan-alan-sroufe/

Ogden, P., Minton, K., & Pain, C. (2006). *Trauma and the body: A sensorimotor approach to psychotherapy.* New York: Norton.

Rizzolatti, G. & Craighero, L. (2004). The mirror-neuron system. *Annual Review of Neuroscience, 27,* 169–192.

Rothschild, B. (2021). *Revolutionizing trauma treatment: Stabilization, safety and nervous*[[Tab]]*system balance.* New York: Norton.

Schore, A. N. (2022). Right-brain-to-right-brain psychotherapy: Recent scientific and clinical advances. *Annals of general Psychiatry, 21*(46). https://doi.org/10.1186/s12991-022-00420-3

Schwartz, A. (2018, July 21). *Somatic psychology and the satisfaction cycle.* Center for Informed Therapy. https://drarielleschwartz.com/2018/07/#.YPGaUi1h0Us

Schwartz, R. C. & Sweezy, M. (2020). *Internal Family Systems* (2nd ed.). New York: Guilford.

Shapiro, F. (2018). *Eye Movement Desensitization and Reprocessing (EMDR) basic principles, protocols and procedures* (3rd ed.). New York: Guilford.

Siegel, D. J. (2020). *The developing mind: How relationships and the brain interact to shape who we are* (3rd ed.). New York: Guilford.

Siegel, D. J. & Payne Bryson, T. (2020). *The power of showing up: How parental presence shapes who our kids become and how their brains get wired.* New York: Ballantine Books.

Stern, D. (2004). *The present moment in psychotherapy and everyday life.* New York: Norton.

Stern, D. N., Bruschweiler-Stern, N., Harrison, A. M., Lyons-Ruth, K., Morgan, A. C., Nahum, J. P., Sander, L., & Tronick, E. Z. (1998). The process of therapeutic change involving implicit knowledge: Some implications of developmental observations for adult psychotherapy. *Infant Mental Health Journal, 19*(3), 200–308.

Tronick, E. Z. & Gianino, A. F. (1986). Interactive mismatch and repair: Challenges to the coping infant. *Zero to Three, 6*, 1–6.

Vaish, A., Grossmann, T., & Woodward, A. (2008). Not all emotions are created equal: The negativity bias in social-emotional development. *Psychological Bulletin, 134*(3), 383–403. https://doi.org/10.1037/0033-2909.134.3.383

van der Kolk, B. A. (2014). *The body keeps the score: Brain, mind and body in the healing of trauma.* New York: Penguin.

Winnicott, D. W. (1960). Ego distortion in terms of true and false self. In D. W. Winnicott (Ed.), *The maturational processes and the facilitating environment: Studies in the theory of emotional development* (pp. 140–152). New York: International Universities Press.

Winnicott, D. W. (1971) *Playing and reality.* London: Tavistock Publications.

Part V

Synthesis and Integration

Playing with the Elements Needed to Promote Change in Trauma Treatment

Chapter 9

Playing with Change

So far in this book, we have established why, and how, infusing our playful spirit into trauma treatment is scientifically supported to accelerate and facilitate healing. We learned how to infuse playfulness to create and use a sensorimotor-sensitive space that promotes exploration. We discovered how embodying and enacting our attuned-on-steroids stance further catalyzes the earning of relational security and opportunities for change. Now, in this chapter, we will explore the natural outcome of this academic and clinical journey—change itself. We'll address what change is and how it can lie hidden in plain sight with severely traumatized clients. We will examine what primes clients to be ready to embrace change, infusing playfulness into this process. Finally, we'll explore how to deepen, expand, and elevate the experience of change to help our clients live a healthier and more balanced life.

What Is Change?

The "change" I am referring to throughout this chapter is change for the better—and "better" is what feels good and right (Fosha, 2013, 2021). In trauma treatment, change is the process and outcome of removing and transforming the trauma-induced processes meant to promote survival only.

The process of change in trauma treatment can be thought of as having horizontal, vertical, and spiraling movement. First, the horizontal and vertical movements resolve the corresponding trauma-induced brain splits in sensory information flow and functioning (discussed in Chapter 2). Horizontal change synthesizes opposites and dialectics between the right and left hemispheres (Laub & Weiner, 2013). This enables trauma memory networks and their related states of fear and aloneness, negative affect and cognitions, to shift into adaptive networks with related states of safety and connection, positive affect and cognitions (Laub, 2014). Play capitalizes on this horizontal synthesis. Vertically, the process of change integrates or links (Laub, 2014) the functioning of different brain structures—subcortical with cortical—enabling trauma memories to be brought into awareness, relationship, and be unburdened. We effectively

DOI: 10.4324/9781003509493-15

differentiate or unfuse trauma-linked autonomic nervous system (ANS) pathways, uncoupling trauma-related sensations and movements from emotions and cognitions. Our body and mind integrate as the multiplicity of parts works cooperatively with our whole Self, enabling us to move readily among intrapersonal, interpersonal, and transpersonal or spiritual connections.

Transformation results from therapists mining the recursive spirals of positive change (Frederickson & Joiner, 2002) experientially (somatically and emotionally) and cognitively. This means we help clients *have* an adaptive change experience and *know* they've had it (Fosha, 2021).

Therapists facilitate the process of change by creating mismatch or juxtaposition experiences which pair the opposites of trauma with self-righting/adaptive energies. This is why bringing trauma and play states together is so powerful. Mismatches unlock old trauma neural networks allowing new adaptive memory networks to form (see Chapter 5 and Ecker, 2018). Through mining and bolstering our clients' always-present, adaptive energies of the Self, therapists promote healing, foster growth, and create the opportunity to flourish. This is the ultimate outcome of change for the better.

Since the experience of trauma is isolation, the process of change must be relational. When clients feel and know they are safe, seen for their true Self, and affectively soothed by their therapist, they can more readily face their trauma memories (with related behaviors, emotions, thoughts, etc.). No longer alone, clients can show up with a sense of belonging, meaning, and purpose to affect change which enables their appraisals and experience of trauma memories to become tolerable and resolved—or resolved enough. Their appropriate sense of control and agency in relation to the trauma gets restored. Change *un*does the six UNs of trauma and promotes affect regulation which enables integrative brain functioning and the earning of intrapsychic and relational security. Clients' boundaries become healthier, appropriately protective, and flexible. Clients learn from the reparative relational experience with us, their therapist, to attune and meet their own and others' needs in just right, or right enough, ways.

When change is embodied, Self is experienced with its qualities of the eight Cs and five Ps (see Chapter 8 and Schwartz & Sweezy, 2020). Clients experience greater intrapsychic and interpersonal flow, harmony, and cooperation. In Accelerated Experiential Dynamic Psychotherapy (AEDP) terms, clients can connect with their core state marked by acting adaptively, naturally, with flow, vitality, ease, well-being, openness, relaxation, empathy for others and self, and generosity of heart and mind (Fosha, 2005, 2021).

While positive healing moments of change can be obvious and expressed explicitly by our clients, we are focused on experiences with traumatized clients whose movement toward change for the better shows up as symptoms or protectors in disguise. Calli offers us an example of this.

Calli's Hair Nest: A Metaphor to Guide Change

Calli returned to treatment at age 23 after a four-year break from therapy. She and I had previously worked together for five years during her early to late adolescence on sexual abuse by peers, social isolation, bulimia, consequences of her learning disability, and crippling separation issues. Her parents deeply loved Calli but had styles of dismissiveness and enmeshment due to their own unresolved traumatic relational histories. Their parents—Calli's grandparents—had disorganized styles due to alcoholism, divorce, the Holocaust, and other relational traumas.

Since Calli and I had last met, she experienced more sexual abuse, significant financial hardship, domestic violence, divorce, substance abuse, and, while unmarried, gave birth to an unplanned child that nearly caused her family to disown her. She was isolated. Calli lived in an apartment, paid for by her parents, with the once-heroin-addicted father of her baby. He was unemployed and reliant on the marijuana he grew in their closet. She was hijacked by deep despair and barely left her bed. Her child was growing up with a mix of deprivation, neglect, and love. Child Protective Services did not deem her child's case bad enough for ongoing services because they were overwhelmed and overrun by "more dire, severe" life-and-death cases, all heightened by the COVID lockdown.

When Calli entered my office, she plopped with a thud onto my couch, barely making eye contact. My eyes were drawn to the crown of her head, on which sat a mangled, matted, unwashed knot of hair; if let down, her full head of hair fell midway to her waist. This knot was a visible, complicated, weighty mess. Even now, recalling the sight of such a beautiful soul weighed down by this "mess," I cry. Calli announced, "I haven't showered again in over a week, and my hair is so tangled, I can't even get a comb through it. It's too painful. It's like a bird's nest, but there are no birds in it." With heaves of despondency, she said, "Look what's happened to me."

Yet, Calli had walked into my office. She had lived walking distance from my office for years, but needed to feel ready to walk through the door where part of her remembered change had once happened and was perhaps possible again. "I know you won't judge me," she said. Relationally, our bond had always been strong and loving. Calli had come back to find a way to unravel, detangle, and comb through the painful, complicated mess of her life. This small step—arriving—was monumental, which we explicitly bolstered and explored relationally and affectively through metaprocessing (discussed further in the next section). As I scaffolded her brave movement toward life-for-the-better, she expressed deep sobs of shame and self-loathing. Crying with overwhelm, Calli said, "What do I do? Where do I begin? I can't see myself getting out of this, and I have a child who I brought into this hell!" We breathed together and explicitly acknowledged the messy nest; it was real and there for us to hold together.

Then I acknowledged, "Notice where your nest rests." Calli had slowly been growing her connection to spirituality through work with her higher powers, experimentation with psychedelics, tarot and oracle cards, and crystals. She knew what I was getting at.

With a slight lift of her head, looking straight into my eyes, Calli said, "My crown chakra."

"Exactly," I responded. She had taught me that the crown chakra is all about spiritual connection and transformation, connecting a person to the divine and to the divine in one's Self. A glimmer of hope flashed across her face. My reflection spoke to her truth. I tried to stretch out Calli's intuitive knowing by slowing down and deepening her felt sense of it, because we need to both *have* (feel) an experience *and* know (cognitively) we've had it (Prenn & Fosha, 2017). Calli had awareness of her insight and felt the optimism of having it.

However, Calli's protectors were now triggered by the hope causing her to feel a scary, suffocating pressure to perform in a way parts of Calli felt incapable, inexperienced, and unready. Yet, the momentary, shared relational experience was real. I said with sincerity and a wink, "I appreciate that connecting more with your deep wisdom about hope and change feels too much to manage for many parts of your mind, AND, we know it's real and there." Calli nodded and quickly moved to the painful impossibility of things getting better.

For months, we were guided by her crown chakra hair nest. It mirrored her small yet huge steps of change. Calli shared efforts to shower more often and the resistance of her hair nest to receive any combing through. Her protectors were present between and among her strands of hair, just like in her mind and in therapy. When we talked about using extra conditioner, she realized, "I didn't even try conditioner yet!" The implied metaphor: while the detangling work of therapy would be hard, we would bring ease to it however we could. By letting in my support of her, Calli, in turn, could start to support all parts of her mind.

Each time she came to session—and she came regularly despite parts of her not wanting to show up—Calli would show me her nest's progress. It was getting smaller, less matted, and knotted. Her head literally felt lighter. The unraveling work of her hair nest and therapy as a whole was slow, yet hugely significant. Her hair nest was a visible barometer for both of us to gauge her movement. After at least three months of deep, attachment-oriented, experiential, playful, and spiritually informed work, her nest disappeared. Calli's nest mess had experienced an earned security with me and Calli: it had been and felt safe, seen, and soothed. It offered evidence of and hope for more change. The nest protector had served its purpose.

Calli's hair nest was the beacon illuminating the path of change. Just like we learned to welcome symptoms as our allies in Chapter 6, Calli's hair nest was a protector part in disguise. It visibly manifested her darkness and pain along with her wisdom, spiritual energies, and past experience that hope and change were possible. Calli taught me that we need to experience light to see and appreciate darkness and experience darkness to see and appreciate light. The healing work which includes making space for change with Calli is ongoing. It is nonlinear, challenging, and rewarding to her and to me.

Calli's hair nest is a metaphorical reminder for us to be gentle in supporting change—especially with chronic trauma survivors—and to always attune to our client's readiness and tolerance for positive affect. Just like play, positivity leads to recursive cycles of more positivity, which can feel extremely threatening to the internal system of a trauma survivor wired to survive, not thrive. Calli's hair nest symbolizes how our clients' visible and internally experienced mess reflects their efforts to hold and manage what is wrong, while communicating an innate hope and wish to have things feel and be more right and better.

Inviting Change

For change to occur, we need to create literal and figurative space in mind, body, emotions, and spirit to grieve and let go of what has been lost or no longer serves us. This includes grieving and letting go of all adaptations that helped us once survive but now block us from embodying our Self-at-best. Even updating our adaptations can trigger grief. "Something needs to die so we may live. When we are no longer alone, unguided, unmirrored, unverified, a new consciousness, visceral confirmation, awareness, internal ally and inner acceptance emerges" (Bakur Weiner & Simmons, 2009, p. 17). In this way, grief work is healing and allows transformation to unfold—we need to grieve to heal. Let's now examine how we invite opportunities for change by saying goodbye, letting go and grieving, and playing.

Inviting Change by Saying Goodbye

When we invite change into our experience, we are saying goodbye to our attachments to people, places, things, values, internal working models and scripts about self, others, and the world with related adaptation patterns, identities (ascribed to oneself or by others), future possibilities/dreams, hope, or past innocence. Saying goodbye to our attachments causes suffering, pain, and loss, even if the attachment itself was abusive or neglectful.

The reason goodbyes are hard from the perspective of the therapy process is that these attachments have functioned as our protectors. Goodbyes to adaptations that once served our traumatized clients are like severing bonds with dear and loyal buddies despite the harm or self-sacrifice they may have caused. These buddies helped our clients survive. That's why when we try to update younger protector parts (and their scripts), their fears of rejection, abandonment, or being replaced may emerge. Similar fears may appear when death, separation, or breakups force us to let go of toxic relationships. Trusting we will make new, safe, connections eases this process, as does engaging playful creativity.

There are two types of goodbyes that trauma therapists encounter, which influence how we can facilitate creating space for change. First, a complete goodbye, which is possible when a loss is final, finite, and in the past—like the death of a loved one. In chronic and complex trauma, especially unresolved relational trauma, we often deal with the second type: an incomplete or ambiguous goodbye due to an unclear loss that continues without resolution or closure (Boss & Yeats, 2014, p. 63).

In ambiguous goodbyes, there can be physical absence with psychological presence or there can be physical presence with psychological absence (Boss & Yeats, 2014, p. 64). Examples of the first kind might be leaving without a good-bye, missing soldiers or civilians during war, kidnappings, a missing person in the aftermath of natural disaster, a loved one moving to a care facility, or a miscarriage (Boss & Yeats, 2014, p. 64). Psychological absence with physical presence might include people "leaving" due to cognitive decline, terminal illness, chronic debilitating mental illness, brain injury, comas, addictions, and autism (Boss & Yeats, 2014, p. 64). Cycles of leaving and returning may characterize each type of ambiguous goodbye when psychological and physical reconnection occurs, even if temporarily. Examples might include rallies into life before death or cognitive clarity amidst episodes of complete disorientation.

Creating space for change is easier when losses are complete. However, this is not possible for many of my clients who care for loved ones with dementia, cancer, and degenerative conditions. Other clients have been in the confusing and complicated position of caring for or becoming dependent on those who historically abused or currently abuse them. Others have needed to cope with ongoing and unresolvable war affecting family and friends, long COVID, and societally baked-in discrimination.

For clients with incomplete loss, the healing work focuses on sitting with and containing the impact of the continued and cumulative losses by creating space for celebrating the joys of life. Juxtaposing playing with grandchildren, growing curiosity with new hobbies, listening and dancing to uplifting music, watching shows that bring laughter, playing in and exploring nature, and discovering wonders in the little things all help contain the pain of their out-of-control, ongoing losses. Saying goodbye, while continuing to be playful and creative, allows clients to preserve their life force and hope; soften the pain and blows of goodbyes; tap into their resilience; and regulate their ANS, which helps soothe their loved ones too. For example, one client mourning her husband—now unrecognizable due to the physical and mental ravages of Parkinson's disease—found joy and the strength to get up every day when planning her daughter's wedding and babysitting her first grandchild.

Inviting Change by Letting Go and Grieving

Once goodbyes have been said, or the need to say goodbye has been recognized, we can help clients let go and grieve their (misattuned, abusive, or neglect-filled) attachments to open up space for change. Letting go is part of the saying good-bye process and is central to healthy change. Letting go opens up energy so we can welcome new possibilities for enrichment, fulfillment, and connection to our Self. *Knowing* we are letting go (Prenn & Fosha, 2017, p. 29) deepens and inte-grates the emotional change experience (and is discussed in the deepening and expanding change section below). At a neuronal level, letting go means our brain prunes old networks that no longer serve us and then either rewires or wires in new circuits that serve us best now. Letting go means old, procedurally learned action patterns, and related affects that were once adaptive to surviving trauma are updated or created anew with ones that promote thriving.

We can support our clients to let go of and grieve their attachment by infusing the process with playfulness and creativity. We can borrow from rituals related to death like wakes, funerals, sitting Shiva, and memorials, which often include forms of play and creativity like singing, music, storytelling, dancing/move-ment, and sharing photos or poetry. Such play-informed and creative rituals can help clients of all ages grieve and offer rich metaphors to bring treatment themes and healing full-circle. When creating goodbye rituals, using the elements of earth, water, air, and fire can be grounding and can tap into the powers of meta-phorical play. Therapists need to be mindful of the metaphors the ritual conveys to prevent accidentally contaminating the healing work. For example, while a client may want to bury memories in the form of written words, pictures, photos, or objects, doing so before processing the related affect or sufficiently telling the trauma story connected to them may metaphorically and inadvertently suppress them. So, it is important to relationally and experientially explore the ritual's healing value for clients of all ages before enacting them. By staying attuned on steroids, therapists can somatically track their felt sense and insights to discern the authentic, cathartic value of burying objects.

Eighteen-year-old Darshan bragged about smashing and burying his older, favorite cousin's kaleidoscope—which he got at age 10 as a "trade" for per-forming a hand job on him. He told me that he buried it at the local park, where he loved to hang out with friends, skateboard, and play basketball. As a child, Darshan had coveted the mesmerizing kaleidoscope. His cousin, a sexual abuse victim and closeted gay teenager, taunted Darshan for many months, "How badly do you want it? What would you do to get it?" For a long time, Darshan wanted to be rid of the memory, but not of the kaleidoscope. He also had not sufficiently grieved the loss of his favorite cousin after disclos-ing the abuse. The unprocessed, complicated shame and grief had been buried prematurely. His resistance to working on what's "buried and gone" required more self-patience and compassion before we could literally and figuratively unearth and work through it.

By contrast, a healthy burial metaphor includes putting painful material in its final resting place. Symbolically, the material unearthed in trauma treatment can be put back in the earth in its worked through form. The physical act of digging a hole, placing the objects in it, filling it again, and saying goodbye with compassion and love can serve as a beautiful metaphor of trauma memories getting unearthed in therapy, put in order and metabolized, and returned to the earth as they are let go with peace. Clients have talked about letting "Mother Earth," "God," or "nature" hold, compost, and transform the once toxic to nutritive organic matter. Therapists need to ensure the burial site feels and is safe, soothing, and secure. If there is repeated curiosity or preoccupation with exhuming the materials, it is likely the burial was premature and/or the site was not a good fit.

Instead of burying, clients may prefer to rip up, burn, or flush materials when saying goodbye and making space for new connections to form. For example, some children and adults gain closure or resolve conflictual feelings with deceased loved ones by writing notes on little pieces of paper, folding them up, and putting them into an uninflated balloon, filling it with helium, and releasing it into the sky, heaven, or to their higher power. Other clients have put a message in a bottle and set it out to sea. For those familiar with Diane Spindler's "Slaying the Monster" EMDR technique, clients of all ages can playfully let go by blending drawing, storytelling, bilateral stimulation, and positive cognitions to help regain the power depleted by the trauma. Finally, Schwartz (2021) suggests asking exile parts if they want to give up their burden to the light, fire, water, earth, air, or anything else.

Inviting Change by Playing

Engaging playful creativity opens space for change as it restores aliveness—living with vitality, joy, and connectedness (Malchiodi, 2023, p. 12). Engaging our playful spirit supports healing trauma and metabolizing and integrating change. Once we have found ways to help our clients say goodbye with love and compassion and grieve those losses, their SEEKING system (Panksepp, 1998) can activate to help them explore new possibilities safely, without fear and say hello to new possibilities with curiosity. Said differently, the other side of a goodbye is a hello. The process of changing for the better includes saying goodbye to old patterns which no longer serve us and embodying new attuned ones which promote our best Self. We can imagine change, mixed with goodbyes and hellos, as an experiential process through which trauma is healed and transformed. Healing transformation is the mirror image of mourning (grief). In mourning, resolution comes about as our psyche comes to terms with *not having*—loss and deprivation—while in healing, it comes to terms with *having*—positive experiences that disconfirm the negative, painful, and isolating ones (Fosha, 2007). Let's explore how to make the most of positive change experiences.

Deepening and Expanding Change through Metaprocessing

Trauma therapists can magnify healing moments of positive change, and expand and deepen enlivening affects to support thriving, by using AEDP's powerful, transtheoretical technique called metaprocessing and metatherapeutic processing (Fosha, 2000; Fosha et al., 2019). While metaprocessing refers to our moment-to-moment tracking of our client's reactions that hold glimmers of positive change, metatherapeutic processing refers to us exploring an important piece of therapeutic work in which positive change occurred. For ease of reading, I will use the term metaprocessing to refer to both. Similar to play, metaprocessing can be used with movement, imaginal, metaphorical, energetic, or emotional channels and mines positivity.

What Is Metaprocessing?

Metaprocessing enables therapists to broaden and build the transformative moments of positive change with our clients to create upward, recursive spirals of positive emotions (Fosha, 2007; Fredrickson & Joiner, 2002). Metaprocessing enables suffering to transform into flourishing by turbocharging the positive emotions of change (Fosha, 2000; Fosha et al., 2019). The technique relies on the therapist's ability to detect and amplify our clients' positive vitality affects connected with transformance—innate biological drives to change for the better. Akin to self-actualization, transformance drives us toward self-righting and self-expansion (Fosha et al., 2019, pp. 567–568), maximal adaptability, vitality, authenticity, relatedness, and meaning (Fosha et al., 2019, p. 585). Transformance strivings are appetitive like play—they feel good and we want to do more of it. When we fully embody transformance, we are in core state (Fosha et al., 2019, p. 585) discovering something we have always known (Yeung, 2021, p. 368) and recognizing who we've always been. This means the transformational process of healing change leads us to our inner truth, our essence of knowing and being our full, embodied Self.

Yet is not enough for us to *have* this transformational experience, we also consciously and explicitly need to *know* we are having it. When we metaprocess with our clients, we affectively, relationally, and experientially harness and investigate what is healing about healing. We explore what happened by making the implicit explicit (Prenn & Fosha, 2017) to identify and clarify what contributes to the healing change. Metaprocessing explicitly and intentionally brings together left- and right-hemispheric functions. The right-brain relational, somatic, and affective change experience gets uploaded into the left brain where it is languaged, symbolized, and integrated into self-reflective functioning (Mendes Amaro, 2018, pp. 15–16; Prenn & Fosha, 2017, p. 29). Metaprocessing is an integrative, whole-brain experience that helps us feel and know we've experienced a transformation. It facilitates quantum leaps of change or "change in a heartbeat" (Fosha, 2006). Trauma therapists focus relationally on positive quantum change: from trauma and fear to healing and excitement. (Negative quantum change is in the opposite direction).

So, what does metaprocessing look like in action? We slow down, as if frame by frame, these quantum change experiences. We magnify and explore the transformational experience with our clients. Together we bask in the awe and power of change, healing, and flourishing. We luxuriate and delight in our client's thriving.

We intentionally slow down to make space for our client to embody the transformational feelings using the four micro-steps of *staying with, savoring, spreading,* and *saturating* the transformational energy (Yeung, 2021, p. 353). This means we support our clients to:

1. *Stay with* the sense and energy of the positive experience, which builds positive receptive affective capacity;
2. *Savor* with all their senses, welcome, and embrace the experience of change for the better;
3. Allow the transformational energy to *spread* throughout their body and hold it for about 30 seconds; and
4. Allow this energy to *saturate* or fill their whole physical body and radiate beyond its boundaries for about 30 seconds (Yeung, 2021, p. 353).

These metaprocessing micro-steps help our clients be most fully in and with the transformational experience.

A number of components can aid the therapist with the deeply relational and experiential practice of metaprocessing, too. These include (compiled from Halliday, 2022; Mendes Amaro, 2018, pp. 26–27):

- Seeking permission and checking in with the client to ensure their consent, responsibility, and control
- Having the client focus on and explore their current experience and its related felt sense and somatic aspects
- Self-disclosing, verbally and nonverbally, how the client impacts or touches them
- Affirming interventions that acclaim, appreciate, and acknowledge the client's qualities, abilities, or achievements
- Invoking sincere positive emotions about what happens in the dyadic interactions
- Encouraging patience to let the process have all the space it needs to let what needs to happen, happen (see Fosha et al., 2019, to learn more about how to use metaprocessing)

For me, including the four micro-steps, plus mindfully blending the therapist components of metaprocessing, has invariably allowed deeply hidden, beautiful aspects of my clients' authentic Self to reveal themselves. It feels as if Snow White, our client's essence and Self, has been lying in wait for the "kiss" of a safe relationship to awaken being felt, seen, and known again—or seemingly for the first time.

Let's consider an impactful example of metaprocessing with 52-year-old Len and his Eeyore part of mind, whom we first met in the introduction. When Len entered treatment, he was frequently hijacked by his fight protector—his family described him as often angry and self-absorbed. Growing up, prior to his brain injury, Len's family of origin was supportive, yet not particularly emotionally expressive. While his mother was empathic, neither she nor his father encouraged Len or his siblings to reciprocate empathy or mentalize. His brain injury then magnified his self-focused style of relating.

Over years of our work together, Len invited his wife and kids, in different constellations, to address relational conflicts. He worked hard to grow his capacity to safely feel and express vulnerability, care, concern, and closeness. Each year when the New Year approached, his wife encouraged Len to write me a New Year's card. In one session, I shared with Len that I had kept his New Year's cards from previous years and metaprocessed this sharing. The therapist's role of offering metaprocessing components and the four micro-steps are added in parentheses in italics.

Me: Len, I keep each of the cards you've given me. The one you gave me a couple of years ago sits on my desk at home. I look at the cute picture on the front and reread it. It touches me and gives me inspiration to keep writing my book and not give up. (*Self-disclosing verbally and nonverbally.* I started to tear up.)

Len: Really? (Looking shocked)

Me: Yes (tears falling). Len, what you write in your cards is so meaningful to me. (*Self-disclosing; affirmation.*) How do you feel when I share how your cards affect me?

Len: (Laughs.) I hope this year's card is as good the one from a couple of years ago. (Realizing he didn't answer the question he continued.) I mean, I didn't know I was a good writer. I never thought I could do something that was so meaningful to you. (He gets teary.)

Me: Yes, you can, and did. I see your eyes starting to tear up. What does it feel like to see me so deeply touched by your words and cards? (*Self-disclosing; affirming* impact; *invoking* positive emotions; and *focusing* on the present relational and intra-relational moment.)

Len: Wow. (Pausing, and then appearing a bit puzzled.) I guess everyone feels vulnerable at some time. (Growing mentalization.) I'm glad my card could support you like you have supported me and my family. (Now seeming more present and embodied.)

Me: (Realizing I said "your card and words" not "you," I now want to reflect directly about Len's impact on me.) What does it feel like to know you gave and give me support and inspiration, too? (*Invoking* positives and the relationship; *affirming*.)

Len: Surprising. I didn't realize I could, or I was.

Me: Yes, Len, you can and you are! (*Affirmation.*) Just notice what that's like inside. (*Staying with; savoring.*)

Len: Yes, I *am*! Wow.

Me: You *are*! (More *affirmation.*) I am so proud of how much you've grown. (*Self-disclosing*; more *invoking* positive emotions.)

(Len smiles and I return the smile—*nonverbal self-disclosure.*)

Me: When you and I first met, feeling how you have touched me deeply would have been so hard for you. Do you remember what you mainly felt?

Len: Anger?

Me: Yes, anger. You have worked so hard and have grown comfortable feeling the vulnerability of deep grief, joy, sadness, fear, and self-pride. (*Affirmation.*) Now, notice and feel how well you can give and receive in deeply meaningful, emotional ways. (Building on growing empathic reciprocity; *staying with*; *savoring.*)

(Len nods and I mirror the nod and smile, *nonverbal self-disclosure.*)

Me: Your words, cards, and our relationship bring me comfort and inspiration (*invoking* more positive emotions; *self-disclosing*; *affirmation).* (I pause, to slow down and *stay with* the experience.) I need to slow down and just stay with this feeling (*staying with*; *savoring* I breathe). Now, can we sit with this together for another moment? (*Asking permission* to *stay with* and *savor.*) What do you notice as you drop into your body? (*Saturating.*)

Len: Wow. It's powerful. I'm going to have to think about this more. (Growing tolerance for positive emotion.) Thank you for everything you've given me and my family, Monica.

Me: (Putting my hands over my heart, with new tears rising—*nonverbal self-disclosing.*) You're welcome, Len. And thank *you* for everything you've given me.

Metaprocessing Len's transformational change experience of growing empathic resonance and reciprocity around emotional vulnerability was potent. He grew his capacity to feel and know he could safely connect with deep relational presence, have meaningful impact on me, and connect with profound gratitude and humility—all formerly challenging for Len.

While engaging our playful spirit in trauma treatment can facilitate our clients to safely move into and through vulnerability, in the case of Len, it wasn't needed. If clients can safely tolerate emotional vulnerability, being playful may distance them from staying with their deep affective and relational connection. In this instance with Len, it would have raised defenses. Other times, my playfulness helped ease Len's defenses. Inviting our playful spirit needs to be intentional and attuned to each client and their need at the moment.

Children Metaprocessing through Play

Colleagues and I who use play therapy with young children have noticed that it naturally lends itself to metaprocessing. The recursive positive spirals of change seem to spontaneously unfold and deepen as we play with the different objects (e.g., dolls, sand figures), medium, or sensorimotor experiences (e.g., dance/movement, music, drawing, clay). We speak with and through the characters and the creative arts.

The following is a snippet of metaprocessing with 4-year-old Kat, who has an early history of parental abandonments. She brought her stuffed animal mouse, Bert, into our play together. Notice how, through play, we metaprocessed Kat's newer ability to access and feel her sadness of early deprivation by using Bert to personify a part of her. Metaprocessing grief for healing (called "mourning the self"/"emotional pain" in AEDP, Fosha, 2000, 2021) is important for Kat, who tended to disconnect from her pain. After living for nine months with her stable, loving, and caring aunt and uncle, Kat was adopted and then, in play therapy, started safely visiting her losses. Therapist components of metaprocessing and the four micro-steps are added in parentheses in italics.

Me:	Oh, Kat, Bert has no more cheese! Poor Bert. I wonder how he feels? Would you ask him? (*Focusing* through Bert; *asking permission*.)
Kat:	Sad (said with a sad face).
Me:	Oh, Bert. I see you feel sad too (*focusing* through Bert; *invoking relationship*—mine and Bert's). (I nod at Bert, helping Kat distance, to better tolerate the new experience of feeling grief.) Kat, that's so sad for little Bert (*Focusing* more through Bert). (I pause, *staying with* Kat's new experience of grief.) Can you let Bert know *you see* how sad he feels that he has no more cheese? (*Permission seeking*; *invoke relationship* between Kat and Bert.)
Kat:	Bert, you look sad. (Kat tilts her head to the side and pats Bert on the head.)
Me:	Awww, Kat. That's so caring (*Self-disclosure*). Bert likes that you see him and how he feels. I think he's smiling (*Affirmation* of her empathy to Bert and herself). (I breathe audibly and pause. More *staying with* and *savoring*.) Bert must have been hungry a lot. I wonder what he needs now?
Kat:	(Spontaneously states) Bert needs hugs and lots of cheese!

Me: Wow, Kat. It seems like you know just what Bert needs! (*Affirming* her attunement to Bert and herself. I smile. *Self-disclosure.*) What does Bert feel when you hug him? (Prompt to have Kat *focus*, by *invoking* her relationship with Bert.)

Kat: Good.

Me: (To help Kat grow her feelings vocabulary of positivity and safety, I offer her new word choices.) Yea. I see that feels good (I say with a nod: *self-disclosure* and *affirmation*). Bert seems calm and safe when he gets your hugs. He looks happy too (*Focusing* on Bert; *affirmation*). Can I hug Bert, too? (Growing Bert/Kat's positive receptive capacity for care from others.)

Kat: (Nods yes and hands me Bert.) Dr. Monica, don't squeeze him too hard. He likes hugs like this (she shows me by hugging herself gently and rocking side to side).

Me: (I mirror the same with Bert.) Like this? (Kat nods yes). Thanks, Kat (*affirmation*).

             Kat, you really know what Bert needs. He calmed when I hugged him the way you showed me to. You're a great and loving hugger! (*Affirmation* of her attunement. The word "loving" is me stretching Kat's positive receptive affective capacity, which she tolerates.) Bert must feel so good (Kat's word), safe, and warm (my additions) inside his little furry body when he feels your loving care (*Spreading; affirmation*).

At the end of the session, we engaged in metatherapeutic processing:

Me: Kat, today you listened to Bert so well and helped him feel his sad and being loved feelings. Now he's not hungry. He feels safe and calm (piling on *affirmation; invoking relationship*).

Kat: (Blurts out) And hugged!

Me: (Laughing—*self-disclosure*). Yes, and hugged! I feel warm in my heart that we could help him together. (*Self-disclosure; invoking relationship; savoring; spreading; and saturating*).

Kat: I feel warm all over. And so does Bert!

Elevating Change through Spirituality

As we've seen, using metaprocessing and our playful spirit to invite healing change is deep and expansive. As one client put it: "My change has been like a beautiful tree grows—my roots have spread deep and wide to hold myself more steadily, my trunk has grown bigger, more solid, strong and protective, and my branches have grown complex and expansive with more color and beauty to benefit and hold others." Others have described how change for the better can feel transformative, leaving them more connected to their soul, spirit, essence, truth, and the rightness of their unique being. They also share feeling more expansively and peacefully connected to a universal oneness and the presence of a higher power.

Based on three-and-a-half decades of experience, I see playfulness and change as inextricably connected with spirituality. Embracing a playful spirit helps healing professionals tolerate and be open to a client's unusual (for the therapist) or societally unconventional forms of healing. If they speak to my clients' truth, I've become open to the many vehicles that can support change, including many forms of wise, appropriate, playful, and creative media to effect change and flourishing. I've learned to integrate healing work with their religious texts, prayer, meditation, yoga, Buddhist practices, crystals, and their shared experiences with Kundalini and other energies, past-life regressions, Reiki, acupuncture and Chinese medicine, psychedelics, oracle cards, and channeling spirits of the deceased. Our playful spirit grounds us to nonjudgmentally welcome the sometimes-out-of-this-world or woo-woo beliefs and practices clients share that spiritually ground them. Play therapists embrace the out-of-the-box creativity of children, especially as it lends itself to safely benefitting them. I believe that when trauma therapists for clients of all ages support the creative, personal expression of change in the ways that best fit them, recursive spirals of transformational energy and integration unfold. In most cases, clients then report connecting more deeply with personal truth and interconnecting more expansively with universal truth. "Creative acts . . . are a mixture of instincts, emotion, and also an early experience of deity" (McCarthy, 2007, p. 20).

Our individual, spiritual systems consistently guide and direct our search for the sacred (Pargament, 2007, p. 92). Our PLAY circuitry orients us to heal and become our best selves. Integrating the two is powerful and profoundly humbling. Integrating playfulness and spirituality can usher in new or renewed faith, hope, trust, and vitality. Believing that something greater and good is possible connects us with sacred and spiritual qualities of transcendence, boundlessness, and ultimacy (Pargament, 2007, pp. 38–39). "Spiritual states connect us through a felt sense to something bigger than oneself, a oneness, or strong force which may be experienced as an energy, force, higher power, G-d, deity or transcendent figure or consciousness" (Miller et al., 2019). Something sacred exists in all of us, in our inner core, our essential being, our soul, and in relationships (Pargament, 2007).

Experiencing a felt sense of sacredness and transformational change share a paradoxical quality of being simultaneously calming and intense, light and profound, and security-enhancing and wordlessly incomprehensible. They both feel powerful, enriching, embodied, and balanced. They both provide spiritual uplift and enlightenment to client and therapist that is rooted and grounded and stands in stark contrast with the intoxicating highs that characterize addictive substances or mania. My 84-year-old client Robin expressed both in a moment of deep and expansive clarity when, for the first time, fear was replaced with comfort about her age. She poetically said, "How old am I? The same age I've always been: My essence—it's timeless. Embodying my essence can protect me, I don't have to guard against my essence being hurt (anymore). It brings me truth, contentment, and calm. When I connect with it, I can sleep through the night." Robin illustrates how our spirituality enables us to connect with lightness, joy, humility, and sometimes awe.

We need to mindfully gauge and help clients balance and tolerate these positive, spiritual, and transformational states. For example, three different clients who described Kundalini awakenings explained how hard it was to balance states of enlightenment with the human experience. Clients have shared that Kundalini states of awakening can feel energizing, deeply pleasurable, blissful, and even manic. Human cares and worries may drop away, as may the need to eat, sleep, or work. Kundalini awakenings also can feel crazy-making, destabilizing, and challenging to one's humanity. They can unhinge a person somatically, emotionally, behaviorally, and cognitively.

Blending enlightenment with the rootedness of human experience *is* the work of the trauma therapist. We can help clients prevent themselves from replaying toxic attachment dynamics with self and others while honoring and supporting their spiritual or energetic rightness and truth. Engaging a playful, creative mindset grounds therapists to flexibly hold all possibilities that can healthily support transmuting or change.

In play, we move below the level of the serious, as the child does, but we can also move above it—into the realm of the beautiful and the sacred (Huizinga, 2016, p. 19). Playfulness fosters change, creating space for hope to re/emerge, joy to re/awaken, and faith to be strengthened. The therapist's playful mindset supports trauma states once characterized by feeling fear, terror, loss, hopelessness, helplessness, pain, lost, stuck, or unseen to unfold into states of possibility, connection, forward movement, positive affect, attunement, and validation. Clients of all ages shift their internal working models and related beliefs about themselves, others, and the world. They develop a spring in their step, a sparkle in their eye, and the ability to breathe more deeply and exhale more fully. What seemed impossible becomes possible; what felt unmanageable becomes manageable; and what seemed irreconcilably ruptured becomes reparable. Playfulness lends itself to express and embody deep and meaningful change.

Playing with the Elements Needed to Promote Change in Trauma Treatment

This chapter has defined what positive, healing change is and how the transformance energy behind it can be disguised as symptoms or reveal itself more obviously. We can welcome change by saying goodbye, letting go and grieving, and being playful. We have learned to slow down, deepen, and expand moments of transformational change in therapy through metaprocessing, spirituality, and playful practices. Now equipped with the know-how to make change transformational, we can shift into the rest of Part V which explores how to playfully engage the different elements that traumatized clients need to heal but lack. These include regulating ANS and affect, embracing the dialectics of multiplicity and contradictions, growing connection and earning security through boundaries, and telling the trauma story.

References

Bakur Weiner, M. & Simmons, M. B. (2009). *The problem is the solution: A Jungian approach to a meaningful life*. New York: Jason Aronson.

Boss, P. & Yeats, J. R. (2014). Ambiguous loss: A complicated type of grief when loved ones disappear. *Bereavement Care, 33*(2), 63–69.

Ecker, B. (2018). Clinical translation of memory reconsolidation research: Therapeutic methodology for transformational change by erasing implicit emotional learnings driving symptom production. *International Journal of Neuropsychotherapy, 6*(1), 1–92. https://doi.org/10.12744/ijnpt.2018.0001-0092

Fosha, D. (2000). *The transforming power of affect: A model for accelerated change*. New York: Basic Books.

Fosha, D. (2005). Emotion, true self, true other, core state: Toward a clinical theory of affective change process. *Psychoanalytic Review, 92*(4), 513–551.

Fosha, D. (2006). Quantum transformation in trauma and treatment: Traversing the crisis of healing change. *Journal of Clinical Psychology, 62*(5), 569–683.

Fosha, D. (2007 Summer). "Good spiraling:" The phenomenology of healing and the engendering of secure attachment in AEDP. *Connections & Reflections, the GAINS Quarterly*.

Fosha, D. (2013). Turbocharging the affects of healing and redressing the evolutionary tilt. In D. J. Siegel & M. F. Solomon (Eds.), *Healing moments in psychotherapy*. Chapter 8 (pp. 129–168). New York: Norton.

Fosha, D. (Ed.) (2021). *Undoing aloneness & the transformation of suffering into flourishing: AEDP 2.0*. Washington, DC: American Psychological Association.

Fosha, D., Thoma, N., & Yeung, D. (2019). Transforming emotional suffering into flourishing: Metatherapeutic processing positive affect as a trans-theoretical vehicle for change. *Counselling Psychology Quarterly, 32*(3–4), 563–593.

Fredrickson, B. L. & Joiner, T. (2002). Positive emotions trigger upward spirals toward emotional well-being. *Psychological Science, 13*(2), 172–175.

Halliday, K. (2022, March 13). Experiences Teaches Meeting #3. AEDP Experiential Learning Online Course.

Huizinga, J. (2016). *Homo ludens: A study of the play-element in culture*. Brooklyn, NY: Angelico Press.

Laub, B. (2014). Dialectical Perspective in EMDR Therapy European EMDR Conference, Edinburgh, Scotland. https://www.ifemdr.fr/wp-content/uploads/2014/10/brurit-laub-2.pdf

Laub, B. & Weiner, N. (2013). A dialectical perspective of trauma processing. *International Joural of Integrative Psychology, 4*(2), 24–39. https://integrative-journal.com/index.php/ijip/article/viewFile/72/57

Malchiodi, C. A. (Ed.) (2023). *Handbook of expressive arts therapy.* New York: Guilford.

McCarthy, D. (2007). *"If you turned into a monster": Transformation through play: A body-centered approach to play therapy.* London: Jessica Kingsley.

Mendes Amaro, I. M. M. (2018). *Processing the experience of change: A systematic analysis of the metaprocessing task.* Integrated Master's in Psychology [Thesis University of Lisbon, Portugal]. https://repositorio.ul.pt/bitstream/10451/37882/1/ulfpie053294_tm.pdf

Miller, L., Balodis, I. M., McClintock, C. H., Xu, J., Lacadie, C. M., Sinha, R., & Potenza, M. N. (2019). Neural correlates of personalized spiritual experiences. *Cerebral cortex (New York, N.Y.: 1991), 29*(6), 2331–2338. https://doi.org/10.1093/cercor/bhy102

Neural correlates of personalized spiritual experiences. *Cerebral Cortex, 29*(6), 2331–2338. https://doi.org/10.1093/cercor/bhy102

Panksepp, J. (1998). *Affective neuroscience: The foundation of human and animal emotions.* New York: Oxford University Press.

Pargament, K. I. (2007). *Spiritually integrated psychotherapy: Understanding and addressing the sacred.* New York: Guilford.

Prenn, N. & Fosha, D. (2017). *Supervision essentials for Accelerated Experiential Dynamic Psychotherapy.* Washington, DC: American Psychological Association.

Schwartz, R. C. (2021). *No bad parts: Healing trauma and restoring wholeness with the Internal Family Systems Model.* Boulder, CO: Sounds True.

Schwartz, R. C. & Sweezy, M. (2020). *Internal Family Systems* (2nd ed.). New York: Guilford.

Yeung, D. (2021). What went right?: What happens in the brain during AEDP's metatherapeutic processing. In D. Fosha (Ed.), *Undoing aloneness & the transformation of suffering* (pp. 349–376). Washington, DC: American Psychological Association.

Chapter 10

Playing with Safety
Navigating Waves of Affect

In this chapter, we will explore how to practically integrate our playful spirit to promote and support our traumatized clients in regulating their affect. Using a playful metaphor of "navigating waves" to guide our regulatory work, we shall examine how Polyvagal Theory underlies the therapist's actions to return clients to safety, stability, and connection, as well as how to use playfulness with regulatory sensitivity to encourage client independent functioning. Finally, we will explore how play exercises our vagal brake to contain and expand affect, helping us increase ANS (autonomic nervous system) regulation and affect tolerance in clients of all ages. Because of the fundamental importance of establishing and returning to regulated states for all therapists practicing any modality, we will first focus theoretically on the many and detailed ways therapists can bring sensitivity to and model playful regulation. Then, we will shift our attention to practical exercises that apply regulatory theory and sensitivity.

A Playful Frame for Trauma Treatment: Green, Yellow, and Red Waves

Like the ocean, our ANS has rhythms that influence our affect—our basic, non-conscious, unconditioned emotions, and mood that link to bodily states and arousal (Panksepp, 2009, pp. 1–2)—which play a role in regulating cognition, behavior, and social interactions (Niven, 2013). When our ANS detects safety, our ventral vagal (VV) branch engages, allowing us to experience an ease and flow of body, mind, emotion, and spirit. The waves are gentle, inviting, or even calm. Our affect is regulated: we feel internally buoyed. It's as if an internal green light goes on, signaling us to "go"—go safely explore and SEEK experiences internally and with others with curiosity and openness. These are our *green waves*.

By contrast, when the sympathetic nervous system (SNS) branch of our ANS detects threat, we are mobilized into fight and flight. We experience discomfort. Our affect becomes dysregulated and mobilizes us. The ocean waters become choppy, and the currents become somewhat tremulous and uneasy. They are still

DOI: 10.4324/9781003509493-16

navigable, but we struggle to regain our sea legs. We may sense a change in the tides at any moment: will we restabilize as the waters settle or will we get swept up and away in an increasingly unstable current? In this state, we stay alert and vigilant to any shift in the flow toward increasing safety and stability, or danger and instability. These are our *yellow waves*. Successfully navigating these waters feels rewarding and helps us return to calm, green waves. However, losing our center or direction is highly destabilizing, leading us into even more challenging waters and affective dysregulation.

Unsuccessfully navigating the SNS yellow waves back to green ones activates the dorsal vagal (DV) parasympathetic branch of our ANS. We move to further protect and disconnect. We are immobilized into states of freeze, faint, flop/shut down, and dissociation. The currents feel like strong rip tides and even escalate to tidal waves and tsunamis. As we are overpowered by these forces, our sense of stability, identity, or life is threatened. Our affect is dysregulated, causing collapse and shutdown. We submit and surrender, relying on the most evolutionarily primitive parts of our ANS and brain to enable our survival. These are our *red waves*.

We see that all regulatory work involves ANS and affect. For conciseness, throughout this chapter, I will use the term "affect" to refer to the waves of emotion, mood, and behaviors with their underlying polyvagal ANS states.

Return to Green Waves for Safety, Stabilization, and Connection

When navigating affect waves in trauma treatment, we must remember what Polyvagal Theory (Dana, 2018; Porges, 2011) teaches: if our ANS does not neurocept safety, all bets are off for repair work or genuine connection. The safe relational connection and milieu of therapy is a *precondition* for healing work, setting it apart from our clients' historic traumatic relationships and experiences. Relational and situational safety serve as the secure base from which our clients can voluntarily and bravely experiment when moving into more affectively turbulent waters. Therefore, we must start the healing process by guiding our traumatized clients to move into VV green waves of safety and connection. Here, they can affectively feel and cognitively deal (handle), relate to their Self and others (the therapist) in mindful and embodied ways, and balance their needs for independence/dependence with appropriate boundaries.

Teaching clients how to move into green waves of safety and stabilization or their window of affect tolerance (WOT) (see Chapter 2 and Siegel, 2020) also fosters their (and our) trust in the therapeutic relationship, encouraging them to do increasingly challenging trauma work. Trauma therapies for children and adults agree that safety, stabilization, and engaging the attachment system are essential to begin the healing work (Courtois & Ford, 2013; Gomez-Perales, 2015; Herman, 2022; Rothschild, 2021; Warner et al., 2020). Rothschild (2021) reminds us that monitoring and modulating a client's dysregulated nervous system is one of the practitioner's best lines of defense against traumatic hyperarousal and hypoarousal (my addition) "going amok," risking dissociation, decompensation, and/or them abandoning treatment.

Promote Intentional and Independent Navigation of Affect Waves

First, we need our client's commitment and intrapersonal (all parts of mind) and interpersonal (between us and them) agreement to grow their affect regulation and tolerance skills. When we explicitly ask, "Is every part of you on board with doing this practice?" we encourage internal consensus between all parts of the client's mind and highlight the importance of client consent.

Then, we provide psychoeducation that waves of dysregulation and related symptoms are allies or trauma-time protectors (see Chapter 6) that need updating to function in present-time relevant ways to help clients better regulate. We teach clients that our practice in returning to green waves—whether effective or not—will help us learn something to benefit the healing work. We encourage curiosity, openness, and exploration using an experimental attitude (Ogden et al., 2006) by asking "Can we try something?" "Are you up for a little experiment?"

We guide our clients to move from a place of absolute regulatory dependence, to relative dependence, and then toward independence (Winnicott, 1960). For example, early in treatment clients may lack self-trust to affectively navigate turbulent waters, but gain trust in us to lead them. We implicitly and explicitly communicate messages like, "I can handle this. Come, try this with me. Even though you may not like it, I trust you can handle it with me." When our clients seem ready, we move to relative dependence by stepping back or to the side, encouraging them to sit with and gain more comfort with discomfort. We step in if needed. Just like wise caregivers, attuned therapists instinctively "Know how to fail their child [their client] in ways that will facilitate and stimulate psychic growth and development" (Levine, 2023).

Having internalized our support and believing they can independently handle affective discomfort, clients will say, "I've learned that it's uncomfortable, but it won't kill me, and what doesn't kill me makes me stronger!" The more we encourage and trust our clients to independently handle their regulatory challenges, the more capable, adaptable, and resilient they become. With attuned support, clients of any age can learn to navigate the challenging waves.

Handling red and yellow waves grows a person's unique creativity and spontaneous flexibility. Navigating these waves playfully can make this learning more fun by privileging positive affect (Fosha, 2021) to broaden and build resources for navigating the seas of life, trauma, and all (Fredrickson, 2006). We can then metaprocess (see Chapter 9) the green waves of regulatory success to deepen their resiliency and resourcefulness.

The Playful Therapist Navigates with Regulatory Sensitivity

While being playfully spirited might feel fun for therapists, we must attune to our client's comfort with this style. We must be playful with regulatory sensitivity.

Be Sensitive to Play as a Medium of Abuse

Play may trigger clients whose perpetrators used play as the medium of abuse. Clients abused by "trusted" others may have experienced gradual boundary-blurring from playful states of connection, safety, and fun, to "playful" states marked by disconnection, danger, and fear. This was true for 4-year-old Min, whose fun babysitter molested her when playing doctor, and 20-year-old Alan, who got drunk with his friend and was then raped by him.

Taking a play history (see Brown, 2009; Dana, 2018) can alert us to these unsafe "playful" interactions. However, gaps in memory or self-blame for playful times going awry may leave clients, and subsequently their therapists, unaware of playfulness triggering yellow or red waves. We may only discover this in session when the memory network is triggered. Therefore, we must be cautious when being playful with our clients by acting attuned on steroids (see Chapter 8) to minimize these types of dysregulation.

Be Sensitive to Unconscious Playful Ruptures

Even when attuned on steroids and play has not been a medium of abuse, we can cause relational ruptures with playfulness. This happens when our playfulness emerges from unconscious countertransferences and reflects enactments (Maroda, 1998) or dissociative attunement—unconscious countertransferences in which we synchronize by being out of synch and misattuned (see Hopenwasser, 2008). Here are examples of two types of playful ruptures and repairs to which we can grow sensitivity.

Dysregulating Jokes/Humor

Owing to mirror neurons and therapist-client right brain-to-right brain synchrony, we may consciously or unconsciously act playfully to relieve our own discomfort and/or that of our client. However, our misplaced playfulness may inadvertently communicate: "I can't tolerate your discomfort either."

Shareen, a 28-year-old client on the autism spectrum with visual and physical disabilities, held me to account in one session after I punned that her co-workers and family must be wearing "the wrong prescriptive lenses, because they can't see you clearly," and "are blind to your disability."

Shareen directly confronted me. "That's not funny, Monica. I don't even feel seen by you. You don't live with my experience. Your comments are insensitive to others who struggle like I do!"

My intention to empathize with Shareen and lighten the heaviness of her mood instead left her feeling more misunderstood and alone. She accused me of being, "Just like my parents and dismissive boss who make light of all my limitations!"

Acting attuned would have required me to sit with her pain. I took responsibility and said, "Shareen, I appreciate you letting me know how I missed what you needed from me. I'm sorry. I acted insensitively. What I said left you feeling more misunderstood and alone." Shareen calmed. I breathed, paused, and then continued, "It is hard for me to hear and feel how painful this has been for you. I don't want you to keep having these hurtful experiences. I feel helpless and deeply sad for and with you. And what I did was wrong."

Then I asked, "What does it feel like to you to hear my regret and apology?"

Shareen paused, scanned my face, and nodded. "Yeah, that feels right. And it sucks." Then, we sat together silently with the sucky feelings.

It is consoling to know there are ways to repair these ruptures—and that the repairs have their own healing worth. Shareen reminds us that therapists need to show up mindfully and get consultation to gain awareness of our own regulatory edges and expand our tolerance.

Dysregulating Best Intentions/Interventions

In therapy, an important part of regulating and growing affect tolerance rests in finding the silver lining when things don't work out as hoped. Even with the best of intentions to expand negative and positive affect tolerance, therapists will intervene in ways that fall flat or are more dysregulating. This can happen when therapists adhere rigidly to protocols and procedures and downplay the importance of exploring the relational process itself. I experienced this when first learning Eye Movement Desensitization and Reprocessing (EMDR, Shapiro, 2018) when I tried to install a Safe Place/State which felt light and playful, yet two of my highly dissociative clients became *more* dysregulated.

At these times, we need to help our clients and ourselves reanchor— remember, we both are navigating affect waves! As Internal Family Systems guides us, rather than push away hijacking parts and their related symptoms, we intentionally embrace their wisdom and meaning intended to protect the most vulnerable parts of mind (Schwartz, 2021). Therapists need to guide protectors out of red waves into yellow-greenish ones and earn their trust to cooperatively and wisely protect deep vulnerability.

Be Sensitive to Play and Different Attachment Styles

While our playfulness is intended to promote safety and connection, it can trigger relationally traumatized clients for whom connection was fraught or dangerous. Knowing our clients' attachment styles helps us adapt our playfully spirited interventions to better and more sensitively fit them.

For example, clients with avoidant attachment styles are characterized as having disembodied minds (Wallin, 2007, p. 80), relying more on left brain–based dealing and not feeling. Safe, playful relationality is geared to downregulate (calm) their over-functioning minds, and upregulate (energize) their bodies and emotions. We can help these clients tolerate and integrate right brain–based embodiment by using attunement, sensorimotor, object, and cooperative social play.

By contrast, clients with anxious-ambivalent attachment styles are described as having mindless bodies (Wallin, 2007, p. 80), relying more on right brain–based feeling and not dealing. Safe, playful relationality focuses on downregulating these clients' over-functioning bodies and emotions and upregulating their wise minds. Over time, we can support these clients to tolerate and integrate more left brain–based problem-solving and organizational skills through attunement, imaginative/pretend, creative, and narrative play forms.

Finally, clients with disorganized and chaotic attachment styles vacillate between acting with mindless bodies, disembodied minds, or mindless disembodiment (extreme dissociation). They may neither feel nor deal. These clients adapted an upside-down circuitry of safety and connection. Familiar traumatic and toxic attachments are experienced *as if* they are green states, while unfamiliar safe attachments like the therapy relationship are experienced *as if* they are red states. Safety feels dangerous, and danger feels safe. We use safe, playful relationality to help these clients un-fuse and rewire their upside-down connection circuitry. In session, therapists must continuously track, attune to, and regulate the client's rapidly changing part of mind and related affect that shows up.

Be Aware of Extreme Waves

Extreme states of mobilization, like aggressive fight (SNS yellow waves) and shutdown (DV red waves), can feel destabilizing to client and therapist. The former can raise concerns for the physical safety of the therapist and others in the treatment space. When dealing with danger and possible life threat, we might need to distance, call in others (family members, security, and police) for help, or physically restrain the client. By contrast, when we face our client's crippling hypoarousal—collapse, shut down, catatonia, or complete disconnection—we may get hijacked and feel at a complete loss, stuck, and not know what to think or do to reach our client. We do not feel unsafe, per se, but in a mirrored DV red-wave state of immobilization with fear.

Managing our clients' extreme dysregulation often induces our somatic, emotional, and/or cognitive countertransferences. The most expedient intervention requires us to practice what we preach and self-regulate (e.g., breath work). Then, we can re-access our wise therapist self and trust our clinical intuition and experience. Prayer or calling on a higher, wiser power can help us feel less alone. We can do the best we can with what we've got when all else is inaccessible or ineffective. (This will be discussed fully in the "Improvising, aka Scrambling" section.)

Model Co-regulation

Therapists can use sensorimotor mirroring and hypnotic language to model and regulate affect. Since this practice is interactive and affects both therapist and client, I refer to it as co-regulation. All therapy work is co-regulatory since client-therapist right brain-to-right brain processes are reciprocal and mutually influential (Schore, 2021).

Leading by Example

Intentionally navigating affective discomfort is strengthened when therapists relationally and experientially process personal mistakes that trigger our clients. We can lead by example in dealing with dysregulation by naming and taking responsibility for our relational misattunements as I did with Shareen. We can share what the ruptures have taught us and check whether that fits for our client. We remind clients they do not have to sit with red or yellow waves alone—differentiating the current healing relationship from past traumatic ones.

As a team, therapist and client can objectively explore what went awry or right, brainstorm how to work more effectively and efficiently, and flexibly and creatively tweak or discover out-of-the-box ways to calm the red and yellow waves. If and only when appropriate, we can sarcastically, transparently joke that, "I *meant* for that to not work; this was an exercise to build perseverance and mental strength!" Finally, we highlight that failures are examples of success in progress.

Sensorimotor Mirroring

In all therapist-client interactions, implicit right brain-to-right brain processes are at work by which we move into sync with one another (see Chapter 8), which we can then explicitly process with left brain-to-left brain communication. When we intentionally or spontaneously model sensorimotor regulation, our clients can internalize and mirror it with themselves and others.

For example, to help our clients slow down, we may purposefully exhale deeply, shift in our seats, or drink some water to signal self-calming, which our client may inadvertently mirror. We can first mirror and match their rate and rhythms and then slow down ours. When speaking, we can insert pauses and audible slow breaths. If our client speeds up their rate of breathing or speaking, we can intentionally do the opposite with ours. We can use calming and soothing gestures, like stroking one hand slowly with the other or putting our hand over our heart. Often, clients notice or comment on these soothing gestures and we can explore its meaning and intention.

On the other hand, to assist clients in speeding up, we might use mobilizing gestures like speaking slightly faster or louder with a deeper tone. We can sit more forward or erect in our seat, roll back our shoulders, or stretch/puff out our chest to nonverbally communicate a readiness to act. We can explicitly discuss and process these behaviors with our clients, even inviting them to join us and try it out.

If instead, we notice we've unconsciously mirrored our client as they self-regulate, we can explicitly process this too. We can sincerely state how impressed we feel by our client's self-soothing and ask permission to continue mirroring them to see what it feels like. For example, I have commented about how clients intuitively know how to calm themselves by repeatedly stroking their sideburns, smoothing their eyebrows, or rubbing their fingers together with circular movements. When I try it out and verbalize its effects, clients literally see and reflect upon their intuitive skills and sometimes find ways to tweak and improve them. Whether we intentionally model or reflect self-soothing behaviors, we support our clients' awareness and growth of self-regulatory skills.

Clients may even comment on our unconscious behaviors in return. One client asked, "Am I scaring you away?" as I pulled my head back as if to gain distance from their disturbing story of victimization. Curiously reflecting out loud on my movement revealed powerful themes. I realized I felt overwhelming sadness and unconsciously wanted distance from their pain, while my client revealed how dissociated they were from their emotions. Explicitly processing this re-regulated us both. My client got more in touch with their feelings and mine became more tolerable, enabling further exploration.

Hypnotic Language

We can also use hypnotic language to co-regulate our clients and ourselves. By using words like "calm," "let up," "ease," "slow," "lighten," "down," etc., we linguistically downregulate flight and suggest what the nervous system needs to do. For example, Jermaine was increasingly rageful, speaking in a booming voice with clenched fists about how his alcoholic father humiliated him. I first matched his intensity with my hands and tone. With my clenched fists on either side of my neck, I said, "Yeah! Yeah. (Pause.) I hear you. (Pause.) I get that." Unclenching my fists, and resting my open palms on my legs, I continued: "Jermaine. Hmmmm. (Pensive and slowing down more.) This can get exhausting (suggestive of heaviness and fatigue.) Your father never lets up. (Pause.)

He's stuck." (Long pause.) Then I said forcefully, "You're not. You can shift (downregulate) out of this script. What a relief (unburden) to have a choice (wise fight) to live differently!" Jermaine quieted and looked up and to the right as he pondered a different way of showing up in the future.

By contrast, when hypnotically and linguistically upregulating immobilized states in our clients, we might use words like "move," "flow," "act," "choose," "up," "energy," etc. Liz sat folded in half at her waist and leaned and propped up her right side on pillows. She said, "It's impossible. I will never get out of this marital hell. I imagine I only have 20 or 30 more years till one of us dies."

Joining with and mirroring Liz I replied slowly and carefully, "I hear you Liz, (pause) this has been hell for you." Speaking with more energy and trying to engage her curiosity I asked, "And you know what?" Awaiting a response, I saw and heard Liz sigh big and loudly. With increasing energy, I said, "Yeah. I saw that deep exhale. As you know, exhaling slows your heartrate and breathing. Yet I wonder if part of you took that exhale to ready yourself (suggestive) for something (word implying change)?"

Liz still collapsed, looked up at me and furrowed her eyebrows (SNS mobilization and VV engagement emerging). I asked, "Did I say something confusing?"

She responded with slight irritation (a sign of more SNS mobilization), "Yup, I know every exhale is followed by an inhale (acknowledging she knows and senses possibly feeling pushed by me to mobilize)."

Then, I energized my stance. I rolled my chair closer to her (hoping as I moved, she would too and join me in green waves). Speaking faster I said, "And (implies building on, because I trusted Liz could hold this possibility), it seemed like you were getting ready (more movement) to take a bigger (increased size) inhale to increase your heart and breathing rate."

"So?" Liz replies with more impatience (SNS activation increases).

"So (I replied, verbally echoing Liz to stay connected), maybe part of you (keeping possibility of change contained to only part of Liz's mind so immobilizing protectors don't feel invalidated or challenged) was gearing up (upregulating language) to see a different outcome (crediting her with envisioning change), not just hell."

"Maybe," Liz replied, sitting up. And off we went, exploring the possibility of slowly dealing with other parts that were afraid to change and thus ending her hell.

I invite the reader to mindfully experiment with different ways to use your relational intuition to practice embodying ways to regulate your clients' (and your own) affect with hypnotic language.

Now that we can identify different affect waves and understand the importance of relationally, intentionally, and wisely navigating back to green-wave zones of safety and connection to enable trauma healing, we shift our focus to playing with vagal braking to increase affect regulation and tolerance. Then, we can explore different exercises that translate theory into playful practice.

Playfully Exercising Vagal Braking to Grow Affect Regulation and Tolerance

As we learned in Chapters 2 and 5, exercising our vagal brake grows our affect modulation skills to prevent regulatory hijacking. We can playfully teach clients to intentionally do a number of things with their brake to contain and/or expand affect.

Practicing Vagal Braking through Playful Containment and Expansion

When we apply the brake to slow down hyperarousal (yellow SNS states), we *contain* dysregulating affect, preventing it from overtaking a person. It is not an exercise of avoidance, but one of holding psychic material just as a container holds liquid.

When we release the vagal brake to speed up hypoarousal (red DV states), we *expand* constricted affect. Expansion creates space or broadens boundaries, promoting literal and figurative movement. We release pressure and intensity to make affect manageable.

When we pump the brake by applying and releasing pressure with different speed and force—we *contain and expand* or balance the activation of the always-on VV, SNS, and DV pathways and related affect. All vagal braking practices are intended to return affect to green or greenish-yellow waves of safety and connection.

We use containment and expansion in tandem—in alternating and complementary ways—to manage hijacked states and reestablish safety and connection (VV states) intrarelationally and interpersonally. Together they help our clients navigate the edges of their WOT where change is made possible. Both containment and expansion help our clients control and tolerate too much or too little negative and positive affect, thoughts, feelings, memories, information, or sensation. In turn, this increases protector parts' cooperation to unburden and update the most vulnerable exiled parts of mind. Containment and expansion in therapy give clients real-time practice regulating significant dysregulation and increasing their sense of safety, agency, and responsibility.

Play with clients of all ages functions as a tool of containment and expansion. It neurally exercises (Porges, 2015) their vagal braking ability as we move together through different affect states, encouraging clients to face what needs to be processed. Let's explore how.

Playful Containment

As a container, play helps us gain distance from and acquire a nonjudgmental perspective about triggering material, which calms our affect, supports a here-and-now presence, and brings the prefrontal cortex online. Being play-ful enables a mindful stance so we can be "next to, not in" (Gendlin, 1981, p. 70) what disturbs us, while still feeling it without overwhelm. As Bakur Weiner and Simmons (2009) state, "The paradox of feeling is that it needs grounding in awareness and detachment" (p. xix). Play helps children and adults personify their themes and symptoms (and related parts of mind), ena-bling them to automatically gain distance, "unblend and disidentify" (Fisher, 2017, p. 140) from them. We can personify by using objects (i.e., dolls, blocks), dance or movement, and metaphors and creativity (e.g., drawing, storytelling, role-playing, stand-up comedy). Engaging playfully helps us avoid becoming the problem, increase affect tolerance, and gain bravery to face issues. Playful containment shrinks highly dysregulating traumatic material into more manage-able, controllable, and mastery-promoting forms. Playful containment is func-tional and fun.

But containment without expansion is limiting. I have met clients who learned containment exercises in cognitive-based therapies which gave them great relief to calm. But they sought out a different type of therapy when their containment exercises either failed or more was needed to help them function. For example, 12-year-old Lucy had learned to write down her "problems"—anxiety-filled thoughts and feelings—on little pieces of paper and then put them in a box before bed. The box served as her literal container—an especially help-ful intervention for younger clients. Initially, this helped her sleep, but over time, she said the box overflowed, as did her mind, and her sleep problems returned.

When we literally or metaphorically box up disturbing material, put it up on a high shelf in our minds, or send it away to an outer galaxy, we may hope it never returns. However, continued containment without release acts like a pressure cooker, inevitably causing material to leak or explode. The contained material needs to be digested and metabolized. Lucy had not learned to work through the anxious thoughts, emotions, and sensations on those little papers. Containment is the first step needed to allow the working through of dysregulating material. If a client only desires ways to hold and compartmentalize traumatic material, containment meets their needs. But while containment helps us prevent being taken over by dysregulating arousal, we must also safely approach and move through what gets held to the side. Many clients, like Lucy, long to work through the dysregulating material to disabuse it of its hijacking powers and meaning.

Playful Expansion

Playfulness can help expand constricted intolerable affect, sensations, thoughts, and movements by safely increasing autonomic arousal and flexibility (Kestly, 2018). Many of my clients with chronic and complex trauma histories have asserted they will "not go there"—meaning they fear negative affect will flood them and become intolerable, while positive affect will be too painful to bear because it will inevitably vanish and leave them back where they started. I find sensorimotor-based playfulness particularly helpful with these clients as it lends itself to physically symbolizing or representing disturbances for containment and expansion practices.

Object play can provide an example of playful expansion through containment. We can gain permission to metaphorically or concretely represent what's intolerable (e.g., emotions, affect, sensation, thought) with pieces of clay or Play-Doh. We ask our client to rip off a tiny piece of it, put it to the side, and leave it there—containment. Then, with grounding breaths, we can just notice it and sit with that awareness. We repeat these steps with additional tiny pieces of the intolerable material. Finally, we add the pieces together and ask the client to breathe mindfully and notice how they visually and physically tolerated the big clump—expansion.

Playful Modulation: Both Containment and Expansion

Playful containment and expansion practices work in lock-step and involve pumping the vagal brake to effectively modulate the extremes of too much or too little feeling, dealing, and connecting. The disembodied becomes embodied, the mindless becomes mindful, mind-body-emotion flows, and connection grows. Modulated playful vagal braking is necessary with our most traumatized clients who are highly dissociative or present with an unformed sense of Self. It requires us to use strategies that deal with the tiniest drop, teaspoon (Medbo, 2023), or Tip of the Finger (Mosquera, 2020) of dysregulation. Carefully diluting the intense dysregulation helps us promote affect tolerance bit by bit. As clients learn how to return to, wade and swim in green zones of safety and connection, they grow trust in self-regulating and expanding their WOT.

Playful Exercises for Navigating Waves of Affect

The containment and expansion practices discussed in this section represent a small sample of exercises therapists can use with clients of all ages and all parts of mind to move into the green-wave zone of safety and connection. The exercises include attunement, sensorimotor, object, social, imaginative/pretend, narrative, and creative playfulness. Like many clinicians, I have modified and integrated various techniques learned over many years of practice, attending workshops, and reading. If I do not cite and credit the original creator, I ask the reader's and originator's forgiveness for any oversight. I invite the reader to modify or create your own affect tolerance practices which encourage safety, build mindful awareness, embodied presence, and intrapersonal and interpersonal connection, control, and choice. The more regulating, appealing, and fun the practice is, the more easily the client will resonate with and implement it when most needed.

Exercises for Containment Related to Parts of Mind

In this section, we focus on containment exercises that promote affect regulation for all clients but can be particularly useful with dissociative clients and their conflictual, intrapsychic system.

Imagery and Metaphors

When we create imagined or concrete containers with clients of all ages, we can promote green affect waves of safety, holding, and stabilization. In session, we can create containers using arts and crafts. Whether physical or imagined, containers need to safely hold and be opened and closed, allowing access to stored thoughts, feelings, emotions, memories, etc., when the client feels ready. Here is a loose script to use in session to conjure containment and the image of a container.

> After taking a few breaths to settle, I invite you to imagine creating a safe container. One that will hold all that you need it to for safe-keeping. It can be made of any material (glass, wood, iron, gold, plastic). It can be any color you want. It can be see-through or not. You can decorate your container with anything you'd like. Gems, stickers, feathers—Or not. (Give your client time to create this container in their mind's eye).
>
> This container needs to be safe and stable. Whether you create it with your hands, mind, or both, you need to protect it and make sure only you can access it when you need.
>
> Your container needs a way to close to keep its contents safe. You can add a lock, a forcefield, a latch, a deadbolt—whatever you want to keep its important contents secure. You will be the only one who can open it.
>
> You need to check that you are not overfilling it. If your container is too stuffed, it may not close or stay closed. You will need to make it big enough to hold what you put inside.
>
> You will need to check on your container to make sure its contents are held carefully and securely.
>
> Now, when you're ready, inhale and scan your body. Notice anything which feels like too much to hold.
>
> Then, as you exhale, send that which is too much into your open container. As you send it along say with care, "I am sending you to stay in this box for safe-keeping. To be held and protected. I will check on you. And when it's time, I will take out and take care of what needs to be. If something else needs to go in, I will make sure there is room and put it in. And with that too, I will check on it and take it out when it's time."

When working with highly dissociative clients, containment techniques are geared to organize their internal system of parts and place a safe frame around the process of treatment. For example, techniques like Conference Room (Schmidt, 1998) or Fraser's Dissociative Table Technique (2003) help clients describe and organize an often-chaotic internal system to better work with them. These can be considered the client's safe workspace (Forgash & Copeley, 2008) for communication and cooperation between ego states. When we ask clients to develop internal safe spaces—like a house on a remote, private beach, a log cabin deep in the woods, an amusement park with different sections and rides, a heavily guarded fortress, or a castle with a drawbridge—we lean into their creativity to make a safe and secure area for their ego states to live and play (Forgash & Copeley, 2008).

These safe, imagined places differ from real-world places where clients experience vulnerability and even life threat. They are boundaried safe spaces that promote VV green-wave states. Younger clients often spontaneously develop safe spaces with doll houses, in sand play, and drawing, while older clients may prefer imaginal activities. Both physically created and imagined spaces can effectively promote safety and soothing since both activate mirror neurons and related sensorimotor neural networks (Rizzolatti & Craighero, 2004, see Chapter 8). Returning as needed to their safe spaces in therapy and everyday life empowers clients to bring green waves of calm, comfort, and relaxation to their nervous system.

Even clients without significant dissociation may feel too internally chaotic or overwhelmed to calm and move into green-wave states. Others may jump from emotion to emotion, rapidly shift topics, or switch their body position, eye gaze, etc. This may reflect competing triggered protector parts keeping vulnerable parts at bay, ambivalence, or lack of readiness about diving into the trauma work. In these cases, many clients find the metaphor of a teacher (wise mind) and their class (parts of the mind) helpful to settle their intrapsychic system. You can see this metaphor as a script here:

Do you remember what it was like in school when you had a noisy, rowdy class with only one teacher? Sometimes a few kids were calling out at the same time, "Teacher, teacher! Oooh, oooh, it's my turn. Call on me!" Other students were wiggling in their seats, wildly raising their hands. Others were jumping up and down, getting out of their seats, and roaming around the classroom. Others were tapping their pencils loudly on their desks.

Why were they doing this?

Clients respond, "To get the teacher's attention."

The therapist responds, "Exactly! It's the teacher's job to manage the classroom. Really skilled teachers are great at this. They figure out whose needs are most urgent." Next, they tell students, "I know you each have something important to share. In order for me to hear you and help you best, I need you each to sit down. Take a moment to quiet and settle. Trust I will get to each of you, in turn. If I pass you by, by accident, please gently remind me. Each one of you will have your turn to be heard, seen, and soothed."

This metaphor usually resonates with clients of all ages as they recall parents, teachers, and even bosses who had real competence at managing crises and competing needs. Clients also remember those who completely lacked this skill. I emphasize that those whom we most admire for managing chaos do not act out of fear or instill it but evoke respect and fairness. Clients find this metaphor helpful to triage the affective needs of parts.

The metaphor also helps clients increase intrarelational trust through the promise of return to dysregulated parts. Once forgotten and hidden, vulnerable parts gain trust that the wise Self will consistently check in on them and provide needed soothing. We need to remind our clients that intentionally returning to unmet needs takes practice. We can encourage clients to schedule a regular check-in time with all parts before—not just when—they are triggered. Not only does this practice grow internal trust that all their parts are important and deserve care, it is also emotionally corrective for clients who lacked caregivers who regularly checked in about their needs and strived to meet them.

Parts Language and Role-Play

Parts language helps contain affect dysregulation, supporting our clients to return to green-wave zones. We remind clients that dysregulation is an alert signal that something is not okay—a "save our souls" (SOS) communication from protector parts that something is out of balance.

Using narrative and creative playfulness, we can role-play or act out the messages from the protector parts, similar to how emotions are personified in the movie *Inside Out*. For example, when I become the part, I physically animate and change my voice tone and rhythm to best reflect how I sense my client's anger, fear, shame, etc., part might show up. I tend to weave in some sarcasm—implying a part's frustration in not being seen or heard unless they really hijack the person's functioning. When I speak, I look up, toward the ceiling as if I'm talking to the current day wise Self. The "I/me" language refers to the part of mind that's speaking, the "we/us/our" to all parts of mind, and the "you" to Self.

For example, as a panicky part, I might say shakily,

> Are you there? Haven't you noticed me making our stomach nauseous or our palms sweaty? I'm trying to let you know I'm feeling scared about facing the judge. Should I make us throw up or have palpitations, or did you get my point?

As a rageful part, I might assertively say,

> Damn it! I'm gonna make us blow. Notice our fists and jaw. If mom slaps us again in front of our friends, I'm gonna make us go off on her. She humiliated us! I need help to manage not losing my shit!

Or as shame, I might bow my head, look down, and meekly and tentatively say,

> I don't know how I'll ever handle this job. It's too much for me. I'm taking away our energy and will make us stay in bed again tomorrow. Can you maybe help me out? Or do I need to make us feel even more worthless and depressed?

Then I check in with my client, "Does this feel similar to what it feels like inside for you?"

Clients often laugh and respond, "That's exactly what I feel is going on!" The laugh reflects how much easier it is to see one's own dysregulation mirrored back and personified by someone else in a playful and contained way. If a client says I missed it, I ask them to share what would be more accurate. Then, I might briefly act out the part with the correction. Playfully acting out a part and its related affect can grow the client's self-compassion and the therapist's attunement and return us to VV green waves.

This playful exercise reminds therapists and clients to "assume all distressing thoughts, feelings, and body responses are communications from trauma-related parts" (Fisher, 2017, p. 11). Therefore, when our clients present as hijacked by panic, depression, rage, fear, confusion, inadequacy, hopelessness, insecurity, etc., we must remind them that their feeling, sensation, or thought is a part of their larger, full being. It doesn't reflect their essence or Self which is good, kind, compassionate, caring, and loving. We are not our symptoms. We teach clients they are not depressed but have depressed parts, feelings, sensations, or thoughts. Symptoms are framed as intended helpers which have a specific role in relation to a specific context and trigger. Even when clients assert they are "unlovable and disgusting," we track moment-to-moment verbal or non-verbal communications that reflect different, emergent protectors and their related affects (e.g., anger, anxiety, calm, etc.) and movements. This languaging and process help clients contain dysregulation and return to green waves of safety and connection intrapersonally and interpersonally.

Some clients, like Mindy, do not resonate with parts language. She refuted my statement, "It sounds like part of you feels depressed." This is what followed:

Mindy: "No, *all* of me is depressed!" (My parts language left Mindy feeling invalidated and dismissed the way her family had.)

Me: I circled back, respectfully, "I hear you," and breathed to slow down and let Mindy take this in. I continued, "I see your slumped shoulders and hear your very quiet voice. Is that your depressed side (instead of 'part') showing itself?" (This acknowledged both me seeing Mindy as depressed and me noticing her depressed expression in parts of her body.)

Mindy: "Yes," she responded and nodded (conveying a sense of being seen).

Me: "Yeah, I can see that." (To reinforce her sense of being seen, I paused to let Mindy take in my seeing her and I nodded.) I then continued, "Mindy, I also am noticing your clenched fist and jaw. Would you notice that with me? I wonder if your fist and jaw are feeling depressed or something else?" (Experimenting to see if Mindy takes in this variation on the concept of parts: body parts [not all of someone] can hold different affects, thoughts, etc.)

Mindy: "Well, maybe they feel tense or even angry." Her depressed symptoms, once acknowledged, stepped to the side.

Me: "It seems like your shoulders and voice are holding depressed feelings while your fist and jaw hold angry ones."

Mindy: "Maybe you're right. I didn't even notice I could hold different feelings at the same time in different parts of my body." (Once Mindy acknowledges her different feelings [expressions of different protector parts] have been seen, she spontaneously uses parts language.)

Me: "Your body is pretty talented. It holds and says so much about the different symptoms you've shared. That's pretty cool, huh?"

Mindy: "I guess so," Mindy says in a noncommittal way, with the faintest of smiles.

Me: (Providing some psychoeducation and explicitly establishing boundaries between dysregulated parts.) "Even though it might feel like all of us is depressed, the depressed feelings and symptoms are only an aspect of our full being. It's like what happened when you stepped back to track and notice that your angry fight and depressed/submit sides expressed themselves through different parts of your body. In fact, I just saw the faintest smile when you said, 'I guess so.' To me that didn't feel like a submit or angry fight response. What do you sense it was?"

Mindy:	Smiling wider, "It was a fight response, but different. Not anger. More like irritation."
Me:	"Irritation?"
Mindy:	"Yeah, like, 'Damn it, Monica, you proved your point. I didn't want to agree with you, again!'"
Me:	"Aaah, like you didn't want to hear me say, 'See Mindy, your smile shows that not all of you is depressed?'"
Mindy:	"Exactly! I got it, you don't have to rub it in!" Mindy and I laughed together as we both enjoyed her ribbing me and not having the same "see I told you so moment" with me like she did with her sanctimonious parents who criticized her mistakes with ease.
Me:	"Mindy, you are a quick study. I know that! And thanks for your patience with me because I have been known to repeat myself to drive home a point that you may have gotten ten minutes earlier. Obviously, I may not be as quick a study as you!"

We later teased apart how her fight emotional parts (EPs) of the personality (see Structural Dissociation in Chapter 2), like all EPs, can express themselves in different somatic, affective, and cognitive ways. For example, depending on the trigger, a fight EP can communicate with a clenched fist, snicker of defiance, or by completely hijacking us with yelling and punching. This practice helped Mindy return to VV green waves of safety, stabilization, and connection.

Unlike Mindy, some of my clients have been tremendously and consistently resistant to parts language. Each has been extremely dissociative and experienced deeply wounding chronic relational trauma. I hold awareness that what feels like resistance is a fight protector sensing challenges to their control, relational trauma adaptations, and internal system organization/functioning. I acknowledge their discomfort and ask if different words like "sides," "facets," or "aspect" feel better. I offer using words they prefer even in their mother tongue. Often, clients have replied that they do not agree with the entire concept of parts.

To relationally traumatized clients, speaking parts language may feel like a minimization of their whole emotional experience—triggering memories of past relationships in which they felt invalidated. I explain it is not my goal to change their comfort with parts language and I will try not to use trigger words. I also share that I've been using this language for decades because I believe in the importance of parts work in my personal therapy and as a therapist. I preemptively confess I may slip up and ask their patience and grace in my speaking this way. This respects their boundaries and mine. It also gives clients practice holding my mistakes compassionately—which paves the way for them to do the same with theirs. As our relational trust has grown, some of these clients have become more tolerant of parts concepts and language and have started using it too.

Exercises for General Containment and Expansion

The following playful containment and expansion exercises are for clients of all ages and are infused with attunement, sensorimotor, object, imaginative/pretend, narrative, creative, and social playfulness. They are intended to shift yellow SNS states and red DV dysregulated wave states back to green and support affect regulation. Each practices vagal braking and grows comfort with discomfort, expanding the WOT.

Breath

Inviting clients to mindfully breathe is a popular go-to and can be thought of as sensorimotor play with breath. Therapists can teach clients how inhaling increases heart rate, respirations, and activates fight and flight (e.g., SNS) responses, while exhaling decreases heart rate, respirations, and activates the parasympathetic, slowing down and resting response.

We can suggest our client inhale for a count of two to four then exhale for a count of four to six and notice what this feels like. We can invite clients to take deep belly breaths or balloon breaths. With their hand on their belly, the client will inhale, causing their belly to expand like a balloon and their hand to rise. On the exhale, their belly will deflate and their hand will lower.

Different forms of yogic breathing, like alternate nostril or *ujjayi*, can calm the ANS. Lion's breath is a form of playful yogic breathing that involves sound and sticking out the tongue, stretching it down toward the chin. We can encourage clients to play with pace and depth of breaths, like panting or take short shallow breaths, to see how to raise agitation and then calm it. Children and some adults love using breath to blow bubbles.

A mindful, regulatory breathing game that kids love and adults find curious is one I call Keep It Up. One version includes the client (alone or together with the therapist or family member) keeping a balloon or feather from touching the ground using only their breath. A different version is when a client holds a piece of paper up against a closed door or blank wall, lets it go, and with their breath must keep the paper up against the vertical surface (Greenland, 2010). While the second Keep It Up game is particularly challenging, both share a fun quality. These playful breath exercises allow therapists to make hypnotic suggestions and metaphorical comments. For clients whose positive receptive affect capacity is limited, instead of commenting on their skill as a whole, we can comment about parts of them—their technique is skillful or their lungs are powerful. For clients more tolerant of positive feedback, we can say they are "so creative" or "show incredible perseverance with a challenging task." While attuning to their receptive affective capacity, we take opportunities to metaphorically privilege the positive in the context of the breathing games.

We use playful, sensorimotor breath exercises to increase our client's awareness of and connection to their body, and their sense of somatic control and agency. As clients play with breath, we ask questions to strengthen their sense of embodiment: "Do you notice a slowing down in your mind or body? A speeding up? More or less tension?" If the client reports they feel good, or, "It worked—the thought (emotion, feeling, etc.) that upset me is gone," we remind them, "Wow, you calmed your nervous system. Just notice how well you did that. Now, since the intention is to help you connect safely and calmly with your anger, overwhelm, panic, shame, (etc.), would it be okay to check back in with that part now?" Remember, once the client is better regulated, we can circle back to the part or symptom that needs our attention—it has lots of wisdom to mine.

Movement

There are many ways we can invite clients to playfully use objects and body movement to increase their self-awareness and tolerance of discomfort. When we physicalize—express or put the felt dysregulation into physical form—clients gain distance to figuratively step back and witness what and how they are playing with an object or their own body. Psychodrama (Moreno, 1946) therapists are familiar with the concept of acting-in or acting-through by which the dramatic context is used to create "role distance." In fact, role distance is "the essential component of imaginative play and the basis for the most natural way to learn" (Blatner, 1996, p. xiv). Sensorimotor psychotherapists also help clients physicalize their difficult-to-tolerate affect.

I guided Sasha, age 28, to physicalize her emotions through her body using playful movements. The intention was to enhance her mindful awareness and curiosity, while containing and distancing from her dysregulated affect. I noticed aloud, "Sasha, your clenched hand looks mad. If it could make a sound, what would it sound like?"

She growled.

Then I asked, "If it could speak, what would it say?"

Sasha burst out, "Asshole!"

"Now, Sasha, give your hand permission to move however it would like. How does that movement feel?"

While punching the air, Sasha replied with a broad smile, "Powerful!"

Physicalizing might feel silly to some adults, yet over time it yields curiosity, intrigue, and appreciation of one's body's wisdom and strength.

Cathy demonstrated a different way to physicalize by using an object, in this case the tassels on the pillow of my couch. My clients frequently play with these tassels, sometimes braiding, pulling, twirling them, or stroking their hand, arm, leg, or face with them both to self-regulate and express feelings. When 17-year-old Cathy talked about her unsupportive and self-absorbed stepfather, she unconsciously started yanking one tassel so hard that it ripped off the pillow.

Like a deer in the headlights, Cathy immediately quashed her anger (SNS activation), moved into a red wave of DV shame, dropped her head, and averted my gaze. She feared she would be yelled at by her stepfather because I'd charge him for a replacement pillow.

But I said, "That was perfect!"

She looked up, confused, with the hint of a smile. "Huh?"

"No worries," I said, "I can sew that back on. Now, imagine that tassel is your stepfather, what would you like to do with it?" Without skipping a beat, she threw the tassel on the floor. Stepped on it. Kicked it a few times. And then squished it with her foot. I said, "Clearly your foot has a lot to say to him. Would you give your foot words or sounds to express itself to him?"

Cathy said, "You're such a narcissistic asshole! If you can't see I have needs and feelings, then I'm kicking you to the curb." And with that, we left the ripped-off tassel in the corner of my office until the session ended, at which point she picked it up and handed it back to me with a smile of feeling understood. Channeling her rage into the tassel and her foot was a form of safe containment that allowed Cathy to playfully tolerate, express, and expand her intense affect.

Time

Timers and clocks are great tools for playfully returning clients to safety and connection and growing their WOT.

If clients report feeling too flooded to sit with their sensations, emotions, or thoughts, I ask if they are willing to try for a few seconds. I have a decorative clock with a second hand that we both can use to keep track. Often clients don't even look, but just go inward to sit with what they are experiencing. I increase the time increments of "sitting with" their experience by 5, 10, 15 seconds, up to a minute or two. I always give clients permission to stop the exercise. Intentionally switching in and out of the states of discomfort and comfort is a form of pendulation (see Levine, 1997) or oscillation (Ogden et al., 2006). It brings control to a previously out-of-control experience. I sometimes make the switch between discomfort and comfort more dramatic by suggesting the client shift away from the discomfort to focus on something fun or something that brings pleasure—like looking at a photo of their pet. This practice further increases their vagal brake flexibility and stretches their zone of affect tolerance.

As clients sit with discomfort for longer increments, we explore what happened internally to make this growth possible. We also celebrate their increasing tolerance of discomfort. For example, going from 5 to 25 seconds is a 500% increase in handling feelings of inadequacy, fear, aloneness, etc. In my experience, when clients can consistently tolerate discomfort for a couple of minutes, their phobic or flighty protectors have grown soothed and intrarelationally secure enough, allowing them to sit with once-hijacking material with more stability.

Little kids enjoy this clock exercise too. The face of my clock has a star at the 12, squiggle at the 3, crescent moon at the 6, and another squiggle at the 9. I will announce, "Wow, you sat with that until the minute hand got to the moon!" Children spontaneously challenge themselves to sit with discomfort until the second hand makes it to a shape a second time. It becomes a game. The shapes anchor kids as they dare themselves to try a new affect tolerance goal. They learn to believe: "I can feel discomfort in a tolerable way and beat my old record!" "I can handle this!" Therapists can share encouraging words along the way: "Wow, look at how you can feel these feelings and you've reached the moon! The star! The second squiggle!"—a fun, metaphorical message addressing their affect tolerance efficacy and that their growth has no bounds.

Distance/Space

We can encourage clients to contain their discomfort through literal and figurative distancing. Distancing exercises support clients to mindfully and intentionally discover adaptive ways to contain their dysregulation for the purpose of resolving it. This contrasts dissociation which is an unconscious process intended to split off and shut down dysregulating thoughts, feelings, emotions, sensations, etc.

For instance, we can ask clients who are feeling really upset to breathe and imagine they are their favorite kind of bird. They can envision themselves flying up onto a hidden and stable perch, like a tree branch. One 55-year-old client loved this distancing image and would spend the first few minutes of every session in this imaginal practice to ground herself. Clients can also pretend they are a bat flying up to the rafters or a mouse scurrying up to the top of the highest, unreachable cabinet of a room. From this vantage point, clients are encouraged to access their objective wisdom—and Self—and watch what is happening from a distance. Clients have commented that this type of imaginative distancing is like depersonalization and derealization, except it is intentional, controlled, and grounded—the opposite of unconscious dissociative experiences. In fact, one dissociative client commented, "No wonder I'm good at this. I'm taking an automatic skill I've used my whole life and making it purposeful to help me deal with, not cut off, my emotions. That's pretty cool!" This containment skill is empowering, helping some heavily dissociative clients purposefully modulate and manage something that had once been out of their awareness and control.

I also use sensorimotor distancing exercises for containment and expansion in family and couples' sessions. To couples who trigger each other, I might playfully say, "I know therapy is supposed to be about bringing you closer together. What about if we practice literally moving you apart?" I invite the members of the family or couple to experiment with moving to different seats or change their body posture or eye gaze to help them return to green waves. Giving permission to create and establish boundaries through physical distance or closeness helps clients become more regulated and embodied in partnership.

Similarly, once getting permission from all family members to grow personal comfort by experimenting with taking space, I ask parents to stand or sit in one place and let their children or teenagers move to where they feel most comfortable, even if they move out of the consultation room into the waiting room or hallway. Caregivers get this literal message of how safe their kid feels in physical proximity to or distance from them. We need to explore these boundaries with therapeutic sensitivity and without shame. I also invite kids to stay in one place and tell their caregiver/s to come closer or move farther away, turn toward or away from, look directly at them, or slightly avert or fully avoid their gaze. This control feels very powerful to children who feel unseen, powerless, or ineffective.

While small, these sensorimotor suggestions and exercises, made in playful ways, generate a wealth of information, while regulating affect.

Interruption

When the emotional temperature increases in individual, couples, or family sessions, I will pause the process and ask, "Am I the only one noticing some growing emotional intensity?" By making the implicit explicit, we encourage awareness of self and others. Whether they answer yes or no, I will track, narrate, and explore similarities and differences between what I felt in my body, observed in theirs, and the clients' experience of the same.

Also, I will invite clients to connect to their emotional and sensory experience and say, "Oh, now that you're noticing what this feels like in your body and emotions, would you like to stay with it, make it bigger or smaller?" Clients often look bewildered by this question because, in real-life relationships, especially toxic ones, we don't have or give ourselves this option. The question highlights their ability to engage personal choice, control, responsibility, and agency. It interrupts the escalating pattern of dysregulation and introduces playfulness, which is both antithetical and paradoxical to the disturbing experience. It is wholly unexpected (see the juxtaposition experience discussed in Chapter 5) and introduces the possibility of wiring in new thought-action patterns when dysregulation arises.

Taking a time out to play catch with a ball or tissue, hot potato with a pillow, doing jumping jacks, or freezing all action in place are examples of containing high arousal using interruption in a therapy session. We can suggest clients get up and pick a different seat, which literally and figuratively gives them a new perspective. When clients sit in "the therapist's chair," they seem to immediately assume a wiser and more objective and embodied perspective. You can't make this up, try it! After using these playful sensorimotor interruptions, we can re-assess the emotional temperature. We might use a scale from 0 to 10 (as in EMDR's Subjective Units of Disturbance, SUDS), hand signals from low to high, a thumbs up, down, or in the middle, or have them describe whether they feel in a wave of red, red-orange, orange-yellow, yellow, yellow-green, or green.

Before returning to the previously activating topic or dynamic, we can ask clients if their ANS is "ready" or "ready enough" to resume. If a client says "yes," we can reframe it by saying, "You're voluntarily choosing to return to the upsetting issue?" Or "Wow, who would have thought you're actually giving me permission to bring up this issue?" We can make explicit how this reflects their greater comfort in handling dysregulation and further processing.

Embodied Mirroring

As we learned earlier in this chapter, therapists can use right brain-to-right brain processes to model containment somatically, which clients may unconsciously mirror and internalize. As a twist on this concept, therapists can intentionally *with the client's permission* mirror their dysregulated state to help bring them into a WOT. This practice is the basis for the embodied mirroring technique (see Blum, 2015), which emerged out of me dealing with relational impasses in red DV wave states—particularly disconnected, shutdown, or dissociative ones. Embodied mirroring borrows from the sensorimotor psychotherapy technique of consciously "taking on" (Ogden et al., 2006) a client's physical state with the client's permission. The technique relationally and somatically unfolds therapy impasses through a mirroring process, while promoting affect regulation and deeper connection. When we mirror a client with their permission, in essence we are saying, "Teach me your 'you' in this experience by letting me walk in your shoes, and maybe I'll learn something." Invariably, I have gained insights that help my clients better regulate.

For example, 17-year-old Lindsey would dissociate, become wordless, and stare off at streams of sunlight pouring in from my office window when the topic arose of her sexual abuse by her once loved and trusted perpetrator. Hoping to bring her back into her WOT, I used embodied mirroring and joined her in staring off. I then noticed dust particles in the streaming rays of light. I got up and started playing "catch the dust." We became competitive to see who could catch more particles. This mirroring intervention helped Lindsey regulate and gain comfort connecting with her emotions and me in future sessions.

By contrast, I used embodied mirroring with primary process language quite differently with Luenell, a 41-year-old desperately trying to leave a ten-year co-dependent relationship replete with interpersonal violence, substance abuse, and trauma to her two daughters. Luenell had found a way to lie on the floor and partially ground herself with music. However, her mother, also in the office, retriggered her when speaking about moving, a job interview, and getting the older daughter into therapy. Luenell started thrashing while screaming, "I can't do this. Just give Grant (the partner) my kids, and I'll kill myself. This is impossible. I'm terrified of raising them alone!" Then Luenell crawled into a fetal position and closed her eyes to shut us out.

Having worked with Luenell for years, I knew she'd feel safe with me joining her on the floor. I mirrored her position, used the slowest, quietest voice, and said, "Can you hear me, Luenell?" I paused, she nodded. I said, "Open your eyes and just look into my eyes. I'm only going to speak with my eyes to yours. You'll know what I'm saying." I breathed and imagined energy from my heart center going straight to hers through our eye-to-eye gaze. I meditated on the phrase: "You can do this. I believe in you." I nodded my head softly and wordlessly and smiled slightly. We went through four rounds of this as I kept my body mirroring hers. She eventually nodded in kind and smiled too—she was starting to engage her yellow-green SNS waves. Within a few minutes, she accepted my invitation to sit and continue the mirrored practice.

A minute later, she stood up, announcing, "Yeah, I *can* do this." I reminded her she was not alone in her movement toward her self-at-best. Luenell had returned to her green-wave state.

Improvising, aka Scrambling

This is the fly-by-the-seat-of-pants type of containment exercise that requires therapists to lean into our gut and creativity. Let me give you an example of spontaneous containment that could only be described as doing the best we can with what we've got.

Irwin, my wheelchair using 63-year-old client with dissociative identity disorder, a very extensive traumatic brain injury, and legal blindness, was hijacked by red waves due to multiple triggers. Unfortunately, due to Irwin's deteriorated health and COVID restrictions, I had to shift from face-to-face to phone sessions—he was unable to use Zoom comfortably. This made tracking his red-wave states terribly difficult, to say the least. Having worked for years with Irwin in person, I knew one of his red-wave states was characterized by his eyes crossing, one eye closing, head tilting to the side, becoming unresponsive, seemingly losing all muscle tone, and breathing in barely audible ways. This state seemed to conjure the two-month coma state Irwin's spouse had described he had been in following his skiing accident. Another distinct red-wave state was marked by Irwin becoming incoherent and disoriented. Sometimes, these DV states co-occurred.

During one particular call, Irwin was perseverative, spoke inaudibly while moaning, and went completely silent. There was a slight hint of panic evident in his heavy breathing. He seemed unreachable, inaccessible. To boot, he dropped the phone a few times. I would later find out that this presentation corresponded with Irwin having a severe urinary tract infection, which caused disorientation and agitation. At the moment, I found myself panicking, fearing Irwin might be having a stroke. After grounding myself and moving out of shock, I found myself in a state of fear scrambling to do whatever I could to rouse connection. First, I started to use a sing-songy voice, "Irwin, oh Irwin. Are you there? Are you sleeping? It's Monica. I'm here. Can you hear me?" I listened carefully for any response. I sang, "Irwin. Irwin. I need you to come back to me." When he didn't respond, I asked, "Do you like my singing?" He still didn't answer, so I switched tactics to reestablish connection. Since we were speaking landline to landline, I quickly grabbed my cell phone and called his. Irwin re-oriented himself to answer his cell. Bingo! He scrambled to reach his cell phone and reacted to my voice. I assessed his safety and worked to orient him. I told him to stay on the cell phone, but I would hang up the landline to call his wife and live-in nurse who had stepped out briefly. Irwin and I stayed connected on the mobile call until his nurse returned and got the necessary medical interventions started. Irwin reminds us to do whatever works to reestablish green-wave safety and connection if we can.

Highly dissociative clients may also move into preverbal red-wave states, requiring therapists to use primary process language, attunement play, and sensorimotor channels to access their very young parts of the mind. Therapists must find ways to connect to their own Self (intrapersonally) and with others (interpersonally) to effectively navigate these red waves. We can lean into our personal grounding abilities, spontaneity, creativity, and sensorimotor playfulness to soothe our own nervous system in times of client crisis. We also need to create a team of supports like other professionals or our clients' family members and friends who can assist in the work to swim through the red waves into yellow and green ones.

Navigational Lessons Learned

In this chapter, we've learned how through playful containment and expansion practices we exercise the vagal brake to help our clients navigate out of yellow SNS or red DV waves back to green VV waves of safety, connection, and affect regulation. We must remember that navigating affect waves involves complementing containment with expansion practices.

As we close this chapter, let's return to 12-year-old Lucy, who stuffed her little container with her "problems" but never took out them out. With me, she put a 0 to 10 rating on each piece of paper to denote her SUDS. When regulated enough, Lucy was taught to return to her little sparkly box, open it, and pick one paper at a time—the least dysregulating first. She was taught to close the box and tell each of the other little pieces of paper, "I'll be back to take out each one of you and take care of you." Lucy processed fears of darkness, being alone, then memories of her house being robbed, and finally her mom's cancer. Lucy returned each week with her sparkly container and having pre-selected the topic of the session, she'd direct me to the sensations, emotions, thoughts, and memories to process. Eventually, the box stayed on a high shelf on her bookcase at home because "I don't need to put anything in it anymore. But it's there if I need it." Lucy gained confidence to feel dysregulated affect. She expanded her window of tolerance as her confidence and competence to handle discomfort grew.

For Lucy and all clients, we can playfully exercise the vagal brake to flexibly regulate activation. As clients gain comfort with discomfort, their window of tolerance expands. Their fear of approaching and moving through yellow and red waves shrinks as they strengthen their ability to return to green waves of safety and connection. They trust that change for the better awaits their discovery and exploration.

As we witness our clients' expanding WOT, we need to reflect it back and make it explicit. By metaprocessing it relationally, we help clients identify: (1) what made the change possible; (2) how showing up in regulated ways—around formerly dysregulating triggers—can be experienced somatically, emotionally and cognitively; and (3) how to savor and deepen the change intrapsychically and relationally to integrate hope, genuine pride in accomplishments, self-trust, and other possibilities of transformation.

Here are a few examples of metaprocessing prompts:

- To address cognitions/self-appraisals we might ask, "What does this mean about you (fishing for a positive self-appraisal or cognition) that you sat with this feeling today for so long?" "What do you now believe about your ability to deal with this discomfort?"
- To help our client emotionally and somatically reflect upon their growth and change we can say, "You used to say, 'I can't go there,' or, 'I can't handle it,' and shoot me a death stare if I invited you to sit with this. Now notice what you can handle. What is this like? How does this feel emotionally and in your body?"
- To relationally mirror how we see and are affected emotionally and viscerally by our client's change, we might ask, "Can you see in my eyes or face how proud I am of your growth?"
- To help a client notice the relational and internal work involved, we might say, "You so openly shared your deep vulnerability and allowed me to accompany you in this work, today. How did that feel to you?" We can share how that felt to us. Then we can remark, "How did it feel that all parts of mind cooperated and worked together so well?"

Relationally savoring the accomplishments of playfully navigating the affect waves and their ANS states is an important testament to the hard work.

This chapter has taught us how to help clients playfully navigate affect waves to establish the precondition for all trauma healing work: safety and connection. The next chapter builds on these playfully infused skills as we learn to relationally play with another element needed to support change in traumatized clients—the dialectics of multiplicity and contradictory experiences to wire-in change for the better.

References

Bakur Weiner, M. & Simmons, M. B. (2009). *The problem is the solution: A Jungian approach to a meaningful life*. New York: Jason Aronson.

Blatner, A. (1996). *Acting-in: Practical applications of psychodramatic method* (3rd ed.). New York: Springer.

Blum, M. C. (2015). Embodied mirroring: A relational, body-to-body technique promoting movement in therapy. *Journal of Psychotherapy Integration, 25*(2), 115–127.

Brown, S. (2009). *Play: How it shapes the brain, opens the imagination, and invigorates the soul*. New York: Avery.

Courtois, C. & Ford, J. (2013). *Treatment of complex trauma: A sequenced, relationship-based approach*. New York: Guilford.

Dana, D. (2018). *The polyvagal theory in therapy: Engaging the rhythm of regulation*. New York: Norton.

Fisher, J. (2017). *Healing the fragmented selves of trauma survivors: Overcoming self-alienation*. New York: Routledge.

Forgash, C. & Copeley, M. (Eds.) (2008). *Healing the heart of trauma and dissociation with EMDR and ego-state therapy*. New York: Springer.

Fosha, D. (Ed.) (2021). *Undoing aloneness & the transformation of suffering into flourishing: AEDP 2.0*. Washington, DC: American Psychological Association.

Fraser, G. A. (2003). Fraser's "Dissociative table technique" revisited, revised: A strategy for working with ego states in dissociative disorders and ego-state therapy. *Journal of Trauma and Dissociation, 4*(4), 5–28.

Fredrickson, B. L. (2006). Unpacking positive emotions: Investigating the seeds of human flourishing. *The Journal of Positive Psychology, 1*(2), 57–59. https://doi.org/10.1080/17439760500510981

Gendlin, E. T. (1981). *Focusing*. New York: Bantam Books.

Gomez-Perales, N. (2015). *Attachment-focused trauma treatment for children and adolescents: Phase-oriented strategies for addressing complex trauma disorders*. New York: Routledge.

Greenland, S. K. (2010). *The mindful child: How to help your kid manage stress and become happier, kinder and more compassionate*. New York: Free Press.

Herman, J. L. (2022). *Trauma and recovery: From domestic abuse to political terror*. London: Basic Books.

Hopenwasser, K. (2008). Being in rhythm: Dissociative attunement in therapeutic process. *Journal of Trauma & Dissociation, 9*(3), 349–367. https://doi.org/10.1080/15299730802139212

Kestly, T. (2018). A cross-cultural and cross-disciplinary perspective of play. In T. Marks-Tarlow, M. Solomon, & D. Siegel (Eds.), *Play and creativity in psychotherapy* (pp. 110–127). New York: Norton.

Levine, H. B. (2023, March 23). *On the necessity of failure*. Presentation at the Michigan Council for Psychoanalysis and Psychotherapy (MCCP).

Levine, P. (1997). *Waking the tiger: Healing trauma*. Berkeley, CA: North Atlantic Books.

Maroda, K. (1998). Enactments: When the patient's and analyst's pasts converge. *Psychoanalytic Psychology, 15*(4), 517–535.

Medbo, A. (2023, July 14–17). *Rescuing the SELF: From no SELF to core Self*. [Online Live AEDP Advanced Skills Module training sponsored by AEDP Institute.]

Moreno, J. L. (1946). *Psychodrama* (Vol. 1). New York: Beacon House.

Mosquera, D. (2020, March 1). *Treating dissociative disorders with EMDR Therapy.* [In-person presentation New York City.]

Niven, K. (2013). Affect. In M. D. Gellman & J. R. Turner (Eds.), Encyclopedia of behavioral medicine (pp. 49–50). New York: Springer.

Ogden, P., Minton, K., & Pain, C. (2006). *Trauma and the body: A sensorimotor approach to psychotherapy.* New York: Norton.

Panksepp, J. (2009). Brain emotional systems and qualities of mental life: From animal models of affect to implications for psychotherapeutics. In D. Fosha, D. J. Siegel, & M. F. Solomon (Eds.), *The healing power of emotion: Affective neuroscience, development and clinical practice* (pp. 1–26). New York: Norton.

Porges, S. W. (2011). *The polyvagal theory: Neurophysiological foundations of emotions, attachment, communication, and self-regulation.* New York: Norton.

Porges, S. W. (2015). Play as neural exercise: Insights from the Polyvagal Theory. In D. Pearce-McCall (Ed.), *The power of play for mind brain health* (pp. 3–7). mindgains.

Rizzolatti, G. & Craighero, L. (2004). The mirror-neuron system. *Annual Review of Neuroscience, 27,* 169–192.

Rothschild, B. (2021). *Revolutionizing trauma treatment: Stabilization, safety and nervous system balance.* New York: Norton.

Schmidt, S. J. (1998, June). *Internal conference room ego-state therapy and the resolution of double binds: Preparing clients for EMDR trauma processing.* EMDRIA Newsletter.

Schore, A. N. (2021). The interpersonal neurobiology of intersubjectivity. *Frontiers in Psychology, 12,* Article 648616. https://doi.org/10.3389/fpsyg.2021.648616

Schwartz, R. C. (2021). *No bad parts: Healing trauma and restoring wholeness with the Internal Family Systems Model.* Boulder, CO: Sounds True.

Shapiro, F. (2018). *Eye Movement Desensitization and Reprocessing (EMDR) basic principles, protocols and procedures* (3rd ed.). New York: Guilford.

Siegel, D. J. (2020). *The developing mind: How relationships and the brain interact to shape who we are* (3rd ed.). New York: Guilford.

Wallin, D. J. (2007). *Attachment in psychotherapy.* New York: Guilford.

Warner, E., Westcott, A, Cook, A., & Finn, H. (2020). *Transforming trauma in children and adolescents: An embodied approach to somatic regulation, trauma processing, and attachment-building.* Berkeley, CA: North Atlantic Books.

Winnicott, D. W. (1960). Ego distortion in terms of true and false self. In D. W. Winnicott (Ed.), *The maturational processes and the facilitating environment: Studies in the theory of emotional development* (pp. 140–152). New York: International Universities Press.

Chapter 11

Playing with Dialectics

Multiplicity and Contradictions

As we continue to explore how to practically infuse our playful spirit into trauma treatment, we get to dig into a dialectical challenge: how can we help clients hold the multiplicity of trauma-related sensations, emotions, and beliefs in their whole being and deal with related opposites or contradictions? In this chapter, we will examine how to playfully engage traumatized clients of all ages to hold the multiplicity of "both/and" as well as the different-yet-linked opposites of "either/or" trauma-related material. Encouraging our clients to sit with these dialectics grows their flexible thinking, resourcefulness, creativity, sense of interconnectedness and, most importantly, supports their transformational change.

Embracing Multiplicity and Contradictions: The "Both/And" and "Either/Or" Mindsets

When we invite our traumatized clients to consciously practice holding all sides of an experience, resistance may emerge. A client's push-back isn't necessarily to bust our chops but reflects trauma-related adaptations.

For example, Jaysun may have trouble believing their father can love them if dad is financially supportive, yet emotionally absent. Objectively speaking, the presence of contradictory behaviors—parental support and absence—can both be true of one person. Jaysun struggles to hold the multiplicity or "both/and" aspects of their father's actions: part of dad can give easily physically/financially, but as a whole, he struggles to give and be present emotionally. Also, Jaysun believes *either* dad loves me *or* he doesn't. Jaysun grapples to experience all aspects of their relationship with dad because they are hijacked by their trauma-induced unresolved feelings of abandonment. Jaysun only notices dad's hurtful behaviors (not the whole of dad's actions) and the all-or-nothing qualities of dad's presence or absence.

We as therapists would support Jaysun to *synthesize* (horizontally across left and right hemispheres) and *integrate* (vertically across brain structures) (see Laub & Weiner, 2013) the belief that "My dad loves me the best way he can, yet expresses it in misattuned ways that leave me feeling unloved and abandoned."

DOI: 10.4324/9781003509493-17

To enable Jaysun, and all clients, to have this experience which integrates part/whole relationships and synthesizes contradictory material, we encourage their mindful dual awareness—the ability to notice, validate, and hold their past-triggered internal distress in the context of the present safe healing relationship (Laub & Weiner, 2013; Shapiro, 2018). We need to highlight how opposing and diverse parts (expressed as different cognitions, emotions, and sensations) are interrelated to their whole being, always interactively moving toward resolution and unity (Linehan & Schmidt, 1995). We would help Jaysun experience all aspects as true for them, while feeling and being safe, seen, and soothed in the therapy relationship.

Linking trauma-time sensations and emotions with present-day relational safety and validation enables dual-attention awareness, affect regulation, self-reflective functioning, self-validation relationally (between therapist and client) and intrarelationally (between client and all parts of their mind), and memory reconsolidation. As a result, a client's self-questioning about whether their experience and feelings are real lessens while connection to a safe other and embodiment of their truth and Self increases.

In therapy, when we introduce the mismatch of our playful mindset to trauma content and process, the client's challenge to hold complex and contradictory experiences is exaggerated. Our goal in playfully spirited trauma treatment is to help clients consciously and in regulated ways: (1) differentiate separate parts (boundaries, sensations, emotions, and thoughts) and link them into a larger, coherent yet complex whole, and (2) develop new ways to hold contradictions.

Understanding Trauma's Age of Onset Effects on "Both/And" and "Either/Or" Mindsets

Before introducing our playfully spirited interventions, we need to learn when developmentally, our client's trauma occurred because it impacts their ability to master "both/and" and "either/or" mindsets. Specifically, the postformal stage of thinking develops in adulthood (and for some never) and allows a person to think flexibly and adaptively, hold multiple realities, examine the dialectic or multiple sides and understand paradoxes, and combine analytical and intuitive thinking (see Koehler, 2021, explaining Piaget). Let's briefly look at trauma's impact on this ability in childhood- and adult-onset trauma.

Childhood-onset Trauma

Clients who were preverbally traumatized may not have achieved the developmental milestone of holding "both/and" and "either/or" abilities because their left-brain and higher-order thinking abilities had not yet come online. Even those abused in later childhood cannot hold complex incompatible beliefs about their trauma.

For example, 9-year-old Katrina, who had been raped by her father, could not believe that bad things happen to good people. She would have been unable to function in a world where victimization was random, especially if caused by those you love and depend on to survive. To "make sense" of her trauma, Katrina adopted the belief, "I did bad things, that's why dad did this to me." To control and prevent further harm, she became the perfect, rule-following child. However, even when Katrina behaved with complete compliance, the incest continued, challenging her belief that her bad behaviors caused the abuse. To explain this confusion, Katrina further adapted by "reasoning" that, "I am bad" ascribing this belief to her essence, not just to her behaviors. Even into young adulthood, Katrina struggled to see herself as worthy and good, impairing her positive receptive affect capacity.

Adult-Onset Trauma

When trauma occurs in adulthood and the postformal stage of cognitive development has been achieved, "both/and" thinking can be challenged as well. For example, clients traumatized as adults in interpersonal violence dynamics often struggle to hold the contradictory realities that their perpetrator simultaneously loves and hurts them. These clients often self-question their personal truth and reality and accept being gaslit to maintain their dependence or connection. Adult trauma victims may also struggle to hold "both/and" thinking because their victimization may reactivate younger parts of mind and related scripts or deeply threaten their established integrity of mind, body, emotion, and spirit (see Boulanger, 2007).

By contrast, sometimes adults are programmed to have absolute thinking in fear-based dynamics. For example, soldiers are militarized through behavioral conditioning and deconstructing personal identity to dehumanize others, which leads them to kill the perceived enemy (Schrader, 2019, p. 158). In effect, they are programmed into black-and-white, either/or, dichotomous thinking: we are good, they are bad. We are the victims; they are the enemy. Adult-onset, us vs. them, absolutist thinking also occurs in radicalization that creates extremist views and actions with respect to race, religion, politics, etc. and fosters blind obedience to authority. Deprogramming these deeply held beliefs is extremely challenging, as with cult survivors.

Cultivating the "Both/And" and "Either/Or" Mindset through Playfulness

Cultivating a playful "both/and" plus "either/or" mindset requires therapists to intentionally create an open, curious space that allows our client (and us) to non-judgmentally hold multiple possibilities at once, even if paradoxical. We help clients believe that both, or many, things can be true simultaneously. As always, our intentional mindset must be attuned on steroids (see Chapter 8), which takes precedence over all else, including techniques or protocols, no matter how well evidence-based and effective they may be. Therapists must be present, embodied, and *with* our clients so they can be and feel fully safe, seen, and soothed: this is a precondition to all interventions. We can use many forms of playfulness to achieve this goal. Some playful sensorimotor, imaginative, narrative, and creative examples follow.

Creating Space

I'd like to share a meditative practice (inspired by an Eye Movement Desensitization and Reprocessing [EMDR] workshop taught by Julie Green of Awake Mind) that helps clients playfully engage their imagination in making space to hold a multiplicity of feelings, sensations, and thoughts/perspectives.

> Breathe and imagine a barbed-wire pen that is quite small and tight, maybe 100 by 100 feet. In the pen stand 100 cows, tightly pressed up against each other. They bang into each other when they try to move. They struggle to eat the tiny patches of grass on which the other cows stand.
>
> Imagine how the cows feel physically? Emotionally? How does this affect their milk production? How does each cow react to the others? Take some breaths.
>
> Now, imagine an expansive pasture, as big as the eye can see. A post-and-rail wooden fence surrounds this expanse to keep the cows safe and contained from getting lost. The grass is bountiful for all cows to graze.
>
> In this space, imagine how the cows feel physically. Emotionally? How is their milk-making affected? How does each cow react to the others?

We can change the content to best fit or resonate with each client. Alternatives might include a classroom and students, a home and family members, etc. The key is to create an image that starts with limited space and can be greatly expanded to accommodate what is held within. Once we effectively guide clients to create a spacious and safe holding space, we can support them in growing their skill to internally hold and tolerate "both/and" and "either/or" possibilities.

Holding Differences and Contradictions

For the practice of embracing pluralistic thinking and holding multiple feelings, I love to share lessons from life and simple, relatable children's books, which can appeal to the youngest parts of all-aged clients. When appropriate, I read these books to young clients or suggest older clients read them to themselves. The book *Double Dip Feelings* (Cain, 1990) uses ice cream metaphors to address how we naturally and simultaneously have multiple and contradictory emotions and perspectives. It is simple and self-explanatory.

As a related or separate exercise, we can ask clients to name what ice cream flavors (or candy, types of books, music, etc.) they like. This prompt helps clients define personal preferences and therefore boundaries. Some clients might need some encouragement, because voicing their likes may not feel natural or safe. Usually, clients are open to sharing because we're asking about relatively innocuous things. To foster their curiosity, when they say, for example, "chocolate and butter pecan," or "strawberry and rocky road," we might ask, "And any other?" We might follow up and ask, "Could you ever imagine getting *two* scoops in one cup?" If they say, "No," we can ask, if they could imagine anyone else ordering a double or even a triple scoop of flavors in one cone. Even if it's not okay for them, our client can picture or remember others doing this. The implied metaphor helps clients practice spacious acceptance of multiplicity whose parts (flavors) sometimes mix well together, other times not.

We extend this metaphor to emotions, thoughts, and memories to allow them to be more easily be digested (get the pun?). We can play with concepts like different ice cream flavors have value, yet can be incompatible, like Reese's peanut butter and cotton candy. Returning to this metaphor often helps clients gain comfort with the multiplicity of somatic, emotional, and cognitive states. We can remind clients to create a bigger space—whether cup, cone, classroom, pasture, or universe—to make room for "both/and." Helping clients sense what this experience feels like can broaden, deepen, and strengthen this accomplishment.

I also like to use tactile, sensorimotor channels to practice holding differences and contradictions. Based on Shapiro's Two-Hand EMDR Interweave (2005), clients literally physicalize different and often competing beliefs, options, and ego states and anchor them in their hands—making the concept of holding different/competing parts within one body both metaphorical and concrete.

Specifically, we ask clients to identify two sides of a conflictual feeling, thought/belief, situation, or ego state. We prompt them to breathe and imagine sending one side of the disturbance to be held in one hand and then repeat with the other. As this is an imagination-based practice, clients don't need functioning hands and can send the disturbance to be held or anchored in their left and right feet, elbows, etc. While it doesn't matter which hand holds which side of the dialectic, we can inform them that they might sense a better fit in one side over the other. When we invite them to check for fit, clients often move as if weighing what is in each hand. This action distances, physicalizes, and contains the disturbing material while building body attunement and discernment about fit. As we learned in Chapter 6, physicalizing or personifying our symptoms and disturbances helps us objectively hold and notice rather than embody or be them.

We then ask our client to alternately open and close their hands instructing them to, "Hold and release. Just notice." When they have finished a round of bilateral holding and releasing, we ask what they notice. We can visually track our client's body, noticing any changes in muscle tension or movements. After a few rounds, we can explicitly reflect back any changes (e.g., hand positions) and explore how that might mirror internal emotional and cognitive shifts which, in my experience, are interconnected or go hand in hand (that pun was necessary!). This two-handed holding exercise shows clients that when they intentionally give space to hold and then tune into different parts, their wise Self and related innate healing drives (e.g., adaptive information processing) find solutions and greater peace.

Finally, the children's book *From the Stars in the Sky to the Fish in the Sea* (Thom & Ching, 2017), through stunning illustrations and poetic prose, offers readers practice accepting differences and contradictions that can be challenging or even mind-bending. It chronicles the experience of Miu Lan, a child who can change into any shape they imagine yet can't decide whether they are a girl or boy. The book follows Miu Lan's struggle to be understood and accepted by others and even themself. Child and adult clients with whom I've shared this book have resonated with aspects of its messaging: ambivalence of identity (e.g., religious, gender, and sexuality), the struggle to be seen and accepted for their true Self, and the soothing security that comes when others openly welcome their truth or essence. This book helps clients gain curiosity to embrace their unique and diverse expressions of Self and appreciate the rich, multiplicity of their being.

Gaining Flexibility of Thought

Inspired by the book *That's Good, That's Bad* (Cuyler, 1993), this exercise offers a twist on "both/and" by challenging emotional and cognitive assumptions about what seems obvious and unchangeable to clients. *That's Good, That's Bad* (and other books in this series) is so beautifully illustrated (by David Catrow) that I share it with clients of all ages. The book follows the adventures of a little boy who faces multiple, potentially life-threatening events that seem "bad," but somehow help save his life and are thus "good." By contrast, what seems like "good" circumstances turn into life-threatening ones—presenting a great metaphor for disorganized attachment themes.

Most clients' reactions have been, "That's so clever," or, "Who'd ever have imagined something so scary could be a blessing?" We explore how it feels to openly and nonjudgmentally look at situations, people, and thoughts from multiple perspectives, challenging "either/or," black-and-white, rigid/absolute thinking. The book offers a segue, inviting clients to entertain different self-beliefs, perspectives, or possibilities about others' actions and life circumstances that aren't just negative. In addition, this book offers a reframe of trauma and life's hard knocks. One client spontaneously offered, "Yeah, the tree fell on and destroyed my car, which sucked! Yet the insurance money allowed me to put a down payment on a new car, which I needed for years. It was a gift in disguise!"

Another client said, "*That's Good, That's Bad* shows that nothing is at it seems. You can't trust anything or anybody at face value." Even this relational trauma–based reaction can bear fruit. We can discuss how the little boy's naïve trust in the process and go-with-the-flow attitude contrasts our client's due to their trauma history. Yet, we can highlight how our client's hard work in therapy strives to embolden and empower them to prevent unconscious trauma repetitions.

Countless other playful books, games, stories, songs, etc. can be used or created to strengthen our clients' ability to hold a "both/and" perspective, which by its very nature re-wires extreme, binary, my way-or-the highway thinking. It allows clients to know two (or more) things can be true and co-exist, including different parts of mind, feelings, and sensations.

Let's now turn to the cases in which we help clients decide between dialectics (because both can't be true) yet support multiplicity of mind.

Playing with Mutually Exclusive Contradictions to Promote Change

Sometimes, we as therapists can purposefully reveal contradictions that potentially lend themselves to new experiences for memory reconsolidation in which "either/or" thinking is reparative. Mutually exclusive dialectics can emerge organically or we can intentionally set them against each other—creating juxtaposition experiences (Ecker, 2018).

Playing with Juxtaposition Experiences

Dialectics allow for the juxtaposition of any two related aspects of being (Linehan & Schmidt, 1995, p. 565). We'll now examine different playful ways to create juxtaposition experiences using reality testing, pretend imagery, the earned security of the therapeutic alliance, and paradoxical agreement with protector parts.

Reality testing

Luenell provides us an example of reality testing with juxtaposed contradictions. She claimed, "I can't handle life—It's too much. I'll never succeed." I sarcastically retorted, "You're right Luenell, you *can't* handle life," which gave her pause and grabbed her attention. She seemed shocked at my agreeing with her.

Then I added, ". . . Except you regained custody of your kids from foster care and have lovingly and consistently keep them safe and cared-for 2 years. You got off oxycodone. You got your sonographer certification. Yup, Luenell it sounds to me like you can't handle a damn thing—except seemingly insurmountable tasks, or anything you try!"

Luenell rolled her eyes and smiled. She got the point which we further processed.

Presenting contradictory and incompatible material, like I did with Luenell, disconfirms or mismatches our clients' expectations or schemas which unlock related, neurally linked response patterns (and corresponding beliefs, affects, and sensations) allowing brand new positive memories to be created and consolidated (Ecker et al., 2015). When trauma memories are reconsolidated, the content of the trauma memory remains intact, but the brain's emotional expectation of being plunged into pain when touching it is changed (Ecker, 2018). Thus, the mismatched expectation—an essential and necessary mechanism of transformational change—powers memory reconsolidation (Ecker, 2018). Our client's trauma learnings and related affects are modified and even nullified (Ecker & Bridges, 2020).

We fuel transformational change of trauma with our playful spirit as we juxtapose play and trauma states to create autonomic nervous system (ANS) mismatches. In Chapter 5, we learned how play states activate ventral vagal (VV) circuits of safety and connection with related positive affects/emotions and self-cognitions. By contrast, trauma states activate dorsal vagal (DV) circuits of protection with related negative affects/emotions (e.g., fear) and self-appraisals, and "expectations of absolute disconnection and aloneness" (Ecker, 2018, p. 39). Juxtaposing playfulness in the same field of awareness as trauma disconfirms trauma-related expectations. Something has to budge as clients are made aware of how their there-and-then trauma-time adaptation does not fit their here-and-now experience. This cues up repair as both can't be true at the same time.

We can look for or create mismatches through juxtaposition experiences that focus on the original trauma memory (as is done in EMDR and Flash Technique [Manfield et al., 2017]); current or historic insecure relational attachment patterns (as in Accelerated Experiential Dynamic Psychotherapy [Fosha, 2000, 2021]); and current disturbing sensorimotor experiences (as in Sensorimotor Psychotherapy [Ogden et al., 2006]) that tap into these networks. Once unlocked, we introduce new incompatible and positivity-filled states of affect, sensation, perception, movement, cognition, imagery, and emotions, enabling memory reconsolidation and repair.

Juxtaposition experiences can feel weirdly jarring, cognitively, emotionally, and sensorily, which makes them fun to work with. When asked to simultaneously hold two incompatible truths—"I am worthless" and "I am worthy"—one client said it was like blowing a circuit in her mind. Numerous clients have paused with facial expressions that convey, "This does not compute." That's because it doesn't. It's literally impossible to hold both as true simultaneously.

Imagine embodying the negative self-attribution "I am unworthy" and its DV-linked feelings of shame, a downward head, and slumped shoulders at the same time as the positive self-belief "I am worthy" and its VV-linked feelings of pride and competence, an erect spine, and a forward gaze. To hold mutually exclusive beliefs, emotions, ANS and affect states, and their related protector systems as true, we must switch—sometimes rapidly—between one and the other. Incompatible states are just "either/or" not "both/and."

Returning to Luenell, her belief "I can't handle life or succeed" could not be simultaneously true with, "I have been handling life and am succeeding." The former reflected trauma-time shame-filled protective adaptations, while the latter indicated real present-day functioning. Luenell could not refute her own reality.

It was also true that her life challenges were hard and raised significant anxiety—as they would for most of us. Over time, Luenell learned that "I can handle life's challenges, and while it might feel impossible and really uncomfortable while I'm going through it, I'll feel so proud when I accomplish my goals." Luenell had grown the mindful ability to hold the complexity of positive and negative affect states, without one overtaking the other: both were valid. Luenell's statement reflected her dramatic and deep change in having a positive future orientation, gaining wisdom from experience, growing trust to find attuned and supportive others, and her own resourcefulness and adaptability. Together sharing tears of pride, we metaprocessed (see Chapter 9) her accomplishments and mastery. These gains came from years of hard work and keeping hope alive that her thriving was possible.

Luenell reminds us of the importance to slow down so we can co-create enough space and time to juxtapose trauma-based perceptions and current reality-based facts. This allows incompatible circuits to activate and be challenged playfully to promote memory reconsolidation. With the addition of metaprocessing, transformance strivings can be catalyzed to facilitate deep and lasting change.

Pretend Imagery

We can creatively use humor and imaginative play to set up juxtaposition experiences and memory reconsolidation opportunities as I did with 40-year-old Jannique. Since childhood, Jannique struggled with her mother's enmeshed behaviors and disorganized parenting style. After learning that Jannique's first husband had been sexually and emotionally abusive, her mother's boundary violations became ceaseless and suffocating. Although long divorced and currently in a healthy relationship with her fiancé, Claude, Jannique reported her mother pummeled her about safe sexual practices to protect her, causing Jannique to experience panic attacks.

With a straight face, I juxtaposed humor with Jannique's panic state. I said, "Next time, before you and your fiancé have sex, imagine inviting your mother into your bed so she can really keep an eye on things. Of course, you and your fiancé may need to upgrade your queen to a king-sized mattress."

Using the mother's symptom of boundary violations in this over-the-top way made Jannique and I laugh uproariously to the point of tears, enabling memory reconsolidation. She could not hold both as true, "I will protect my mother from violating my boundary" and "I will invite my mother to violate my boundary." Going forward, Jannique called up this image whenever her mother launched into this topic, which made her laugh and allowed the hurtful relational ruptures and violations to loosen their unrelenting hold on her.

Earned Security

We can capitalize on the safety and earned security of the therapy relationship to highlight unexpected and incompatible experiences, as I did with 34-year-old Michael, who asserted, "You get paid to care about me and, at the end of the day, you go home to your family and forget about me." I replied, with a tone of sarcasm which I knew he could tolerate, "Yup. The many times I've beamed with pride and been delighted in your accomplishments with your boyfriend—yup, that was fake. Or when your suffering has deeply touched my heart, you're right that was just because you pay me. Oh yeah, when we sat here praying together for a clean MRI scan, that was cuz I learned that in my grad school casebooks, not because I wanted you to thrive in health. You're right, feeling my care all those times couldn't be real." Using the data of therapy is hard to refute, especially when there are numerous examples.

I then explicitly juxtaposed both truths, "So Michael, nobody cares about you and your boyfriend and I care about you deeply." We processed these mutually exclusive beliefs. With practice, Michael rewired and updated his protector parts and let in feeling really cared about. He grew to appreciate how his protective adaptations helped him cope with his devoutly Christian, alcoholic parents whose care was absent or misattuned. He mourned his parents' limitations— their inability to accept his homosexuality, show him care, and securely provide for him. He also believed they truly wished for him to live a healthy, happy, and financially stable life. Eventually, Michael integrated the helpful aspects of multiplicity and contradictions to earn relational security. He summed it up well: "My negligent, alcoholic parents cared for me the best they could, which was really misattuned. *And* now I've created safe and loving relationships in which I really am and feel cared about."

Paradoxical Agreement

We can present a mismatch experience with simple statements. First, we must explicitly link different ego states to their related cognitions, emotions, and sensations. Then, by creating space to hold all parts safely, we can notice the contradictions and their incompatibility.

For example, when a client says, "I don't care about living anymore," we can respond, "I hear that and that makes sense," which is disarming to clients who don't regularly have their intolerable angst reflected and held—this is a relational, emotional mismatch.

Believing this statement comes from a suicidal protector part, and because we don't want them killing themselves we can clarify and add, "Of course, part of you doesn't care, because another part of you cares too much—that balances things out."

If a client refutes, "None of me cares," we can provide contradictory information, using evidence from the session.

"Well, if that were true, you wouldn't have shown up to therapy, asked me to turn up the air conditioning or gotten yourself a drink of water. Those are self-attuned, caring actions." Clients may then shift focus onto what they "don't care" about that has felt hopeless. We can empathize, "No wonder this protector part doesn't want to live anymore. The pain and exhaustion have been intolerable for so long. How hard this part has worked to keep you going! That's tireless and committed self-protection. Wow!" Working with the client to appreciate their protector's relentless perseverance, we can add, "Please send along the message inside to your protectors, how much you and I appreciate their efforts to manage your pain," and query, "How much can they feel and take in our appreciation?" to assess receptive affective capacity. We can share similar sincere statements of care and compassion for the protector part itself.

These intrarelational and interpersonal messages present mismatches for clients whose expressed vulnerabilities have been previously dismissed, abandoned, or minimized. These mismatches enable memory reconsolidation through repeated rounds of relational unfolding and metaprocessing.

Like playing with symptoms, when we play with juxtaposition experiences we make space to simultaneously hold both the welcomed and the unwelcomed, invite the presence of what clients want and don't want, bright light to darkness and darkness to light, and welcome trauma-time protectors to be unburdened and updated to serve as wise and helpful present day protectors.

Playing with Contradictory Protector Parts

When we playfully hold and engage contradictory protector parts of mind in a safe space, greater intrarelational communication and cooperation emerge. Narrating and role-playing our clients' incompatible ego states (see the sections on parts language and role play in Chapter 10) is another way to help clients more objectively observe their internal contradictory and confusing dynamics. We borrow this idea from children, who spontaneously express and play out different parts in sand play, dress up, drawing, doll play, etc.

Bernard, a 45-year-old male client with a chronic and complex history of parental chaos, physical and emotional abuse, and abandonments, struggled internally. One day Bernard overheard his 68-year-old mother telling his 10-year-old son, Ralph, "When your daddy was a little older than you, Ralphie, daddy had a bad, bad temper. He would chase me all over the house and hit me." His mom omitted sharing that prior to Bernard's aggression, she had mercilessly beaten him with a belt, called him "the devil," and threw scalding water in his direction. Bernard stormed into the room and told Ralph to get in the car.

Before Ralph exited, Bernard's mother dropped to the floor shaking and screaming, "Bernard, you are possessed by the devil. Jesus has no mercy on your soul. You will be consumed in the fires of hell!"

A day later in therapy, Bernard's teenage parts wanted to yell at his delusional mother and forbid her from ever visiting his son, believing, "The trauma is all her fault." His preverbal and elementary school–aged parts of mind by contrast believed, "I must have made her so upset," and wanted to call his mother to apologize for yesterday's behavior. Seeing that Bernard felt very dysregulated and conflicted, I asked if we could take some breaths and if he would allow me to take on his parts while he brought his wise, paternal, intuitive, objective Self to simply observe. He agreed.

First, I role-played his teenage part. With a loud, deep voice I said, "Man, you young parts don't know what you're talking about. Our mother is unsafe. She's a fucking nut!"

Then I switched into a quiet, timid voice for his young parts, "But she's our mommy and if she said we did something wrong, it must be true."

I then asked Bernard to bring his wise, adult Self to help these parts resolve this deep contradiction. I asked him to speak to me as if I were his teenage self. He said, "I get it dude. You're angry because she *is* fucked up."

Speaking as his teenage part, I said, "Damn straight, she's losing her shit and Ralph cannot be around that bitch!"

Then Bernard said to me as I role-played his very young part, "I hear you too, little Bernie. You must feel so scared and confused. This is your mommy."

I said meekly, "I am. Mommy can't be bad, it must be me."

Bernard soothingly and wisely said, "I am here with you. I'll help you figure this out. It's so hard. Did you know mommies can love their sons and still scare and hurt them?"

I tentatively responded, "Really?"

Bernard continued with deep, paternal care, "Yes. And when mommies are not safe, we need to get safe. I can help you, and so can teenager Bernie. Would you like our help?"

At this point, I said to Bernard, "That's so beautiful. You got this. Protect and guide your little ones and teenage parts to find a way through this together." I encouraged Bernard to drop into his body and with bilateral tapping (from EMDR, Shapiro, 2018), find a path that worked for all parts.

After some time of agitation, tears, and then calm, Bernard said that the little ones knew, deep down, it wasn't their fault and really liked the teenage part reminding them. Meanwhile, the teenager appreciated the little ones reminding him that mom has some kind and loving parts that she shares with Ralph—and Bernard's young ones enjoy being around for that. They also understood that ending mom and Ralph's relationship could significantly hurt Ralph.

Bernard additionally shared that both sides agreed his mother had betrayed them, breaking their trust in the present and past. They also agreed that she was scaring and confusing Ralph and he did not feel safe.

Bernard said, "Adult me told them that I'll sit Mom down and explain how she betrayed us and Ralph. I'll tell her that neither me nor Janet (his wife) would allow visits to continue if this recurred. To build trust, we'll supervise visits and lay ground rules about what she can do and say. My teenage side likes the threat to limit visits—it helps him feel powerful. My little ones like that they and Ralph could spend time with mom safely."

We can also have clients write out the dialogue or draw the contradictions occurring between parts. Then their wise, nonjudgmental, and mindful current-day Self can be accessed to find solutions. Clients often surprise themselves at how resourcefully they generate new scripts, problem-solve, and reconsolidate memories after holding both sides in juxtaposition. In these re-imaginings, clients' resilience and adaptability can grow too.

The Promise of Playing with Dialectics of Multiplicity and Contradictions

As we've seen, when therapists playfully embrace the trauma-related dialectics of multiplicity and contradictions, we frontload juxtaposition experiences. The mismatches between trauma-time expectations and the present-day safe-and-connected positive experiences allow past memories to be unlinked, differentiated from the present ones, forming new neural linkages. As we help clients synthesize horizontal "either-or" and integrate vertical whole/part or "both/and" dialectical processes (Laub & Weiner, 2013, p. 27), they effectively separate old, negative, and wire together new, positive associations.

Positive change through playing with dialectics results in neural regulation and integrative functioning which grows intrapsychic and relational regulation (Siegel & Payne Bryson, 2020). Additionally, the positivity of play broadens and builds our clients' resources, creativity, flexibility, adaptability, and resilience (Fredrickson & Joiner, 2002), resulting in positive recursive spirals of transformation where more (healing) begets more (Fosha, 2010). Consequently, therapy engagement increases as does its enjoyment for client and therapist.

In Chapter 12, we will explore how therapists engaging sensorimotor play-fulness can use literal and figurative movements of separating and connect-ing to help clients repair and create healthier boundaries intrapsychically and interpersonally.

References

Boulanger, G. (2007). *Wounded by Reality: Understanding and treating adult onset trauma.* New York: The Psychology Press.

Cain, B. S. (1990). *Double-dip feelings: Stories to help children understand emotions.* Washington, DC: Magination Press.

Cuyler, M. (1993). *That's good that's bad.* New York: Henry Holt.

Ecker, B. (2018). Clinical translation of memory reconsolidation research: Therapeu-tic methodology for transformational change by erasing implicit emotional learnings driving symptom production. *International Journal of Neuropsychotherapy, 6*(1), 1–92. https://www.coherencetherapy.org/files/Ecker_2018_Clinical_Translation_of_Memory_Reconsolidation_Research.pdf

Ecker, B. & Bridges, S. K. (2020). How the science of memory reconsolidation advances the effectiveness and unification of psychotherapy. *Clinical Social Work Journal, 48,* 287–300. https://doi.org/10.1007/s10615-020-00754-z

Ecker, B., Ticic, R., & Hulley, L. (2015). Minding the findings: Let's not miss the mes-sage of memory reconsolidating research for psychotherapy. *Behavioral and Brain Sciences.* https://doi.org/10.1017/S0140525X14000168

Fosha, D. (2000). *The transforming power of affect: A model for accelerated change.* New York: Basic Books.

Fosha, D. (2010). Wired for healing: Thirteen ways of looking at AEDP. *Transformance: The AEDP Journal, 1.* https://aedpinstitute.org/journal/wired-for-healing/

Fosha, D. (Ed.) (2021). *Undoing aloneness & the transformation of suffering into flour-ishing: AEDP 2.0.* Washington, DC: American Psychological Association.

Fredrickson, B. L. & Joiner, T. (2002). Positive emotions trigger upward spirals toward emotional well-being. *Psychological Science, 13*(2), 172–175.

Koehler, J. (2021). *Who the hell is Jean Piaget?: And what are his theories all about?* Suffolk: Bowden & Brazil.

Laub, B. & Weiner, N. (2013). A dialectical perspective of trauma processing. *Interna-tional Journal of Integrative Psychology, 4*(2), 24–39. https://integrative-journal.com/index.php/ijip/article/viewFile/72/57

Linehan, M. M. & Schmidt, H. (1995). The dialectics of effective treatment of borderline personality disorder. In W. T. O'Donohue & L. Krasner (Eds.), *Theories of behavior therapy: Exploring behavior change* (pp. 553–584). Washington, DC: American Psy-chological Association.

Manfield, P., Lovett, J., Engel, L., & Manfield, D. (2017). Use of the flash technique in EMDR therapy: Four case examples. *Journal of EMDR Practice and Research, 11*(4), 195–205. https://doi.org/10.1891/1933-3196.11.4.195

Ogden, P., Minton, K., & Pain, C. (2006). *Trauma and the body: A sensorimotor approach to psychotherapy.* New York: Norton.

Schrader, B. (2019). *Fight to live, live to fight: Veteran activism after war (SUNY series in new political science).* New York: State University of New York Press.

Shapiro, F. (2018). *Eye Movement Desensitization and Reprocessing (EMDR) basic principles, protocols and procedures* (3rd ed.). New York: Guilford.

Shapiro, R. (2005). The two-hand interweave. In R. Shapiro (Ed.), *EMDR solutions: Pathways to healing* (pp. 160–166). New York: Norton.

Siegel, D. J. & Payne Bryson, T. (2020). *The power of showing up: How parental presence shapes who our kids become and how their brains get wired.* New York: Ballantine Books.

Thom, K. C. & Ching, K. Y. (2017). *From the stars in the sky to the fish in the sea.* Vancouver, BC: Arsenal Pump Press.

Chapter 12

Playing with Connection through Boundaries

This chapter continues our exploration of how to purposefully integrate our play-ful spirit to promote meaningful and lasting change in trauma treatment through its focus on healing relational connections harmed by trauma. Specifically, we will focus on how to heal the traumatic effects of too much or too little connec-tion in which important others *come too close* or *go too far away,* resulting in feeling unbearably alone. Aloneness emerges from boundary violations that are experienced as intrusive and suffocating—as in physical, sexual, or emotional abuse—or absent—as in physical or emotional abandonment and neglect. Some-times, one trauma, like lockdown during COVID, can simultaneously bring both too much and too little closeness and feelings of isolation (from our sense of Self and others). First, let's see how and why adaptations of distance and close-ness emerge before examining three cases that represent how to playfully do this work with clients of all ages.

Sensorimotor Adaptations to Trauma across the Lifespan

We can adapt to trauma at any point in life. As discussed in Chapter 2, at any age, and necessarily during preverbal years, trauma causes brain functioning to shift to right hemisphere and reptilian brain dominance with its instinctive, sen-sorimotor, survival-promoting mechanisms. Related sensorimotor behaviors or procedurally learned action patterns (Ogden et al., 2006) develop and get wired in with repetition.

In response to relational trauma, the sequence of movements that enable us to satisfy our need to re-establish safety is affected—yield, push, reach, grasp, and pull (see Chapter 8 and the satisfaction cycle). For example, we may learn to become submissive and not reach, grasp, or pull effectively and instead yield without our need(s) getting seen or fully met. Or we may learn to become overly aggressive, pushing too hard and grasping and pulling too frequently. These sen-sorimotor adaptations become procedurally learned memories which serve as our go-to way to cope with relationships and circumstances that we neurocept as

DOI: 10.4324/9781003509493-18

similarly threateningly. Eventually, due to internal working models (see Bowlby in Chapter 2), our brain and body may generalize these adaptations to many relationships and situations subjectively perceived as threatening, even if not objectively endangering. The earlier these procedurally learned sensorimotor action patterns get wired in and the more frequently they're used, the more practice clients need to re-wire new patterns and develop healthy, respectful boundaries for connecting securely.

Needed Developmental Skills for Attachment Security

Supporting our clients to form healthy boundaries for safe and secure connection necessitates that they know and feel seen and cared for by others. This enables mastery of the developmental skills of object permanence and object constancy (see Chapter 4). While usually achieved by toddlerhood, we know many of our relationally traumatized clients have not yet achieved these skills leaving them feeling untethered and dysregulated when relational conflicts, inconsistencies, rejections, or abandonments arise. Let's briefly review these developmental milestones and see how sensorimotor playfulness in attachment-informed trauma treatment can re/establish relational security.

Missing Milestones

To review, object permanence refers to the baby's physical interactions with the world and their ability to sense something exists even if it they can't see, smell, or touch it. The internalized sense of object permanence says, "I know you're physically always here/there." The baby who knows the block hidden behind their father's back still exists even though they can't see it has achieved object permanence. The normal emergence of separation anxiety reflects the infant/toddler's practice of internalizing the sense and knowing that a parent's physical separation is not permanent and forever—it is a temporary distance, not permanent absence.

Building on object permanence is object constancy, which refers to the baby's emotional and relational interactions with their caregivers. Object constancy reflects the little one's ability to internalize a constant image or sense of their caregiver's traits, particularly of love and care, even when the caregiver isn't present. "I feel your care/love whether you're here or not." Object constancy helps little ones deal with separation from caregivers because it allows them to experience emotional permanence: the emotional trust that others have enduring traits (hopefully) of valuing and loving them no matter what has happened between them. Emotional permanence enables children to hold a full sense of their caregiver as positive, despite them sometimes acting attuned and nurturing and other times not. As children with object constancy mature, they can relate to others as being a whole being and not just their positive or negative parts. This translates into "I feel your enduring love/care despite the ups and downs that have happened between us." This developmental achievement is part of what facilitates the formation of secure attachment.

These relational developmental milestones are critical to forming healthy boundaries and attachment security in and outside of therapy. Without object permanence, the caregiver's or therapist's separation can feel like a physical disappearance forever, causing a deep and terrifying void. No one can survive without connection. Meanwhile those who haven't achieved object constancy lack a sense of emotional permanence and constantly seek reassurance and soothing from caregivers or therapists that they won't be emotionally abandoned or betrayed. They deal with the caregiver's or therapist's emotional attunements or misattunements through defensive splitting, believing the other is either 100% supportive or unsupportive. They struggle to hold the entirety of the relationship with its ups and downs, instead seeing things as all positive or negative. Consequently, change and relational separations during infancy and later in life feel unsafe and can compromise individuation—visible in anxious/ambivalent and disorganized/chaotic adaptation styles like borderline personality. Avoidant styles present as extremely separate and individuated—being fiercely independent, capable, and tending not to rely on others. (For a fuller review, see Chapter 2.)

Achieving Milestones

Fortunately, if object constancy hasn't been mastered, we can playfully support its growth and integration through the healing therapy relationship. When very young children separate from their caregiver, they will get a hug or kiss and merrily go on their way. For children who have some difficulty, I recommend parents read the book *The Kissing Hand* (Penn, 1993) with them. It is a lovely story about Chester getting reassurance any time he separates from his mother, Mrs. Raccoon, and feels scared. Mrs. Raccoon gives Chester a kiss in the middle of his palm and says to Chester, "With a Kissing Hand, we'll never be apart. Just press your hand upon your cheek and feel that loving glow. It's Mommy saying, 'I love you,' wherever you may go."

Clients have creatively adapted this message for their children. For example, one father told his son, "Whenever we're apart, just look up at the sky and see the sun, stars, moon, and clouds. Remember, I will be seeing the same sky wherever I am. It will connect us, always." Some parents share with their children that their Higher Power (e.g., God) is in the skies and heavens, holding both of them together.

In addition, young children can be given a concrete, transitional object that symbolizes or reminds them of their connection with the caregiver from whom they're separating. Touching, holding, seeing, smelling, or sucking on the object literally helps them *feel* a connection with their caregiver when apart. The transitional object provides comfort, soothing, and security as the child shifts from relying on their primary caregiver as their main, or even sole, source of soothing to an object they can control. Very young children may focus on tactile sensations, like a soft blanket or squishy stuffed animal. By contrast, some school-aged children who have awareness of how others view them may feel embarrassed by having a "baby" thing. They may opt for something more age-appropriate to remind them of their connection, like a watch, piece of jewelry, or marble, which they can put in their pocket and touch or look at. Or they may prefer a note in their lunchbox, which they can read at any time to feel connection.

However, clients who come to therapy with separation issues and struggle with object constancy may not find these practices sufficiently soothing when separated. This may in part be due to fears that when leaving the caregiver, harm may come to them. We need to remember, in the natural order of things, infants and toddlers need and want to explore their world and separate from their primary caregiver. However, those with separation anxiety have internalized the experience from those around them: "We are/I am not safe, or the world outside the home isn't safe, so don't leave."

For example, when relational trauma occurs in the home (e.g., domestic violence, substance abuse), a child may not feel safe to leave, feeling they must stay and protect siblings or even parents. Other times, parents consciously or unconsciously impart messages of feeling alone and abandoned and need the child to stay close to soothe them. By contrast, caregivers can convey messages that the world is unsafe and others can't be trusted, as children of Holocaust survivors have experienced. Finally, when children reach their parents' trigger age, the age the parent was when harmed, the caregiver may feel particular resistance to their dependent's separation and exploration of the world around them.

In an ideal world, our clients will have mastered object permanence and constancy before entering treatment. However, in the real world as a trauma therapist, we work with clients (and their intrapsychic parts) of all ages who have not yet achieved these developmental milestones. This means the work will go more slowly as we work with greater compassion, sensitivity, and patience to establish these milestones. Clients who lack these achievements may get very dysregulated when we go on vacation or cancel a session due to illness. These clients also may need more frequent contact between sessions through texts, emails, short calls, or voicemails. We need to know if we are practically and emotionally capable of providing this consistent, predictable, stable contact and reassurance (within limits), because these clients not only are hungry for it, their youngest, most insecurely attached parts need it. Working with these clients can be extremely emotionally challenging yet equally rewarding because achieving these milestones so positively impacts their healing and transformation.

Fortunately, by targeting our clients' sensorimotor adaptations to trauma, therapists can promote change at its root. The case examples in this chapter focus heavily on showing the reader how to use relational, sensorimotor playfulness to establish and wire in healthier physical boundaries, which translate into healthier social and emotional connections. The three cases—a child, a teenager, and an adult couple—illustrate playful ways to practice and re-wire movement patterns and physical boundaries to ensure that clients' needs are met in attuned ways. We will see how different clients need to strengthen under-used and rebalance over-used movement patterns to help them relate more healthily and appropriately.

Sensorimotor Boundary Practices to Heal Connection

Questions to Guide Our Practice

When working in bottom-up, heavily relational, and/or somatic ways with clients and their boundaries, we need to help them stay mindful of and answer the following questions when relating to themselves and others (e.g., family member, friend, co-worker, and significant other):

- Where do I begin and end in physical space? What is my me? What is your you?
- How do I share space or objects with you? *Is* it and does it *feel* safe and respectful to me and to you?
- How do I/we effectively maintain my/each other's boundaries?
- How do I/we violate my/each other's boundaries?
- How do I/we re-establish healthy boundaries?
- How, when, where, and with whom do I/we need to shift my/our boundaries?

We can observe and reflect back to our clients:

- Which movements are easiest? Hardest?
- How consciously and effectively can they modulate their use?
- How well and with whom do these movements get their needs met fully? Partially? Not at all?

In addition, guided by the satisfaction cycle, we can assess how our clients use movements and language—or others' descriptions of them—related to yield, push, reach, grasp, and pull. For example, overreliance on push can be associated with erect postures, a puffed-out chest, and readiness to pounce, and words like push, strong, demanding, aggressive, controlling, force, etc. In contrast, overdependence on yield may appear with hunched postures, collapsed shoulders, floppy arms, and words like weak, pushover, collapse, submissive, compliant, sheepish, etc. As we heighten our personal and clients' awareness about imbalances or inefficacies with particular movements related to satisfying their needs, we open avenues for playful proprioceptive and sensorimotor practices to promote neuroplasticity and change. Let's see how.

Three Cases across the Life Cycle: Sensorimotor Playing with Boundaries to Promote Connection

Seven-Year-Old Nikki: Establishing Boundaries to Separate

Nikki experienced a double fear. First, she would be forgotten about by her parents, whom she felt deeply dismissed by and wondered whether they really loved her, and second, that harm would befall her from unsafe others in the world. Nikki presented as anxious, with problems self-soothing, separating, and developing friendships.

Her parents described Nikki as extremely clingy and colicky for her first 8 months, which blindsided them since none of Nikki's older siblings behaved the same way when they were babies. For the first year of Nikki's life, her parents felt at a loss, exhausted, and incompetent. They hardly slept and neglected the care of their other children and the house. As a result, they decided to put Nikki in daycare at an earlier age than her siblings.

After a few weeks, Nikki resisted going. She screamed and flailed when put in her car seat. When Nikki was 15 months old and had some words, her parents learned that she was being physically and emotionally abused by one of her daycare workers. They immediately pulled Nikki out and kept her home until kindergarten. Her elderly grandparents watched Nikki so her parents could work. She did not have playdates because her grandparents had limited mobility and noise tolerance. To keep her quiet, they gave her food and an iPad to watch hours of videos. The COVID pandemic happened during what would have been Nikki's kindergarten year; she, yet again, learned the world wasn't safe. When COVID restrictions lifted, going to school or camp became a harrowing and draining ordeal for Nikki and her parents. However, worst of all, her inability to separate from her mother worsened at home. Nikki clung to mom's legs frequently and screamed in panic when mom went to the bathroom and tried to close the door for privacy. In the middle of the night, Nikki often found her way into her parents' bed.

Boundary practice. When starting therapy, Nikki could not separate from her mother to enter my office for play sessions. So, I included mom. I observed the quality of their attachment and noticed mom's explicit and implicit messages. At times, she welcomed when heavy and tall Nikki spontaneously climbed or jumped into her lap. Other times, mom pushed Nikki off, became silent, and stopped looking at her. I worked with mom to make explicit and consistent boundaries about her physical comfort. She told Nikki, "I like it when you sit on my lap calmly. And you need to ask me first if I'm okay with it."

To further help Nikki practice empathy and mentalization, I invited mom to "sit" on Nikki's lap or lean on her heavily without first asking. It got the point across. Nikki blurted, "Ow! That doesn't feel good. You need to ask me before you do that!" We explored how Nikki and her mother could share physical connection in mutually comfortable, appropriate, and satisfying ways in therapy and at home.

The consistency and clarity of mom's messaging and behaviors helped Nikki settle, which I noticed out loud, "Being close in ways that are comfortable for you and mom feels calming." This statement privileged the positive, which I tried to deepen and expand. "You both have big smiles. Your breathing seems in rhythm too." I asked them to breathe into the emotions and asked them to notice "How does your body feels sharing space together this way?"

Nikki nodded yes and said, "Good."

Mom said, "Yah, good." It became clear across sessions that Nikki had an extensive vocabulary for negative, disturbing emotions but not positive ones—based on her fraught history of being criticized. I offered both the mother and Nikki different choices to expand their feelings vocabulary for positive affect.

"Oh, does that mean you feel relaxed? Happy? Safe? Comfortable? Close in your heart?" With practice in sessions and at home, Nikki's positive affect vocabulary expanded—as did mom's and reportedly dad's too, who infrequently attended sessions. Concomitantly, Nikki's teacher shared at parent-teacher conferences that Nikki was acting more respectful of her peers' physical space than earlier in the school year. These generalized effects of our boundary practices were encouraging.

Separation/Object permanence and constancy. We practiced having Nikki separate from her mother in small, playful ways. First, we used a ball toss game. Nikki and her mother alternately tossed the ball to each other. Each time someone caught the ball, they took a baby step back ward, literally creating distance between them. If they missed, they came back together and started again standing toe to toe. The goal was to create as much physical distance between the two that Nikki could tolerate and still successfully catch the ball. We started the game in my office. After a few successful catches, I asked them to take a medium step backward. We were literally increasing Nikki's ANS (autonomic nervous system) and affect tolerance for separating physically from her mom.

When the giant steps took them outside the boundaries of my office, we moved into the hallway where they could experiment with more distance. We practiced throwing the ball in silly ways—underneath the leg, spinning around a bunch of times, and then throwing it forward and then backward to each other. Each missed catch caused them to stay in place, which Nikki found a bit frustrating. She was a competitive child, so not advancing in the game frustrated her more than the growing distance dysregulated her. I chose this game because it was a powerful, paradoxical metaphor: achieving distance felt fun and was a success while staying in place or moving closer was a failure. The game provided a juxtaposition experience because fun and distancing/achieving a goal were incompatible with the anxiety and frustration of staying in place/ not progressing.

In the next session, we continued to play with separation/object constancy through the ball toss game as we proceeded from the office, to the hallway, into the parking lot. I encouraged them to throw in funky and unpredictable ways so catching the ball became harder, which Nikki liked. We practiced throwing the ball backward so the thrower couldn't see the receiver. Nikki loved how catching the ball became even more challenging. More importantly, when mom was "out of sight," Nikki did not equate this with mom's absence. However, when she couldn't see mom, Nikki would yell, "Are you ready?" thus reestablishing auditory connection to soothe herself. Soon I added another challenge: asking each to stay quiet because it would make it harder to catch the ball. They could face each other, but the thrower would have to keep their eyes closed.

When the distance became too far to toss and catch the ball successfully, I invited them to switch to a call-and-response game. We changed from visual, proprioceptive, and tactile channels of connection to a solely auditory one. I invited them to close their eyes, wait to hear each other make a noise, and then echo the same noise in response. If they did, they could take another step back. I stayed by Nikki's side, as a safe anchor. We played on a quiet sidewalk. Eventually, Nikki and I proceeded around the corner and she was too far apart from her mom to see or hear her. I switched the game to a text call-and-response game in which mom sent a text to Nikki on my phone and she replied. This game had now switched from auditory to visual connection using age-appropriate reading. Texts from her mother served as a transitional object to aid her separation. Since Nikki could not see or hear her mother, she had to wait for re-connection through text.

We played with slowing down the text response to further increase Nikki's tolerance of distance from mom, while I made comments like, "Wow, mom is texting back slowly and you are so patient. I wonder what she will text you?" At times, Nikki showed some agitation and wanted to run back to her mother. I'd reassure her, "You know she'll respond. She's not as quick a texter as you. Breathe into your patience. Remember: She's there, even if you can't see or hear her right now. Isn't that pretty cool how you're still connected yet apart? What's that feel like?"

Nikki responded, "Okay, but she's still doesn't text as fast as me."

"True," I responded. "And check inside. How does your body feel as you wait?" I had also helped Nikki identify younger "baby parts" (Nikki's term) and find ways to listen to their needs and soothe them. Sometimes, this meant slowing down with breath, other times jumping up and down or spinning around, other times balling up into a fetal position and covering herself up with a blanket. We practiced tuning into her younger parts in ways that fit each environment she was in.

Over three or four sessions, the ball toss game morphed dramatically and, truth be told, unpredictably. Using attunement on steroids (see Chapter 8), I followed my creative intuition while tuning into Nikki's style and preferences. I stayed intentional and mindful, intent on keeping the playful interventions focused on assisting Nikki to internalize an image and felt-sense connection of her mother while distant.

At this point, I recommended mom read *The Kissing Hand* to Nikki, which Nikki previously dismissed and disliked—perhaps because she had not achieved object permanence and constancy. This time Nikki was receptive and asked mom to send little notes with a "surprise" sticker in her lunchbox. Even when mom forgot one day, Nikki remained regulated at school. She had learned to soothe younger dysregulated parts with her 7-year-old wise Self. When she got home, she appropriately expressed sadness and disappointment, which mom validated and soothed. I reflected and explicitly celebrated this growth and accomplishment to both of them.

Nikki's preverbal and toddler parts seemingly had developed object constancy and moved through the separation anxiety which she had not mastered earlier in life. Her parents also developed greater attunement and patience. I had given them psychoeducation about parts of mind (Internal Family Systems [IFS] Schwartz & Sweezy, 2020) and protector parts related to Structural Dissociation of the Personality (SD) (see van der Hart et al., 2006 in Chapter 2) in relation to Nikki's traumas. When Nikki physically reached for help and support, it was no longer panicky. Her grasp and pull movements no longer had a desperate, dysregulated, or clingy feel. She was able to move through the satisfaction cycle completely and appropriately. Together Nikki and her parents had met a previously unmet developmental need to help Nikki soothe. In addition, Nikki's growing ability to self-soothe served her well when new family traumas arose and her parents could not attune to her needs.

Seventeen-Year-Old Gwen: Establishing Separateness and Connecting to Younger Parts of Mind

Gwen came to her initial session with both parents and asked they stay, which is not typical of teenagers. When I asked Gwen why she was coming to meet me, she said, "My parents thought it would help. They've sent me to therapy since I was 6, yet I still have trouble going places without them." Gwen was making it clear that she had lost hope in the therapy process yet felt forced to attend by her parents.

I continued to ask Gwen questions and let her parents know I'd get to them shortly—since it was apparent they played an important role co-creating this dynamic with their daughter. I wanted to establish boundaries to learn what Gwen's hook was into treatment, separate and distinct from that of her parents'. I made this boundary separation explicit by asking, "So Gwen, what do *you* want, whether or not it's the same as what your parents want?" This allowed for the expression of separate needs, which may or may not overlap with her parents' needs.

She replied, "I get really dysregulated when I try to go to sleepaway camp, a school trip, sleepovers with my friends, or out with my boyfriend. I used to wet my bed, but at least I got over that!"

I said, "No longer wetting your bed is an accomplishment. And it sucks that you can't yet do what *you* want." I then dropped my shoulders and exhaled audibly in a nonverbal effort to connect. "And you used the word, 'dysregulated.' Gwen, you weren't kidding that you've had some therapy! Not many 17-year-olds use that word, much less accurately and easily put it into a sentence!" I said laughingly, trying to establish a sarcastic connection, "You use psychobabble terms like me!"

She smiled and said with pride, and perhaps hidden shame, "Yeah, I've had more therapy by 17 than most people probably have had in their whole lives!"

I enjoyed her smarts, wit, and I felt compassion for her wounded and hopeless parts. All that therapy and not enough to show for it—that's demoralizing. I said, "I can imagine you would have a skeptical part that doesn't believe therapy will help, or won't help much, and another part that has some hope." She nodded. I introduced the dialectic between parts of mind, which I later learned she had no previous experience with.

I turned to her parents, who were ready to share the laundry list of Gwen's diagnoses of separation anxiety, obsessive compulsive disorder, generalized anxiety disorder, possible bipolar disorder, and some possible borderline tendencies. She was on medication since age 10, including Lexapro and Xanax as needed. I watched Gwen roll her eyes (her fight protector) and shrink deeper into the couch (submit/shame protector). I noticed this out loud, "Wow, Gwen. I saw your eyes roll and you sink deeper into the couch."

She seemed to appreciate being noticed and said, "Yeah, I'm a walking DSM (Diagnostic and Statistical Manual) to them!"

"That was funny, in a very sad kind of way," I said, then paused and made a sad face while engaging eye-to-eye gaze. I held it with a head nod, and she droopily nodded in return. I continued and pendulated to an opposite affect state of pride, "And you really know how to use your psychobabble," I said with a wink. Gwen and I were connecting through sarcasm and realism.

I continued with her parents, "You can imagine this might be hard for Gwen to hear."

They both nodded with compassion and turned to Gwen, "You know we wouldn't bring you here unless we thought this could help you and us?" (This seemed an interesting admission.) "We don't think you and we have to live this way forever." (Their struggle was embedded in Gwen's.) They elaborated how they worried that as Gwen approached taking college entrance exams, she would not be able to live an independent life, go to college, or move away to start a career and family. "We know she desperately wants a life on her own, and we want that for her too!" They wanted her to separate and individuate, and they wanted to do the same.

The parents articulated an extensive family history of extreme relational trauma. Both parents were therapy savvy: each attended individual treatment and couples therapy together. Gwen's mother had been hospitalized for dissociative identity disorder-related issues a handful of times. She had an extremely abusive and neglectful disorganized attachment history. Dad had one marked by deep emotional absence and dismissiveness. The parents admitted that because of their histories, they had tried to allay all discomfort in Gwen since birth. Both parents were loving, caring, well-intentioned, and motivated to do better—for Gwen's and their own sake. The dynamics with Gwen were taking a toll on the entire family, including her 13-year-old brother Evan and 11-year-old sister Sarah.

The parents shared how Gwen had been an extremely colicky infant. During her first 6 months of life, her mother suffered debilitating postpartum depression and was often unresponsive to Gwen's cries. The mother would collapse onto her bed and cry while the father came to the rescue. He'd frequently swoop in and comfort Gwen at the hint of her starting to cry. Over the years, both parents recalled trying to rescue Gwen from any discomfort, which they admitted caused them distress. The parents were expressing, perhaps not consciously, that Gwen's dysregulated states triggered their younger parts' distress. To correct their histories, they overcompensated; they tried to quash any hint of Gwen's dysregulation, preventing her from developing self-soothing skills. Additionally, her separation anxiety stage of development was met with her parents frequently staying close to her side: they aborted attempts to leave her and stopped her from going too far away from them, lest harm come to her. This dynamic interfered with Gwen developing object permanence and constancy.

Gwen's first experience of separation anxiety occurred when she was 6 after her very close and loving aunt suddenly died of a heart attack right before joining her and her family for their annual family vacation. Gwen developed obsessive thoughts and compulsions, which caused her parents to bring her to therapy for the next two and a half years. While therapy helped decrease her obsessive and compulsive symptoms, at age 8, Gwen started bedwetting, preventing her from going to sleepovers. She started therapy again and her bedwetting stopped, but her anxiety increased around separations. She was put on medication by age 10, which helped decrease the intensity of her anxiety, but Gwen was not able to stay overnight at her friends' houses—often crying by midnight to be picked up. Overnight camp became a nightmare, causing her parents to pick her up after a week. Brother Evan reportedly felt, "Gwen controls my life and my family's," while sister Sarah withdrew into her world of gaming.

Separation, object permanence and constancy, and intrapersonal cooperation. After a number of individual sessions with Gwen in which we worked on our connection, she learned about her internal system using IFS and SD. She identified parts of her mind and related action systems. Gwen identified a "Baby Gwenny" self-state as the part that hijacked her, causing her to panic when separating from her family. Gwen said her baby believed, "I don't exist if I can't see them [her family]. Or if they can't see me, I am not there."

Gwen suggested we have a family session and include Evan and Sarah. "Even though Evan is only in middle school, he seems more stable and emotionally well-adjusted than the rest of our family combined! He might have some good insights!"

"What about Sarah?" I asked.

Gwen responded, "She's bright but a gaming freak. Who knows, maybe she'll add something to the mix!"

I loved that Gwen was starting to direct the course of treatment, which I reinforced through a metacognitive statement, "You really are a great co-therapist, Gwen. I trust your instincts and direction. Let's do it!"

In the first family session, Evan expressed the irony of Gwen's separation issues: "We ask her to come out to dinner with us, hang out with us at home or at the dog park, but she always finds a reason to hang out with her friends instead. But as soon as she goes away from home, she texts and calls us incessantly. And, when she's with us, she's constantly texting her friends. When our parents tell her, 'No phones in the restaurant,' and she can't text her friends, Gwen has a panic attack."

Sarah added, "And they say I have the problem with screen time. Ha!"

This tension perfectly encapsulated the struggle between Gwen's parts: the one that wanted age-appropriate independence, and the younger ones that did not achieve object permanence, constancy, or healthy separation.

During the session, I first educated the family about parts of mind and then asked everyone to indulge me in a game. I asked Gwen to pay attention to all parts and what they felt. I asked her to take a pillow and play peek-a-boo with her parents and siblings. Fortunately, no one found this game too infantile. Gwen tentatively looked over the top of the pillow and, when making eye contact with everyone, she demanded, "Look more excited to see me!" At this point, her parents and siblings became more animated; they enthusiastically started giggling and cheering when their gazes met. When asked to put up the pillow to disconnect eye contact, Gwen never fully put it up. It seemed her Baby Gwenny part was not comfortable with them being completely out of sight.

To further assess Gwen's overall comfort with separation, I asked if she would walk out to the waiting room with me by her side and leave her family in the consultation room. Gwen went along with the experiment, continuing to scan all parts of mind. Once she closed the door and could no longer see them, Gwen became agitated and began to cry, saying, "I don't know why I'm crying." Her Baby Gwenny self-state was feeling uncomfortable, sad, and anxious at this separation.

I narrated, "Your Baby Gwenny part can't hear, see, feel, or smell your family and might feel that they are gone forever." The agitation increased in Gwen's body, which she acknowledged. I asked Gwen to use the ways she had learned to soothe this dysregulated part. Through breathing, hugging her body with her arms, and looking into my eyes for reassurance, she calmed a bit. However, only when opening the door to see her family, did she fully calm.

We narrated what happened and debriefed. Gwen thought we needed to help her baby part have more practice. Everyone agreed. In the next session, to support the development of object permanence for Gwen's baby state, the intervention was playful, concrete, and tactile. I adapted Katie O'Shea's (2003) heart-to-heart string of connection with Anna Gomez's heart jar (2013, pp. 99–100) practices. While she was seated, I asked Gwen to hold one end of a 3-foot piece of yarn firmly in her hand and place it on her heart. Her parents and siblings, on the couch perpendicular to Gwen, were asked to firmly hold different parts of the yarn on their hearts too. They were instructed to notice the tension in the yarn, which helped concretize the connection between their hearts and Gwen's. Gwen was asked to bilaterally tap, using her left and right hands (bilateral stimulation [BLS] from Eye Movement Desensitization and Reprocessing, Shapiro, 2018) to resource her felt sense of connection. Then, I asked Gwen to send along her sensory experience of connection with her breath and an imagined heart-to-heart string between her heart and Baby Gwenny's. At this point, I suggested Gwen take a few steps away—to start separating—from her family and pull the yarn to its most taught point. Again, I asked her to notice the tightness of connection, breathe, and perform BLS.

I then replaced the 3-foot yarn with a spool of yarn over 200 yards long to allow practice with greater distance. Again, Gwen held one end on her heart, while her family members held other parts of it on theirs. This time Gwen gradually walked away while her family stayed in place, holding the yarn on their hearts. First Gwen walked 8 feet away to the threshold of the office door. Here, she could still see and hear her family. She then moved out the door around the corner into the waiting room where she couldn't see but could still hear them. Everybody commented about the tension in the yarn as it wrapped around the corner of the door frame and was told to, "Notice the heart-to-heart connection you feel with each other through the yarn." I cued Gwen to spontaneously use BLS as her Baby Gwenny needed to calm and strengthen her sense of connection. The family and Gwen playfully tugged at it, cuing each other to mirror back with a tug. Gwen then moved into the hallway, no longer able to hear or see her family, but still feel the tension in the yarn. "Notice how you can feel the connection to them, even though you can't see or hear them." She used BLS as needed. Gwen proceeded to test the comfort limits of her separation by moving out of the hallway and through the door leading to the stairwell. She laughed as she noticed the colorful yarn wrapping itself around the doorway. Then Gwen proceeded up one floor, getting a kick out of the colorful string moving with her around the banister.

I asked if she wanted me to join her and Gwen said, "Nah."

"Okay, I'll stay here," I responded. She no longer needed me to assist her separation.

Gwen then ascended one more flight, to the very top of the stairway. As she called to me, two floors down, I encouraged Gwen to notice her body and emotions, especially Baby Gwen's to being so far away from her family. Gwen said she felt them with her in her heart and it felt good. She used BLS to more deeply anchor-in this feeling. When sitting with this felt sense for about a half a minute, Gwen was asked what she wanted to do—and she spontaneously let go of the string and announced, "I still feel connected to them." BLS was used again. Eventually, she chose to come back downstairs and reconnect with her family. She was joyful and pleased with herself. We reviewed the purpose of the experiment. All the family members shared how "powerful" and "fun" it was. They laughed.

To test how well Gwen had helped her baby part achieve object permanence and constancy through an internalized, felt-sense connection with them, the family was instructed to play peek-a-boo again with Gwen. This time Gwen raised the pillow really high to entirely block seeing her family and them seeing her face. When she brought the pillow down to see them, she moved it fully down and away from her face. She seemed to be at greater ease, even though her family was not particularly animated upon seeing Gwen's face emerge from behind the pillow. This was a win.

To further test her object permanence and constancy and tolerance for separation, I invited Gwen to leave the office with me. We closed the door behind us. I asked her to connect with her baby state and notice what she felt. Gwen announced, "Calm," and added, "I feel she and I are a team. Handling this together." She smiled broadly.

When reentering the room her family asked, "So now what?"

Gwen spontaneously responded, "Florida"—referring to the state where her favorite college was. Her family responded with some disbelief and encouragement.

Interpersonal boundaries. As separation anxiety is a family systems issue, I also needed to help Gwen and her parents, specifically, develop appropriate boundaries to allow for safe distancing. I worked collaboratively with her parents' respective therapists to make sure family session gains were supported. I sincerely shared how much I appreciated the parents' openness to experiments. They admitted to often being perplexed at the games we played but grew to trust they'd always walk away having learned something in a fun way. I explicitly thanked them for their trust in me, the process, and Gwen.

In another session, I asked if they would try another experiment in which Gwen would direct them to do something and they'd follow her lead. They looked at each other and then me and Gwen quizzically, and said, "Why not?"

I explained we would play a version of the Mother, May I? game, called Gwen, May I? in which Gwen would literally direct them to create comfortable physical boundaries of closeness and distance. Similar to early caregiver-dependent attunement play, the rules of the game are dependent-centric, driven by only the child's needs and comfort. It helps the parent/caregiver attune on steroids and get a deeper sense of their child's comfort with proximity/distance while separating out their own needs.

Gwen stood on the far side of my consultation room and one parent stood on the other. She was asked to tell her parent to take one step at a time toward her, pausing to assess her physical comfort with their proximity. She used cues from her repeated internal body scans to decide what distance felt right to *her*—regardless of how her parent might feel. Then Gwen was asked to direct each parent's body position to face toward, away, or sideways from her. She could tell them whether to make direct or indirect eye contact and how to move their arms—whether to reach toward her, rest them by their sides, or put them behind their back. The parent could ask, "Gwen, would you feel comfortable if I . . .?" acknowledging that Gwen had the final say. This game allows client and caregiver to establish, rewire, and encode comfortable and attuned physical boundaries and emotional connection. It gives the dependent full agency and control in directing their caregiver to physically attune in just-right ways, which promotes feeling and being safe, seen, and soothed.

Interestingly, Gwen felt most at ease in her mother's presence when she stood about 3 feet away, had a sideways gaze, with her arms down by her side. By contrast, Gwen felt most comfortable with her father right in front of her, holding eye-to-eye gaze, and reaching out to hug her. These boundaries made sense based on her mother's disorganized and intrusive style of attaching and her father's distant, more avoidant style.

This game beautifully and powerfully spoke volumes without words: Gwen's boundary needs were different and tailored to the dynamics with each parent. I reflected how this fun experiment helped them discover the most attuned, dyadic fit for Gwen's boundary needs. I encouraged them to discuss how it matched their own comfort needs and supported their attunement to Gwen's comfort without disregarding their own going forward. They learned to negotiate how much time they spent together and with what level of physical closeness/distance. Gwen and her family worked and played hard together in treatment and now have a lovely, open, mutually respectful, and healthy-boundaried connection to show for it.

Kurt and Chrissy: Attempting to Grow Connection

Kurt, a 41-year-old VP of marketing at a Fortune 500 company, entered individual therapy at the behest of his wife Chrissy, 38, who claimed he needed "anger management" work. Kurt married Chrissy 15 years prior, feeling she would fit the profile of a good mother and spouse, and, "I thought she was really attractive." Over the course of their marriage, Kurt and Chrissy were a good team in running the household and raising their four children. While others thought they had the "ideal" marriage, Kurt said it felt vacuous, devoid of true joy, deep love, and satisfying sex.

In the first six months of treatment, Kurt became increasingly sullen as he started connecting with what underlay his anger: deep sadness. He started to identify feeling similar to when he was a teenager, "I had no 'corner guy,' someone who I knew would be there for me no matter what." Kurt was an only child. His mother had had three miscarriages prior to conceiving Kurt. He described his mother as a barely functioning alcoholic, who kept a secretarial job but at home was constantly crying and unable to cope. His father was a nose-to-the-grindstone, blue-collar worker who was handy and frugal, raised by Depression-era parents, and had no time for "pansy feelings." His mother followed his father's lead.

Kurt noticed similarities between Chrissy and his mom, who never initiated, only complied. Kurt said even sexually his wife was passive. He felt unseen by her, shamed for his perverted sense of humor, and very emotionally distant. He shared Chrissy's history of being raised by a single mother with post-traumatic stress disorder and flashbacks that triggered psychotic-like reactions. With no father in the picture, Chrissy was protected by her brother, four years her senior. Kurt said she never spoke about her history, leaving many questions unanswered.

Interpersonal boundaries and connection. As therapy proceeded, Kurt felt increasingly disconnected from Chrissy. Without the ability to emotionally discuss things, Kurt struggled to make bids for connection. He contemplated going outside the marriage for attention, sexually and emotionally, and did. Kurt was a man who attended to all details of his life meticulously, and so, Kurt admitted, "I must have left my chat screen on so Chrissy could discover my infidelity." When she did, he asked Chrissy to come into therapy to discuss his cheating and the state of their marriage. She agreed to, though made no promises about repair.

Kurt sat at the corner of the long couch while Chrissy sat at a 90-degree angle to him in the corner of the separate loveseat. They shared no physical or eye contact. They didn't speak to each other. The air was thick. Chrissy looked around my office to orient. Kurt sat facing me and said, "Doc, what do we do?" His trust in me was strong, but I wasn't sure. Attuned on steroids, I somatically and emotionally scanned for any countertransferences from which I could learn and follow. Probably like Kurt, I felt heaviness and pressure to do something. I sat there breathing and opened my mind and body to whatever came up. The next thing I knew, I walked over to the shelf and picked up a 5-inch diameter, clear, plastic ball that held golden glitter water. I gave it to Chrissy and said, "Here's my glitter ball." She laughed, as did Kurt. I asked, "What made you laugh?"

Kurt answered, "I thought you said 'here's a clitter ball.'"

Chrissy said, "I did too."

The sexual tension was front and center as my glitter ball became a clitter (clitoris) ball.

I smiled and said, "Ahh, now I get it." I continued, "I never thought of it that way, but if you'd like to play with the clitter ball together, you're more than welcome to."

Chrissy held the ball awaiting my direction. I invited her to breathe and notice what her body wanted to do with the ball. Without hesitation, she handed it to Kurt. He took it, without any facial reaction. Then I said to Kurt, "Now breathe. Check inside and notice what your body wants to do with the ball." Kurt immediately pulled the ball closer to his chest and held it there tightly. The nonverbals were deafening and so painful to witness.

I began describing the relational dynamic out loud, focused exclusively on the ball to help manage any dysregulation. "Chrissy, it seems like you want to share the ball with Kurt without hesitation. Kurt, it seems like it's really hard for you to share the ball with Chrissy." I let this comment take up some space and after a few breaths into the silence, asked, "What are you each noticing inside?" This prompted a deep unfolding and articulation of pain. Chrissy shared not feeling seen for how she tried to connect with Kurt. Kurt seemed unmoved and responded that it's hard for him to play ball with someone who never sees anything good in him. His fight protector came front and center. Chrissy withdrew. The clitter ball had revealed all.

At some point, Kurt admitted spontaneously that he had ended his short affair. He confessed that, in some way, he was glad Chrissy found out because it brought them together to work on their marriage, which he felt was limping along. In the remainder of the session, I tried to establish what their treatment goals were. I referred Chrissy for her own therapy to deal with her anguish, feelings of betrayal, and decision about going forward in the marriage. She nodded, saying she felt heard and that made sense to her. Meanwhile, Kurt who seemed tense and was gritting his teeth agreed to continue our individual sessions to help him become aware and take ownership of how his behavior affected Chrissy and learn to communicate his needs and empathize with hers. Releases of information were signed, allowing me and Chrissy's therapist to coordinate care.

Intrarelational connection. With his marriage on the line, and not wanting his children to cope with parental divorce, Kurt's fight protector stepped to the side, allowing his 5- and 15-year-old parts to see the light of day. He connected with memories of being alone in his room, screaming, throwing, and breaking his toys, following him losing a tennis championship match due to his poor serves. As an aspiring college tennis player, he felt his future was crushed. Neither parent came to comfort him.

Later that day, he had asked his father if he had heard him. His father dismissively said, "Yeah, I heard something. But figured you'd get over it, and I had to finish changing the oil in my car."

When he came out of his room, he went to the kitchen and saw his mom, "She was completely sloshed, head down on the kitchen table. She picked her head up to see dried tears on my face, red from crying and screaming. She started wailing uncontrollably, 'Look at me. I'm a terrible mother, I burned the roast again'."

Kurt felt pained, desperate, and invisible.

Having suffered many similar incidents since age 4 or 5, Kurt decided, this was my defining moment; from that day forward, "I'll never again be vulnerable. I'll work my ass off and have enough money to take care of everything I need. No one will ever again have the power to hurt me."

We worked with his wise, paternal compassion, a quality he shared effortlessly with his four children. He was patient, empathic, expressive emotionally and practically—a truly wonderful, attuned, and adoring father. We spent many sessions helping his paternal wise Self show up in similar attuned ways for his own vulnerable and hurt exiles. These parts grew to feel and know they had a real "corner guy" in his adult wise mind. Kurt even allowed himself to feel I was a corner guy/gal for him. Kurt learned to rebalance his tendency to push away and fight with a trusting receive and yield movement. His need to reach, grab hold tightly, and pull in without letting go loosened.

Meanwhile Chrissy's therapist reported that Chrissy seemed hurt, quite guarded, and even dissociated. She had a spotty memory of what she herself deemed a traumatic childhood. The therapist couldn't get a real grasp on Chrissy. She described Chrissy as disconnected, compliant, and not reaching for any obvious real or genuinely helpful support from friends or family. We both agreed, though, that it seemed time to have another couple's session to define what they wanted to do with the marriage.

When Kurt and Chrissy returned, Kurt, with minimal encouragement from me, spontaneously took ownership of his infidelity. He leaned into his compassion, owning his betrayal and how it hurt her. He acted with sincerity. Chrissy listened, yet seemed to be playing it close to the vest. She said she appreciated the work he had done and his apology. Neither Kurt nor I could get a read on what she was really feeling, despite me explicitly checking in with her multiple ways.

I decided to get the clitter ball. This time I offered it to Kurt first. I asked him to notice what his body wanted to do with it and follow that. He sat looking at it, as if reflecting that not sharing it was a reflection of their marriage's deterioration. He looked at Chrissy, reached, and gave it to her. Chrissy put it in her lap and let go of it, leaving it there. I asked Chrissy to take a breath and notice what her body wanted to do with the clitter ball. She looked at it, but left it in her lap. Then she looked at Kurt and said, "It's too late." Chrissy was done sharing the clitter ball with Kurt. My heart sank with and for Kurt. The exact hurt his fight protectors feared had recurred.

However, this time it was different. Kurt knew he was not alone. I was by his side, and more importantly, his wise, adult, paternal Self was with him. After the previous couple's session, Kurt and I continued to meet for individual work.

He believed the marriage was probably irreparable way before his affair. He mourned and struggled, yet put his all into being the best father he could. He also wondered whether Chrissy had started her own affair after finding out about his because within months of filing for divorce, she moved in with another man. Most importantly, Kurt was able to feel the pain and internally validate and soothe it. I also did the same. Kurt faced his worst fear. He learned to become vulnerable and love in healthier ways, find a sexually compatible partner, and raise his children into adulthood in cooperative ways with his ex. There were many challenges, yet Kurt became more real and alive. He changed careers, giving him less financial stability but lots of emotional fulfillment.

More Playfully Spirited Practice to Transform Trauma

Throughout this chapter, we've seen how engaging sensorimotor-based relational playfulness with boundaries promotes deep and lasting change in relational trauma. Case examples illustrated how we can creatively and playfully cut to the heart of the earliest unresolved attachment issues and support clients to achieve developmental milestones of object permanence and constancy, healthily separate and individuate, modulate and tolerate interpersonal proximity, grow intrapersonal cooperation between parts of mind, earn relational security, and wire in healthy satisfaction cycle sequences in which clients' needs are met in attuned ways by self and others.

While attuned on steroids, we've learned how our sensorimotor playful interventions can welcome and address all parts of mind, even the youngest, ensuring they feel and are safe, seen, soothed, and secure. Healing attachment adaptations that no longer serve our clients with playfulness makes the repair work more fun and tolerable to us and our clients.

So far, our exploration into transforming trauma's impact on clients of all ages has shown us how to invite our playful spirit to the elements needed to promote change including ANS and affect regulation, constructive use of multiplicities and dialectics to create juxtaposition experiences and promote memory reconsolidation, and sensorimotor boundary practices to earn security within self and with others. The next chapter shows us how to help our clients access, make meaning of, and integrate their trauma story by being playful with the narrative.

References

Gomez, A. (2013). *EMDR Therapy and adjunct approaches with children: Complex trauma, attachment and dissociation.* New York: Springer.

Ogden, P., Minton, K., & Pain, C. (2006). *Trauma and the body: A sensorimotor approach to psychotherapy.* New York: Norton.

O'Shea, K. (2003). *Accessing and repairing preverbal trauma and neglect.* Paper presented at EMDR Conference, Denver, CO.

Penn, A. (1993). *The kissing hand.* Terra Haute, IN: Tanglewood.

Schwartz, R. C. & Sweezy, M. (2020). *Internal Family Systems* (2nd ed.). New York: Guilford.

Shapiro, F. (2018). *Eye Movement Desensitization and Reprocessing (EMDR) basic principles, protocols and procedures* (3rd ed.). New York: Guilford.

van der Hart, O., Nijenhuis, E. R. S., & Steele, K. (2006). *The haunted self: Structural dissociation and the treatment of chronic traumatization.* New York: Norton.

Chapter 13

Playing with Telling the Trauma Story

In this chapter, we will focus on playing with telling the trauma story—whether it is possible and to what benefit for clients. We'll explore playful nonverbal and verbal ways to facilitate this process. Telling the story, which can manifest in myriad ways, brings integration to the unintegrated and meaning to senselessness.

Telling the Trauma Story: What Is Realistic, Possible, and Helpful?

Many of us learned that a full story has a sequenced plot with a beginning, middle, and end. A conflict is presented and then tidily resolved. Our clients' trauma stories contain all of these elements, but they're often disorganized—sometimes even random, chaotic, illogical, and contradictory. We, and our clients, can't make sense of their narrative. The confused trauma story reflects how the brain implicitly and unconsciously encodes the trauma in the right hemisphere in hard-to-access, disjointed, and incoherent sensorimotor fragments (see Chapter 2).

Telling the trauma story supports the integration of the right brain's implicitly encoded sensorimotor trauma fragments with the explicit and conscious left-brain logical functions that bring coherence and meaning. As with all storytelling, we make sense out of "chaotic and seemingly unrelated events ... an essential self-organizing process that facilitates an increased understanding of self and others" (Paivio & Angus, 2017, p. 41). Healing trauma through telling its story involves creating a new, ordered narrative that is embodied (Panhofer et al., 2012, p. 312), (more) coherent, and vital to one's identity (Panhofer et al., 2012). It's a meaning-making process.

Yet, therapists must figure out what is realistic and even possible to bring implicit, sensorimotor story fragments into an explicit, verbalizable, coherent, integrated narrative that helps our clients make meaning of their trauma. We need to ask ourselves: how will focusing on the trauma narrative *serve our client*? Ideally, we support clients to retell and therefore recreate their trauma narrative in

DOI: 10.4324/9781003509493-19

order to have a transformative experience, a premise based on Accelerated Experiential Dynamic Psychotherapy's (AEDP) sense of transformation (see Korn, 2012). This means telling the trauma narrative will help our clients:

1. Feel calm and safe—experience autonomic nervous system (ANS) regulation and affect tolerance (quiet the amygdala).
2. Make the implicit, explicit—bring the unconscious sensorimotor fragments into consciousness and verbalize them (supporting a right-to-left hemisphere shift).
3. Process the explicit, relationally—work on the conscious narrative in the therapy relationship willingly and organically (healing through right brain-to-right brain relationality).
4. Connect experientially with the story—feel embodied and present in the here-and-now (bringing the brain's prefrontal cortex online to enable mindful awareness and embodiment).
5. Experience transformation—find meaning and healing in the newly integrated, coherent, narrative (supporting hemispheric, relational, and intrapsychic integration) and create space to experience positivity, joy, play, and awe.

For this transformational journey, the telling of the trauma narrative needs to be a client-driven and desired process. It unfolds when and how our client is ready. It is their timeline, *not* the therapist's, their family members', or any other related person's (e.g., attorney's). Not all clients can safely and fully have an integrative, transformational, healing, and narrative-creating experience. Let's explore the factors needed to make this possible.

The Need for Safety and a Supportive Developmental-Relational Context

Safety to tell and create the healing story starts with assurance that it will not dysregulate our client's ANS and surpass their window of affect tolerance (Fisher, 2017; Rothschild, 2021). This means we neither want it to trigger hyperarousal, such as flashbacks, or hypoarousal, such as shutdown. Even when clients seem to be explicitly and coherently sharing their trauma narrative, they may be emotionally disconnected or even dissociative. To support a reparative telling, we need to ensure clients have affect regulation, brain integrative functioning, (not split and dissociative), and relational and intrarelational security and connection.

In addition, we must assess our client's developmental-relational-contextual (D-R-C, see Chapter 1) factors, which may affect creating a healing story. These factors could include the client's dependence on the perpetrator, real-life demands/priorities, and access to resources. Let's explore these now.

Dependence on the Perpetrator

When we work with child and adult clients who depend on their perpetrators for survival, accessing, feeling, knowing, and narrating the full gamut of their trauma experience might be intolerable and too difficult to reconcile. It might even threaten their relationship with their caregiver and, therefore, their life.

For example, Darrin, a 38-year-old high-functioning male on the autism spectrum, was paralyzed after being hit by a car. His care rested solely in his widowed mother's hands. While devoted to him, she also sexually abused him. Darrin could not be expected to share the full story of his multilayered trauma unless his mother owned and stopped her perpetration.

By contrast, 13-year-old Laverne had a great grandfather Elias who sexually abused her and generations of family members, including his own daughters, granddaughters, and great granddaughters. Elias used alcohol and drugs to inebriate and somewhat incapacitate them—which caused them to become alcohol and drug-dependent to numb their emotions, sensations, memories, etc. In his small community, Elias generously donated to his church and was a town councilman who had great influence on the police and judges. When Laverne's 16-year-old cousin tried reporting her victimization, the police dismissed her and the church pastor said, "You are a sinner! You have disrespected your elder, a God-respecting, pillar of the community. God will punish you unless you repent and ask for forgiveness!" Reporting and telling her story to child protective services was a nonstarter, so Laverne's cousin ran away.

Laverne and her mother knew the "rules" and kept in their lane. The most Laverne and her mother could achieve in therapy was acknowledge they felt unsafe, find the most creative ways to protect themselves and other family members, while remaining completely dependent upon Elias for food, shelter, and drugs. Telling her trauma story was not safe and likely would have triggered Laverne's pain, stuckness, and hopelessness. Therapy became a long and complicated journey of empowering Laverne and her mother to get sober, access anonymous community supports (in neighboring towns), gain independence, and move away from their enslavement, while neither confronting nor prosecuting their perpetrator. We support our clients' best version of themself to emerge within the constraints of their D-R-C.

Real-Life Demands/Priorities

Balancing trauma healing work with real-life demands, priorities, and necessities is each therapist's challenge. Child trauma therapists prioritize young clients' safety while mindfully supporting enough healing and stability to promote the child's continued academic, physical, emotional, social, and behavioral development. For example, unless severe safety and functioning are impaired, a therapist will not dissuade a child from joining a sports team, acting in the school play, or going on a well-supervised school trip because they will miss therapy appointments. These activities can potentially support skill development and thriving beyond therapy's reach. Their young client's trauma story may remain untold or incomplete. Similarly, when working with adults, we must prioritize helping our clients achieve what is necessary to function well enough in daily life—whether going to work, caring for dependents, or attending to self-care and hygiene—over the complete telling of the trauma story.

Children and adults can always return to therapy to complete their trauma story when life circumstances allow and they are ready. To support this end, therapists can leave clients wanting more (future healing) by providing them with the experience of being in a positive, reparative relationship in which they feel safe, seen, soothed, and secure. Appropriate playfulness in therapy supports this end.

Access to Resources

While clients may be motivated to discover and express their full trauma narrative, they may not currently have the time or financial resources. Insurance companies that manage sessions or payments sadly interfere with the trauma story's completion. Many of my clients realistically joke about how health insurance bureaucracy traumatizes them further, adding stress to the therapy process. Other urgent or traumatic life events may prevent the story's full reparative creation and telling, like a sudden health concern, move, or job loss. We can hope when children grow into young adulthood and live independent of their caregivers that they may be in a more financially independent and emotionally safe space to revisit and return to telling their stories. By contrast, once-independent adults who become dependent on another may lose their ability to explore their story fully. Such D-R-C factors prompt us to ask whether it is safe or the timing's right for our client to create their full trauma story *now*. To help determine our client's readiness, we can ask the following questions. Does the trauma story:

- Feel—and is it—safe to tell and work through now?
- Serve our client now? How will it help or limit them?
- Dysregulate or calm our client (i.e., will they need more resourcing)?
- Open or close our client's access to resources (e.g., family, community, or religious institutions, financial)?
- Result in intolerable and irreconcilable losses (e.g., family, friends, home, community, house of worship, work, financial) and potential isolation?
- Feel complete and sufficient or incomplete for our client?
- Feel driven more by the therapist's (and/or others') curiosity and needs than the client's?

Having asked these questions, therapists are in a better position to know how to proceed. And in the course of therapy, we may need to repeatedly ask these questions as D-R-C influences change.

Awareness of Trauma-Time Cognitions

Telling, unfolding, and creating the healing trauma narrative are affected by the client's age(s) when their trauma occurred and how it was cognitively encoded. Specifically, when a trauma occurs, we unconsciously develop cognitions or self-attributions to make sense of the life-threatening, unpredictable, uncontrollable, intolerable aspects of the trauma. This is what is meant by the "mind narrates what the nervous system knows" (Dana, 2018, p. 35). These cognitive adaptations are affected by chronological age and cognitive development (Laliotis, 2014).

For example, 48-year-old Noor, who identifies as transgender, was incested—from ages 4 to 8—by their father who was an imam until he committed suicide. Noor could only "make sense" of their abuse and father's suicide by believing they were inherently bad and unworthy of Allah's goodness and protection. This reflected the dichotomous, good/bad, black/white thinking of early childhood. Meanwhile, 48-year-old Jenna, initially abused in college by her first boyfriend, attributed her physical, emotional, and sexual victimization to being naïve about how intimate and monogamous relationships worked. Her self-cognition was not about her inherent worth but her experience as a girlfriend: "I don't know anything. I'm naïve and probably wrong." Future incidents of victimization may be internalized or interpreted through this trauma time–generated belief system. Related internal working models (see Bowlby, 1969 in Chapter 2) or scripts emerge which further entrench its intransigence. As is true for treating all trauma, especially chronic and complex, telling the complete healing narrative effectively and productively requires sensitivity to trauma-time attributions and patience.

Respect for the Process

Creating a coherent and full healing narrative is a process. While single incident traumas experienced in the context of loving supportive others may be narrated fully and to resolution in one or a few sessions, chronic and complex trauma narratives will be different. They need a therapist's patience and require many sessions, if not years, to unfold and be told with meaning and relevance. Additional elements may come to light over the course of therapy, filling in holes to bring more unity and sense to the narrative. Therefore, even when it seems like a client created a full and meaningful healing narrative, it may only be complete enough for that time in their life.

For example, as children get older, their cognitive abilities and emotional capacities grow, allowing them to perceive and understand the trauma differently and with more complexity. Nancy, who was neglected by her birth mother and adopted by her mother's cousin, could not understand at age 5 why my "real mommy gave me away." By 15, Nancy had the capacity to understand how her mother's drug addiction and abusive relationship with her birth father left Nancy's life at risk. By 23, Nancy could mentalize and understand how her birth mother's abusive parents left her deficient "to know how to be a mother, since she never had a good one herself." Nancy, while still hurt, no longer felt abandoned but appreciative that her birth mother was wise enough to ensure her safety. Similarly, a young adult who enters treatment and creates a healing narrative may return to therapy and revisit their trauma story when facing major life milestones like getting married, having children, dealing with the death of a parent, or facing end-of-life issues. The healing trauma narrative can grow and morph, developing complexity and different meaning as we mature.

Since creating the healing trauma narrative is a process, we meet clients where they are, inviting them to return to the unfinished process when they are safe and ready. In line with good-enough mothering (Winnicott, 1953), trauma therapists focus on supporting our clients to create a complete-enough and resolved-enough trauma story with reduced-enough symptoms for where they are right now. In this pursuit, let's examine playful ways we can help clients on this journey.

Playfully Moving through the Trauma Narrative

Storytelling as a whole is an "act of externalizing lived experiences" (Paivio & Angus, 2017, p. 41) that gives us objectivity and helps us contain and therefore regulate. Adding playfulness to creating a trauma narrative can further aid healing as it affords clients expression through verbal and nonverbal modalities. Nonverbal narratives may use symbolic language, metaphors, images, music, and poetry alongside play, movement, and dance (Panhofer et al., 2012, p. 319). Let's explore these playfully inspired ways to "tell" the trauma story to make it healing and transformative.

Nonverbal Ways to Tell the Trauma Story: Playing, Movement, and the Body

Therapies that integrate playfulness and expressive arts offer implicit communication "as an innate, yet reparative, form of narration that is not dependent on words alone" (Malchiodi, 2023, p. x). We can playfully use objects (i.e., dolls, puppets, sand figures), arts and crafts (painting, drawing, clay, wood, metal, etc.), creative writing (through poetry, journaling, a memoir, a play), music, technology (making a video or designing a video game), and humor in the repair work. While humor can lighten the gravity of telling the trauma story, it is important to distinguish whether it is defensive anxiety protecting against contact with deeper, core affect. Humor can help us approach painful material and avoid it (Simione & Gnagnarella, 2023)—a sign of overcoming stress or of stress itself.

Using creative playful media can help our clients regulate affect. When we personify the trauma story, we make it more objective and provide containment and distance, helping our clients move through the retelling more easily and mindfully. Using media like cartooning, storyboarding, collaging, sand tray, and doll or stuffed animal play helps clients experience positivity and manage their affect while telling their story.

Also, therapists can provide language and help their clients name what their body knows, holds, and expresses through body movement (Panhofer & Payne, 2011). We can track body movements related to our clients' trauma-related statements and affects, follow and unfold them, and name or put words to the movements made and their related felt sense, emotions, and beliefs. This parallels what a caregiver does with their baby, describing the qualities of their movements. As Baby Bobby raises up his arms, his father says, "Bobby is sooo big," raising his arms too.

Therapists create emotional attunement and an intersubjective experience when they affectively reflect and verbally express the sense conveyed by the movements related to the trauma memory. When therapists safely see, name, hold/support, and soothe trauma's somatic expression through languaging or naming it, we support its transformation. As we guide our clients to use movement, affect, and sensation to safely connect with and calm their bodily-held trauma memories, they self-validate their experience and develop curiosity, compassion, and courage. This intrarelational process allows the trauma memory to be and feel safe, seen, and soothed, enabling its integration into the whole of the client's being.

Embodied mirroring (Blum, 2015), a technique I developed, helps clients give language to and somatically (and cognitively) unfold stuck trauma memories. In order to create movement in therapy impasses and language the trauma narrative, embodied mirroring integrates a variety of somatic approaches (e.g., Dance Movement Therapy, Mind-Body Therapy, Sensorimotor Psychotherapy, and Somatic Experiencing), AEDP's deep, relational, and experiential attachment-oriented stance, and trauma-informed models (including Internal Family Systems [IFS], Structural Dissociation [SD], and sometimes Eye Movement Desensitization and Reprocessing [EMDR]). With the client's permission, the therapist purposefully uses their own body to mirror these somatic stuck states to get a better embodied sense of the client's experience through the somatic countertransferences that emerge. Then, mirrored movements are relationally and playfully unfolded in parallel or guided ways (for more detail see Blum, 2015). Fifty-two-year-old Gail (whom we first met in Chapter 5) shows us how embodied mirroring helps language the trauma story.

Typically, Gail was animated and verbally articulate. However, as she started to touch into a sexual abuse memory from 30 years earlier, she paused, moved her hands under her legs while seated, and froze. As the 22-year-old part of Gail's mind that held her rape memories got triggered, her fear/freeze protector took over to block her from experiencing overwhelming pain and life threat. I purposefully asked Gail to look at me, in my eyes, to reestablish a ventral vagal state of safe-enough connection. I said, "It looks like a lot is coming up." She nodded in agreement, still silent. I asked, "Would you like to try a little experiment in which you can let me hold this for you?" She nodded again.

While I could have mirrored her seated, frozen state alongside her on the couch, I asked Gail if she minded standing up next to me. This literally helped Gail shift out of her frozen state into a mobilized one. I asked if she would guide my body stance to reflect hers—the one in which her hands were under her legs. We moved through many cycles of me checking in with Gail to see if my body position fit her experience. These cycles were accompanied by breathing to help us each grow more embodied and aware of the present, relational connection. A number of times, Gail looked at my hands, then tried it out herself, then told me how to reposition mine. By literally noticing and feeling into her body position, Gail was moving into a place of objectivity, wisdom, and mastery: only Gail knew how to guide me to most accurately "get it."

As I breathed and noticed my tightly clasped hands behind my back by my butt, Gail watched and started shaking—mirror neurons activated an associated memory network. Gail had been drugged and tied up before being sexually assaulted. We slowed down the practice to help her ground and gain more objectivity. I repeatedly checked if she wanted to pause or stop. Gail was determined to continue, because she was now, "Filling in some of the missing pieces and making sense of the story." However, to ensure she stayed in her window of affect tolerance, I encouraged Gail to check what all parts of her mind needed to make this experiment safe and gentle. She said out loud, "College Gail, you are safe now. Look around, it's not happening now. We're okay. This is just me, teaching Monica how to better understand what happened." I encouraged her to tap bilaterally on each of her arms (bilateral stimulation [BLS] from EMDR) to activate right and left hemispheres to integrate her grounding while telling and metabolizing the story.

Gail and I moved through five cycles using embodied mirroring to unfold and narrate different somatic stuck points, each of which was connected to different parts of the previously inaccessible trauma story. I continued to use my body in the service of Gail, objectively working through her trauma narrative in a regulated way. At one point, I noticed my body's wish to push and the simultaneous feeling of being restrained. Before I said this out loud, Gail noticed my body reflect this and smiled. Our mirror neurons were creating a mutual synchrony and empathy. I asked, "Oooh, what do you sense my body wants to do right now?" She told me to slowly free my arms from the binds and move them in front of my body and make two fists. She was showing me how to fight off her perpetrator.

Through my somatic countertransference—now that the perpetrator was off me—I noticed feeling power in my legs for the first time, which I told Gail. She said, "Yeah, they are powerful. Kick the shit out of him!" She told me to keep kicking, punching, and following him until he, "Runs the fuck out of the frat house." I did using slow intentional movements which I now asked Gail to mirror. I wanted Gail to embody her power and experience these acts of triumph (Ogden, 2019)—completing the movements her body wanted to make but had been physically and chemically restrained from doing.

"This feels liberating," I said.

"It really does!" Gail concurred.

We slowed down to breathe into this liberating mastery and used BLS. We also deepened the change through metaprocessing (see Chapter 9). Afterward, her trauma narrative felt more complete, and Gail's body and mind finally felt more at peace.

Verbal Ways to Tell the Trauma Story: Conveying a Felt Sense through Words

"We define words. We imbue them with meaning. We pour ourselves into them" (Koenig, 2022). This is true for everyone, not just authors. We can convey a felt sense using words. In addition, the act of "naming is considered a sacred activity, a recognition and celebration of existence" (Fosha, 2010). In this section, we will explore how to playfully and creatively use words that are made up, in our mother tongue, or pronouns to evoke a felt sense and emotions that can facilitate telling and developing a healing trauma narrative.

Made-Up Words

Many clients have spontaneously uttered a word that expresses their true feelings, yet isn't found in any dictionary. Chaya, an Orthodox Jewish 14-year-old client who did not curse, used her made-up word, *bullshenachas*, to connote the anger of "bullshit" when talking about being bullied by peers or shamed by her teachers for her learning disability. I told her how much I loved her word, and then took it one step further. I said, "Chaya, you're right. This *is* bullshenachas! And I think it's also *bullshetuchen!*"

She laughed and said, "And maybe *bullshlacha* too!"

Over several sessions, we created a religiously respectful vocabulary to safely convey the anger, confusion, and unfairness she felt deeply. More importantly, we celebrated her creativity and found a way for her to be seen and felt emotionally. I've asked Chaya's permission to use her words with others—clients, family, and friends. She looked at me puzzled at first and then smiled a broad smile, "Sure! And make sure to call it the C. W. (her initials) Special!" I reported back how others got a real kick out of her words and loved the emotion they conveyed. We joked how, even with her severe dyslexia, Chaya could create her own new dictionary of feelings words that would put Merriam-Webster's out of business.

Adult clients seem to get more self-conscious when blurting out a word that expresses deep emotion but may not be a "real" word. But I playfully delight in their slips. After many years of trauma-focused and relationally oriented work, 43-year-old Horace started practicing ways to lighten his control and be more flexible with his schedule and more spontaneous in life. He blurted out, "I am living life with more *creativility*!" He paused, and awkwardly asked, "Is that a word?"

I announced, "If it isn't, I love it. Let's make it one! You really have developed true creativility, Horace. Wouldn't you say?"

He laughed, "I really think I have. It's more than creativity, it's an attitude of how I go about my life now!" I was beaming, because his once consuming, insecure parts had grown more embodied and less self-conscious.

Horace saw my big smile and my affective delight in him and asked, "What?"

I shared, "Oh, I'm just absolutely delighting in how you have grown to emanate creativility and connect so beautifully with your true Horace essence!"

He quieted, looked down for a moment, then looked up with watery eyes and nodded, "I really have, haven't I?" This was a moment of pride in his mastery, which we metaprocessed for a few more minutes through explicit, relational, and experiential savoring. Horace was deeply touched by his own progress at unashamedly expressing and embodying his real Self.

Mother Tongue

The playful use of one's mother tongue—the first language spoken and/or heard early in life—can be compelling too. To help clients move more naturally and efficiently to where early trauma fragments are held, I ask them to speak, write, or sing in the language they spoke or was spoken around them at the time of the trauma. This helps clients access states of mind, cognitions, and affect linked to the trauma.

I believe for the use of one's mother tongue to be effective it is not necessary for therapists to understand the content of what is said but get its felt sense—the sensorimotor experience of connecting with it (Bergmann, 2022). Therapists, like caregivers, can grow affective attunement and intersubjectivity by matching the intensity, timing, and "shape" (Stern, 1985) of the client's behaviors. Clients have spoken languages I have no familiarity with—Mandarin, Urdu, Arabic, and Russian—yet somatically and emotionally, I could sense their genuine connection to thoughts, memories, sensations, and emotions surrounding their story. In fact, one client commented, "Monica, I thought you didn't understand Urdu."

"I don't."

They continued, "But your face seemed as if you did." Further exploration revealed how the language of their body when speaking their mother tongue helped me grasp their experience, despite not understanding the words. This is a comforting and powerful tool to use with clients.

Therapists can model the same, sharing words from their mother tongue to convey deep emotion to clients. I have taught many clients, regardless of their background, German and Yiddish words and expressions I learned growing up. I explain how, for me, they convey a lot of somatic truth and many words, especially Yiddish ones, have sounds and rhythms that connote so much more than the words mean. For example, the Yiddish word *meschugah* means "crazy" or "insane," yet conveys "crazy and then some"—it's like a special case of crazy. Or saying a person is a *mensch* goes beyond saying they're a good person but expresses they are a full, honorable, human being with a good soul.

When I use my mother tongue to reflect qualities in my clients, *they* get a stronger felt sense of my experience of them. For example, when clients who historically acted in self-sacrificing or overly deferent ways show assertiveness and gumption, I've said, "Wow, you're showing real *chutzpah!*"—the Yiddish word meaning extreme self-confidence and boldness, with some added gall or audacity. I overemphasize the guttural "ch" sound and try to teach my clients to say it. While we may initially get diverted by the imitation, I return to emphasize how *chutzpah* means, "You've really grown a pair... " I pause and add "ovaries" for women, "balls" for men, and leave it open-ended for non-binary, queer, or agender clients. The tone, rhythm, and embodied emotion behind my word, combined with its novelty and related positivity, help clients internalize the feedback better than if I say: "You're very assertive."

With an expanded felt-sense vocabulary to describe themselves and others, clients can use present language to describe past trauma-related material. Clients develop dual attention—focusing on aspects of the past while grounding in the safe language of the now. Also, words that convey and connect to a felt sense reflect one's voice. Voice is an embodied (self) reflection, uses language that is personal (socially and culturally embedded), and is an instrument of the psyche/ soul, Self, and sense of being: it communicates our experience of what we think, feel, and know (Gilligan & Eddy, 2021).

Different Pronouns

Clients raised with chronic relational trauma histories often adopt behaviors and language that will support their attachment. We know from Neurolinguistic Programming (Bandler & Grinder, 1975) that neurological processes, language, and acquired behavioral patterns interconnect, so changing language can affect the other two. Let's explore how bringing awareness to and changing the choice of pronouns (as one example) can help clients move through trauma and affect how they tell their trauma story. Just to note, I am referring to the use of pronouns in ways unrelated to gender identification, which is an important and separate topic.

Caregivers, bosses, and teachers with personal insecurities stemming from unmet needs in their histories may act in narcissistic ways attempting to fill voids of their unmet needs. They may use pronouns like "I," me," and "mine" more frequently than "you" and "yours." Meanwhile, those who depend or rely on them will more frequently use "you" to attune with and soothe the caregiver.

Similarly, pronoun choice reflects relational boundaries. Those with enmeshed relationships often use "us," "we," and "our." Such caregivers who have difficulty separating from their dependents might say, "When we get ready for school," "We're going to our dance competition," and "Our team needs lots of practice before our game." Rather than healthy joining, this language may reflect difficulty respecting separate identity. On the other end of the spectrum, dismissive caregivers might often use "you" to convey distance and separateness, disavow responsibility for their own actions, or shift blame.

Slowing clients down to choose the pronoun that best reflects their preferred connection and boundaries often gives them pause. For example, Erica financially enabled Charlotte, her 55-year-old daughter. Despite being on a fixed income, she paid for Charlotte's second mortgage to prevent Charlotte from foreclosure. Erica referred to "our debt" and said that "it's hard for us." Erica's rescuing part hoped lessening Charlotte's financial burdens would cause Charlotte to be more appreciative and grow closer to her. It didn't. I repeatedly highlighted, "Notice, Erica, it's *her* financial mess, not yours. Charlotte's choices and actions, not yours."

Over time, Erica realized that making an "us" out of two very separate and disconnected people was an attempt to force a connection. This adaptation was triggered by the memory of her relationship with her parents who behaved in dismissive, devaluing, and disconnected ways. Combined with our relational work, Erica practiced changing her pronouns to "me" and "you," started sitting with a more erect spine, and felt more empowered when she realized she was no longer yoked to her daughter's financial problems. Erica also changed her boundaries when speaking about her deceased parents. Instead of saying "we" and "us," she switched to "me" and "them" to more clearly differentiate their values from hers. The use of different pronouns helped Erica create more peace with her memories of her parents and grow healthier boundaries with her daughter and friends. She grew to enjoy saying, "That's a you problem," or "Not my monkey, not my circus!"

In summary, to create a healing narrative, using felt-sense evoking language simultaneously connects us with the emotion of the right hemisphere and the language of the left—facilitating integration. Our client's use of made-up words, mother tongue, and boundary-supporting pronouns enables their trauma narrative to unfold more organically, personally, playfully, and more efficiently.

Naming and Resolving Trauma: Two Cases

Let's now look at two very different cases—one child, one adult—as examples of how we can support telling the trauma story using playfulness and creativity.

Twelve-Year-Old Laney

Laney age 12, was referred by her parents after becoming a victim of an internet predator. Laney had social and learning difficulties and some features of ASD (autism spectrum disorder), which made her present more like a naïve 8-year-old. Laney was quite socially isolated yet craved being seen and cared about, which made her more vulnerable to social predation or bullying.

To please her parents and the police's request, Laney agreed to help frame the perpetrator. However, she felt extremely mixed, believing that the perpetrator really cared about her, even if he was a 35-year-old man who said he too was in middle school. Complying to frame the one person who "liked" her other than her family caused Laney great discomfort and confusion. Once the sting operation was complete, her parents brought her in for therapy.

Laney was not comfortable with or motivated by any aspect of one-on-one play or talk therapy. At the time, I had only worked with kids coping with siblings who had ASD, not clients with ASD, per se. I found it so hard to reach Laney, much less support her to tell, understand, and work through her story of victimization. I looked for ways to engage Laney and found two: she wished to feel empowered after being so disempowered, and she strived to be more independent and mature. While Laney lacked the emotional and cognitive skills of her same-aged peers, she too was starting the dance of separation and individuation.

I decided to have a few sessions using a game-show format geared to provide psychoeducation about safety, boundaries, trust, and telling the trauma story. Laney was on one team and her parents on the other. The opportunity to compete with her parents delighted her—it was the first time she smiled in treatment. I named the game show "Who Knows More" to motivate confidence- and competence-building through competition. Laney's parents were fully onboard.

I made up rules on the fly—tailoring them to best-fit Laney and the treatment goals. I would ask a question and whichever team was first to raise their hand got to respond. If they responded incorrectly, the other team got a chance to answer. There were no points for wrong answers; easy answers to true or false questions got one point, harder answers to open-ended questions earned three. As the game progressed, I made changes to heighten the competition and strengthen Laney's positive affect of excitement. In turn, this would help her integrate the learning. I added a final lightning round where five points were up for grabs. Laney's parents were intuitive, well-attuned, and knew to provide some challenge yet hang back so Laney could grow confidence. The first game-show session included true/false questions like:

- Anyone who says nice things about us should be trusted.
- If we have the tiniest feeling that something or someone is not safe, we should ignore it.
- If we like someone, we should do anything they ask.
- If someone offers us ___ (candy—Laney's favorite thing—a stuffed animal, money) to do something, we should do it.
- We need to do things that feel wrong to keep a friend.
- If someone will stop being our friend, we should do what they ask to keep their friendship.
- If things feel good in our ___ (heart, mind, or body) but feel bad somewhere else inside, we should keep doing it.
- Others know us better than we know ourselves. (Words the perpetrator had used.)

The next two sessions moved into a retelling of elements of the trauma story that focused on complicated themes. At times, their answers led me to ask follow-up questions that provided more pieces to the narrative. I asked both teams if it was okay for me to give that team an extra point. Sometimes, Laney was hesitant but ultimately was fair in supporting her parents to earn additional points. Questions included:

- Jamie (the perpetrator's pseudonym) was really how old: 13 or 35?
- What was Jamie's real name (parents knew this from the police): Steve or Greg?
- Steve, making believe he was 13-year-old Jamie, said kind, sweet things. True or false?
- Hearing kind, sweet things about us feels good. True or false?
- When we feel good about things people say to us, we like them more. True or false?
- Sometimes people say nice things to us because they mean it. True or false?
- Sometimes people say nice things to us because they want something. True or false?
- What did Steve want from Laney? Each right answer gets a point.
- Why did Steve choose Laney? Each right answer gets a point.
- Can being kind ever be a problem? Yes or no? When? Each right answer gets a point.
- The police can help us be safe. True or false?
- When police help us, we can feel uncomfortable. True or false?
- When we do the right thing—like helping the police keep us safe—we can have mixed feelings. True or false? Name all the feelings you can and get two points for each.
- Protecting ourselves can feel confusing. True or false?

There were more questions that chronicled the sequence of her trauma story, attempted to name related emotions, and make meaning that was developmentally appropriate and helpful to Laney. We focused heavily on Laney's bravery in working with the police to help protect herself from further victimization and other kids from being hurt by Steve, too.

After our sessions, her parents reported Laney seemed calmer, more focused, and was moving on with life. She had developed language to describe her trauma narrative and confidence that she won the "Who Knows More" game—three sessions in a row. To support Laney in making friends, I encouraged her parents to have her join a social skills group at school and introduce her to the Girl Scouts or 4-H Club where appropriate and safe peer interactions could be supervised.

Fifty-Two-Year-Old Camila

Camila, a 52-year-old Dominican woman with a long career as an architect, was raised in the United States by immigrant parents. Her mother had a disorganized attachment style. Her father, with his dismissive style of relating, "divorced the family" and moved back to the Dominican Republic when Camila was in high school. Camila often described how her relationship to her mother, career, and finding a significant other left her like "a deer in the headlights, caught between a rock and a hard place"; she was hijacked by depressive states marked by stagnation and hopelessness. "Why pursue goals or have intentions to improve my life? It leads nowhere."

Camila was very articulate and meticulously detailed her history. In high school, her mother found ways to undermine her softball interests and skills. She prevented Camila from attending important practices or pitching in the all-star game, which college scouts attended. This thwarted Camila from pursing her Division I college dreams. Instead, Camila felt forced and guilted by her mother into using her "gift from God"—her intelligence—and getting a "real education and career" her mother could be proud of. Her father, from a long distance, reminded her to respect her mother.

We explored how adapting to her mother's disorganized style of relating left Camila frequently gaslit. Camila would share some of her mother's voicemails and emails with me, which helped us name the dynamics that would make her head spin and leave her paralyzed, not knowing what was up or down. Camila identified that she was gaslit in her personal and professional relationships, too. Camila also experienced blocks to advancing at the firm in which she worked: she was passed over six times for promotion by white males. She described her two marriages as leaving her feeling empty, childless, and a master at compliance. Doing the right thing for others left her doing wrong for herself.

While she spoke with great detail, Camila often steered away from emotional vulnerability. Camila's kindness, openness, conviction to being a moral person, and intelligence, intrigued me, leading to many cerebral discussions.

While these interactions strengthened our connection, outside therapy Camila continued to loop in her narrative dictated by compliant, rule-oriented behaviors that left her like that frozen deer. Talking clearly wasn't helping shift her stuck narrative or actions.

Knowing how talented an architect Camila was and that she had a great eye for design, I encouraged her to use her computer design software to draw "a deer in the headlights, caught between a rock and a hard place." I invited her to design how the deer could safely and effectively shift its position. She smiled, seeming interested in the assignment. I reminded her that her good little girl was not required to do this as a homework assignment, but her wise, adult Self was invited to get all parts of mind to playfully explore. In fact, I told Camila, if it felt right, she could invite her compliant, good girl part to step to the side and only chime in about the creative side of the practice, like the use of colors and shapes.

When Camila returned for her session a week later, she seemed different. She shared that she had spent a few nights that week making a slide deck that depicted the deer's frozen stuckness. She took out her laptop to show me. Camila explained how she spent time changing colors, shapes, textures (connecting wisely to her good girl part) until it felt right to her (intrapsychic agreement). I explored what that felt like in her body, and she said, "When I felt anger swell to rage, I knew I designed it right." We explored how her creativity helped her connect with and express suppressed rage.

Camila shared how she then created new slides in which she helped the deer move, shifting the headlights out of its eyes and instead illuminating a new unblocked path it could follow toward something better, more promising. I asked if the light was gas-powered.

She laughed and said with a wink, "No gaslighting in this story, Monica!"

I replied, "I figured. Good for you! Knowing you, it's solar-powered light!"

We both laughed and she continued to show me how, in each successive drawing, the rock and hard place were drawn smaller and smaller. Camila's drawings were instrumental in changing her trauma narrative. In one, she placed her deer part of mind in the foreground and her obstacles in the background. She noticed, "Like the deer, I've placed the needs, cares, demands, and expectations of others in front of my own. Look at what happened to the deer when I shifted the perspective by putting it in front and gave it light to lead its way forward: it got bigger, more colorful, and most of all, I felt better."

Camila was feeling stronger, more directed and motivated. She even threw balls at her pitchback for a half hour in her backyard. Camila reconnected with her teenage parts who were competent and skilled at softball. Future sessions leaned into how her nonverbal inventiveness helped her connect with, integrate, and mobilize her sense of what was right—her essence. Ironically, while Camila had words to narrate her traumatic history, it was nonverbal creativity that enabled her to feel, embody, metabolize, and rewrite, so to say, her narrative. As

Camila integrated and rebalanced her left and right brain, she transformed her trauma story and designed a different path forward.

Having Told the Trauma Story ... Now What?

Part V has offered us a host of ways to synthesize and integrate our relational playful spirit with the elements needed to promote change and support trauma's transformation into thriving. In this chapter, we learned how to use playfulness to enable somatic, emotional, and cognitive integration in telling the trauma narrative. To safely support the meaning-making process of telling the trauma story, we noted the importance of D-R-C safety and the role of nonverbal and verbal playfulness to evoke felt-sense language. Ultimately, using our playful spirit helps clients transform their once incoherent, painful, implicitly encoded trauma memory fragments into an integrated, explicit, relational, emotionally meaningful, even spiritually fulfilling narrative that brings coherence and clarity to their identity and supports forward movement.

To wrap up our playfully spirited journey of promoting healing and transformation in treating trauma across the lifespan, we move into our final chapter to help us and our clients figure out: Are We Done Yet? A Playful Conclusion to Trauma Treatment.

References

Bandler, R. & Grinder, J. (1975). *The structure of magic Vol. 1. A book about language and therapy* (1st ed.). Palo Alto, CA: Science and Behavior Books.

Bergmann, U. (2022, November 11). *Recent neural findings and why they matter: Featuring the hidden potential of the body scan practitioners* [Live Webinar]. EMDR Advanced Training and Distance Learning. BeaconLive.

Blum, M. C. (2015). Embodied mirroring: A relational, body-to-body technique promoting movement in therapy. *Journal of Psychotherapy Integration, 25*(2), 115–127.

Dana, D. (2018). *The polyvagal theory in therapy: Engaging the rhythm of regulation.* New York: Norton.

Fisher, J. (2017). *Healing the fragmented selves of trauma survivors: Overcoming self-alienation.* New York: Routledge.

Fosha, D. (2010). Wired for healing: Thirteen ways of looking at AEDP. *Transformance: The AEDP Journal, 1.* https://aedpinstitute.org/journal/wired-for-healing/

Gilligan, C. & Eddy, J. (2021). The listening guide: Replacing judgment with curiosity. *Qualitative Psychology, 8*(2), 141–151. https://doi.org/10.1037/qup0000213

Koenig, J. (2022, January 26). *Author talks: The made up words that make our world.* https://www.mckinsey.com/featured-insights/mckinsey-on-books/author-talks-the-made-up-words-that-make-our-worldhttps://medium.com/age-of-awareness/neuroception-and-the-3-part-brain-b38f482c34b0

Korn, D. (2012, July 14–15). *EMDR the next generation: Finding your way in the dark.* [EMDR Master Class presented in Iselin, NJ].

Laliotis, D. (2014), July 25–27). *Going deeper into personality & character structure using EMDR Therapy.* [A 3-day EMDR master course intensive. Iselin, NJ].

Malchiodi, C. A. (Ed.) (2023). *Handbook of expressive arts therapy.* New York: Guilford.

Ogden, P. (2019). Acts of triumph: An interpretation of Pierre Janet and the role of the body in trauma treatment. In G. Craparo, F. Ortu, & O. van der Hart (Eds.), *Rediscovering Pierre Jane: Trauma, dissociation, and a new context for psychoanalysis* (pp. 200–209). New York: Routledge.

Paivio, S. C. & Angus, L. E. (2017). Why client storytelling matters. In S. C. Paivio & L. E. Angus (Eds.), *Narrative processes in emotion-focused therapy for trauma* (pp. 39–52). Washington, DC: American Psychological Association.

Panhofer, H. & Payne, H. (2011). Languaging the embodied experience. *Journal of Body, Movement and Dance in Psychotherapy, 6*(2), 215–232.

Panhofer, H., Payne, H. L., Parke, T., & Meekums, B. (2012). The embodied word. In S. C. Koch, T. Fuchs, M. Summa, & C. Müller (Eds.), *Body memory, metaphor and movement* (pp. 307–325). Amsterdam: John Benjamins Publishing.

Rothschild, B. (2021). *Revolutionizing trauma treatment: Stabilization, safety and nervous system balance.* New York: Norton.

Simione, L. & Gnagnarella, C. (2023). Humor coping reduces the positive relationship between avoidance coping strategies and perceived stress: A moderation analysis. *Behavioral Science, 13*(2), 179. https://doi.org/10.3390/bs13020179. PMID:36829408; PMCID: PMC9952361.

Stern, D. (1985). *The interpersonal world of the infant.* New York: Basic Books.

Winnicott, D. W. (1953). Transitional objects and transitional phenomena; A study of the first not-me possession. *International Journal of Psychoanalysis, 34*(2), 89–97.

Are We Done Yet? A Playful Conclusion to Trauma Treatment

When Is Trauma Treatment Done?

In theory, we and our clients know that trauma treatment is complete when we've undone the six UNs of trauma—feeling UNsafe, UNseen, and UNconnected, and appraising the trauma as UNbearable/intolerable, UNwilled/unwanted, and UNresolved. As these hurts are healed, autonomic nervous system (ANS) and affect dysregulation, brain disintegrative functioning, and disconnection from others and the Self are dissolved. Clients are no longer symptomatic, indicating they feel balanced- and right-enough. Relational healing and change reveal effective co-regulation, an expanded window of affect tolerance, and an ability to weather situational triggers and ruptures in relationship and return to safety and connection. Brain functioning flows integratively. Intrapsychically, all parts of mind communicate and cooperate. Clients are and feel safe, seen, soothed, and secure. They can nurture themselves and their relationships in all parts of life. Their trauma narrative has been expressed as fully and coherently as possible. Thriving is unencumbered. Play, joy, vitality, hope, and spiritual fulfillment are embodied. As one client put it, "You've helped me achieve what I never imagined. I'm living my best life!" In my experience, this is the ideal ending to trauma therapy. But it is not always possible.

While many of my clients have been fortunate enough to thrive and flourish, others end a course of treatment with many loose ends still in place. This is not bad or good, but the reality of treating real people living in real life. In this final chapter, we'll grow a realistic sense of whether trauma treatment is complete, explore dynamics that interfere with its completion and what to do when it isn't.

Trauma Resolved and Transformed Enough, for Now

Rather than asking, "Are we done yet?" we need to ask, "Is the trauma resolved and transformed enough, for now, for us to close down treatment?" While we can always aspire to achieve the ideal outcome, it is important for us to stay grounded in what is possible, in light of each client's reality and

DOI: 10.4324/9781003509493-20

developmental-relational-context. We must attend and attune to "our trauma-tized client's needs, symptoms, preferences, abilities, [and] current life situa-tion" (Rothschild, 2021, p. xiv). Our grounding mantra needs to be: I will do the best I can with what I've got to help each client promote change for the better that is a right-enough fit for them now. This stance keeps us therapists sober to the fact that when we deal with trauma—especially chronic and complex—just like our clients, we will experience messiness and helplessness. That is the nature of the work and helps us better relate to our clients' experience.

Ironically, while this reality may not feel light, we can still bring play-fulness to the less-than-ideal outcome of a course of trauma treatment. Let's remember that when we intentionally co-create a safe, relational, playful, attuned-on-steroids experience, we provide a juxtaposition experience to the client and their trauma. So, whether treatment is complete enough or not, we can feel assured that we have helped clients wire in a reparative experience linked to positive emotions. When clients have experienced positive relational healing, they know more is possible and can be pursued when ready. Let's look at different ways trauma therapy doesn't go as planned, yet can provide clients a resolved, transformed-enough experience. This last chapter reminds us how even in the most severe trauma cases, the playful spirit can be nurtured and transformative.

When Treatment Kind-of-Sort-of Begins

While this brief section speaks to incomplete and imperfect courses of trauma treatment, it addresses certain important dynamics that can impact the whole treatment process.

Saying Goodbye before Hello

Sometimes, when clients are not ready to commit to therapy due to intrapsychic or contextually-driven ambivalence, we need to say goodbye before treatment can begin. This process parallels that of change when clients need to grieve an attachment to make space for a new, healing one. We also need to gain comfort to graciously welcome a client's return when and if they are ready to commit (or enough parts of them are) to do the courageous work. Some may consider this pre-therapy in which we give clients a taste of what can be. In essence, this process has value and introduces clients to a healing relationship that can be dif-ferent, infused with honesty and positivity.

In the first session, Amy, a 16-year-old, voiced major disgruntlement with me. I offered her a choice to continue with me or look for another therapist. I gave her and her family referrals. Amy returned to treatment with me after interviewing two other therapists. When returning, I asked her, "Wow, Amy. I'm curious. How come you came back? You said you 'hated' me."

Amy answered, "Yeah, I still do. But I hate you less than the other two shrinks I met." I laughed. Then we laughed together. Amy and I worked together into her young adult life on many traumas, including her father's death and the relational impact of her mother's dissociative identity disorder. Ironically, Amy was one of the first clients who, after moving away and terminating treatment, would occasionally check-in. We grew a deep fondness for each other—established through a playful foundation of busting each other's chops.

Inviting clients to try out other therapists and return if they like supports their self-initiation of and commitment to therapy. Therefore, saying goodbye before hello can be framed as a client's use of discernment as they leverage judgment and assess personal comfort in selecting a better-fit-for-them therapist. Since the trauma-healing relationship is one of the most intimate and vulnerable we will ever have, using wise and healthy selectivity needs to be applauded and even metaprocessed.

Working with the Not-Client

Let's take a glimpse at two dynamics that complicate treatment in which a client does not identify as the person needing or wanting therapy.

Backdooring into Treatment

Sometimes the person identified as the client might not be the one whom treatment needs to focus on, per se. Those who refer—children, spouses, parents, and co-workers—are sometimes the ones with the greatest need for therapy. The neediest person thus enters treatment indirectly, through the backdoor, if you will. Family systems theories teach us that one member of the system may be the scapegoat or black sheep—the designated holder but not the original cause of the system's pain. The scapegoat manifestly expresses the pattern of the whole group, signaling that something is awry in the system.

We often see this with caregivers and their dependents. For example, some bold teenage clients have perceptively said, "I don't need to be here; it's my mother/father who does!" Some preschool clients have announced the same, cutting to the heart of a family system issue with the accuracy of a laser. When their assessment is on point and multiple therapists cannot be afforded, we can pivot and target the most receptive person/s whose treatment would help shift the system's unhealthy and unsafe patterns. We creatively adapt to best support systemic trauma resolution and transformation.

At times, such an imprecise identification of who the client should be may require us to say goodbye, for now, to the person we originally hoped to work with. For example, we might prefer engaging the perceptive teenager rather than an ambivalently committed mother. We need to be honest with our willingness to change clients to ensure we can best serve the system and refer out if needed. Sometimes, we can make the identified child, teenager, or partner our co-therapist/consultant to empower their wisdom and guide the repair work. Systems that are open and flexible enough to change will. But when shifting to focus on the client most in need of support is not possible, we work the best we can with the system member most open to change. We'll further discuss this dynamic in the Glass Ceiling section.

Pushed into Treatment

Some clients may enter treatment without motivation or choice. They may be court-ordered, threatened to be left by their partner, or dragged in by family members. How can therapy, particularly trauma treatment, occur without the precondition of safety, connection, and choice being met? It can't, since the threat of abandonment or losing freedom is an underlying condition of these clients' treatment. We must first help them gain choice, control, separateness, and agency to make therapy about and beneficial to them. Sometimes, connecting honestly with one's truth and sharing it openly may not be safe to clients if their records can be subpoenaed and charges can be raised against them.

My early career work with court-ordered offenders and their incest victims was messy and quite imperfect. While the offending parent attended treatment, there were real threats to their full and honest sharing. For one, lifting their dissociative defenses would have caused intolerable and crippling shame when realizing the harm they caused their innocent children and family. Second, telling the truth may have guaranteed their incarceration. Learning to work in a "what if" modality became the compromise. For example, we used imaginal work to grow victim empathy. "Imagine, *if you had* hurt your daughter this way, how would she feel right now? How would this affect her wanting to be with you? What would she need to feel safe and trust you?" Though this approach to therapy is fully understandable and may provide some resolution, it is less than ideal.

When Treatment Ends Too Soon

Life Happens

Trauma treatment is not immune to life outside of the consultation room— actually, quite the opposite. Changes in caregivers, finances, court-involvement, insurance, health, school and work schedules, moves, deaths, and access to transportation and other resources are a few of the life factors that can affect treatment continuity and completion. Sometimes, they cause treatment to pause temporarily or end permanently. We need to respect that life happens. Clients need to put their energies into showing up to meet the pressing needs and demands of daily life—surviving. However, such interruptions may bring up the client's and therapist's futile and hopeless feelings about positive momentum, especially in cases of chronic and complex trauma.

As healing professionals, we can frame the pause or end of treatment as a "goodbye for now." Combining this reframe with a sincere invitation to return in the future can make an ending meaningful and even transformational. We can explore how the therapy relationship and process while unique, is similar to anything else in life: it has ups and downs, gains and losses, completed and incomplete accomplishments, and expected and unexpected hellos and good-byes. We intentionally and explicitly try to identify and metaprocess our client's accomplishments, growth, and change.

If time allows, we can take a session or portion thereof to put closure on what they have mastered to date and explore areas to work on in the future with us or other healing professionals. We can use a known termination date to bring deliberate focus to the relational healing work, as if to say, "Let's make the most of what we have now. Carpe diem!" Doing the best we can with the time we've got helps clients learn from us as we model flexibility, resiliency, and roll with what life sends our way.

Pausing to Practice

Other times, even when more trauma resolution and integration would be prefer-able, clients choose to scale back on or pause treatment to practice their skills in "real life." In a way, this parallels a rapprochement phase in childhood in which the child feels secure enough to separate from their caregiver, yet know they can return for support when and if needed. Relationally, we can identify and troubleshoot red-flag issues and support our client's need to spread their wings, try out their new and fortified strengths, and grow trust in their wisdom through experience. Our letting-go to support our client's practice integrating all they have learned can be extremely empowering and can help clients synthesize and crystallize their Self leadership and wisdom.

Relational Glass Ceilings

On occasion, when working with relational trauma, I've experienced a real para-dox: clients are limited from becoming too healthy by the same person who brings them in for treatment. This mixed message is a great clue that we are working with the presence of a confused, unresolved, or disorganized attach-ment style in the client's system. In the relational glass ceiling dynamic, the person triggering the client's symptoms, unconsciously or consciously, engages the therapist and/or client in a conflict, creating an invisible barrier to our cli-ent's trauma resolution and transformation. If we try to break through the glass ceiling, our client is pulled out of therapy or our interventions are undermined by other members of the system.

I have seen this in some cases of separation anxiety, factitious disorder imposed by another (formerly Munchausen syndrome by proxy), and in the case of Treena (see Chapter 8), whose mother had an unresolved, disorganized parenting style and felt threatened by my attuned care of her daughter. As Treena became healthier and better adjusted, the mother perceived her role was being usurped as the loving, effective, and important caregiver. Treena warned me that her mother would yank her from treatment if she became too asymptomatic. By contrast, another parent with an unresolved traumatic attachment style used to challenge me by trying to expose my limitations, highlighting her superior parenting knowledge and abilities. This mother sabotaged my treatment recommendations, announcing to her children that her failed efforts were "Monica's idea or suggestion." She'd say to them, "I know you better than Monica. I knew you couldn't handle it."

Working toward healthy treatment repair and resolution with clients stuck in glass ceiling system dynamics with disorganized attachment styles can feel like threading the needle. Especially with dependents, we carefully and appropriately buttress the caregiver's competence, while ensuring the dependent's needs are attuned and met well enough. We hold "both/and." Attunement on steroids helps us navigate how to provide good enough, but not too-good therapy, to prevent our dependent client from being ripped out of treatment or further harmed.

In addition, clients can play a role in preserving the relational glass ceiling by self-imposing it to "protect" their caregiver from feeling and being abandoned or seen as inadequate or limited. These clients are overly attuned to their caregiver and learned to sacrifice personal care, growth, healing, and independence-seeking. In one case, a victim of interpersonal violence felt responsible for and guilt-ridden about leaving her alcoholic partner, believing it would trigger his memories of paternal neglect and maternal abandonment and cause him to spiral into alcoholic self-destruction. In a different case, a capable, talented teenage client self-imposed a glass ceiling. She avoided doing her best in school to prevent her mother with limited cognitive functioning from feeling "dumb" or inadequate and being left by her by going to college. Fortunately, despite intellectual limitations, her mother was quite emotionally healthy and told her daughter, "You are hurting yourself and me. Don't hold yourself back from being the brainy kid I know you are." The mom showered her daughter with pride and said, "Don't worry about me. I'm good. Remember, when you do good, so do I!"

Blindsiding: Surprise ... and Goodbye!

Finally, treatment with complex, traumatized clients can end without warning due to our client's internal system getting shaken up. A number of teenage and adult clients—whose internal system of protectors I believed I knew really well—left treatment with little to no warning. For each, a sudden event or trauma occurred in their lives that threatened their managers (see the description of managers in the Internal Family Systems [IFS] model in Chapter 2). Triggers included hard drug and alcohol experimentation, death and losses, and reconnecting with a former significant other or friend which resurrected unresolved issues.

For each of these clients, a rapid intrapsychic deterioration and dissociative fugue state emerged. In IFS terms, their internal systems were hijacked by firefighter parts who tried to abruptly and radically quash the exile's pain from surfacing. The stability in their lives dissolved, causing them to disconnect from friends, spouses, children, and family members and neglect work and life responsibilities. The client's possible shame of me (or them) revealing and dealing with their destructive self-sabotaging firefighter part—who hijacked their lives and treatment gains—may have been "solved" by them abruptly leaving treatment. I felt blindsided, wondering what else I could have done.

Trauma therapists need to accept that sometimes treatment will end with a crash-and-burn because some unpredicted, uncontrollable trigger jolts awake our clients' deeply hidden and exiled pain of unresolved losses and traumas. We may not have warning, nor the permission or access to our client's internal system to work it through with them. We can call, text, email, or mail bids for re-connection or invitations to return in the future. But we may be boxed out of connection.

Such loss reminds us that even when we think treatment is moving in the right direction or toward full integration and/or completion for now, we never know what parts of mind might show up. Novice and seasoned trauma therapists need humility and must wisely defer to our clients as the ultimate guide in leading the work. Healing is directly related to the level of our clients' intrarelational openness and cooperation. Parts of mind unseen by and disconnected from the client cannot be seen or connected with by the therapist. Protectors only work cooperatively when they are and feel safe, seen, soothed, and secure in their trust of the client's wise Self and the therapist's leadership.

When Treatment Doesn't End: Clients Know Best—About Treatment

Staying in Therapy

Sometimes, we think we're approaching the end of a course of treatment, yet our client shows no sign of wanting to end despite consistently accessing and acting from their wise, highest Self. But no client continues the therapy relationship out of boredom. Therapy requires time, money, commitment, and hard work—even when informed by a playful spirit. I've grown to believe that parts of clients unconsciously or consciously know or sense there is more work to be done. It seems that many clients need to experience a period of stability and growth while held safely and securely in the therapy relationship before feeling and being ready to address the next painful or unresolved layer.

We can relationally explore our observations and invite clients to be curious about what might be happening (e.g., a possible shaky trust in their independence). Most importantly, we need to remind clients that we will defer to their inner knowing and wisdom and will be by their side as long as they welcome us on their journey to change. Attuned on steroids, we tune into their pace and honor their route—circuitous, direct, or both—trusting in their innate capacity to heal.

Returning to Therapy

Trusting our client's wisdom and innate drive toward righting what is wrong is especially relevant when a client returns to treatment with new or similar symptoms that we thought had been fully resolved. Some therapists experience or perceive this return as a treatment failure. However, I offer that we see this as a testament to having developed a safe, nurturing, and welcoming healing relationship to which our client feels free to return as needed. While we encourage our client's self-sufficiency, competence, confidence, wisdom, self-directedness, and self-leadership (security), we also teach our clients how to safely reach out to trusted others in times of need (rapprochement). For those with dismissive attachment styles, returning to treatment for more healing work is an incredible success to be reflected, celebrated, and metaprocessed.

Treatment without Resolution—Our Lifers

We have journeyed together through this book learning ways to tap into our playful spirit with the help of my clients' voices and teachings. I wish to honor how even the most traumatized clients, still imprisoned in a living hell, bring playfulness and light to us, inspiring us to continue our healing work with them and others.

Let's return to Irwin, whom we met in Chapter 10. He had dissociative identity disorder and a traumatic brain injury (TBI). At age 58, his life changed following a brain bleed from a skiing accident. He was placed in a two-month, medically induced coma. Owing to Irwin's fierce independence—from being an only child of two alcoholic, emotionally, physically, and sexually abusive parents—he relearned to walk, talk, and feed himself. Despite going on permanent disability, becoming wheelchair-bound and legally blind, he found contentment being in the care of his devoted wife. After 38 years of marriage, she suddenly died when Irwin was 64. His mother became his legal guardian although she was old and frail. Irwin was sent to a long-term care facility where he found purpose in teaching other residents rudimentary computer and word-processing skills and how to be a green thumb.

When cognitive decline—related to age and his TBI—interfered with his memory and communication abilities, Irwin struggled to maintain his friendships. His friends eventually dropped out of his life. At age 66, Irwin lost his elderly father to cirrhosis and his mother was diagnosed with Alzheimer's. She had established a special needs trust for Irwin and, unbeknownst to him, pre-paid for a single room in his care facility guaranteeing Irwin could stay there for the rest of his life—regardless of whether his condition could or would improve. He tried to get guardianship rescinded to no avail. Irwin's cognitive functioning deteriorated significantly after suffering two bouts with COVID and his mother's death. For two years of the pandemic, the nursing home canceled all trips out of the facility. Visitors were also disallowed. Irwin's isolation crippled him, and his depression soared.

My work with Irwin was filled with pain and grief. Irwin and I encountered many people and systems that failed to meet his needs, including his guardian. As he once said, "I am stuck in hell. The hell in my body. The hell in my mind. The hell of this nursing facility from which I can never leave. The hell of having a legal guardian who fails to see me. And the hell of being alone in a world where I've been discarded by friends, orphaned by family, and predeceased by my wonderful wife. I keep losing my purpose. Monica, if it weren't for you, I don't think I'd be here anymore."

Irwin trusted me with his life, which stemmed from me faithfully standing by his side, validating his reality and agreeing: "This shit's pretty fucked up!" We'd painfully laugh and grieve together. The simultaneous burden and hope I held for and with Irwin was monumental. I consulted my supervisor frequently to process my emotions and responsibilities.

As Irwin's 70th birthday approached, I decided to send him a planter containing a few different plants. Irwin had a real green thumb, once tended to a thriving garden, and when attending therapy in-person, used to take clippings from the plants in my office. While his clippings thrived, my plants were never as lucky. We had many conversations in which he would light up as he guided me to help my plants thrive. He reminded me to talk to my plants lovingly, kindly, and gently. He'd remind me, "Give them enough sun, but not too much."

We metaphorically and playfully discussed Irwin's thriving indoor garden. I commented, "Irwin, you have cultivated a beautiful, flourishing world within the world that surrounds you. You, along with all you protector parts, nurture your plants and they nurture every part of you. You have a true gift at growing beauty—anywhere!"

With Irwin, I explicitly noticed and celebrated how his life force, spirit, and positive energy were alive and blossoming despite his "imprisonment."

Irwin's deep love, care, and pride in nurturing the growth of his seedlings transcended his physical and cognitive limitations. Plus, Irwin never gave up. I shared how deeply moved I felt by his resilience. I reflected my felt sense experience of Irwin as someone who embodies his internal, eternal light—always seeking and finding ways to better his life. Irwin responded with a realization, "Wow, that part of me has always been with me." He was referring to his essence.

I magnified his realization, "That is incredible! You have always found ways to connect with your truth, your essence."

Irwin proudly responded, "I know. Not everybody can do this."

"Ain't that the truth, Irwin!" I playfully replied. I expanded upon his insight, highlighting how his adaptation of multiplicity preserved connection to his core Self. "Irwin, it seems like you've grown a profound trust in your protectors' ability to guard your truth, soul, and essence no matter what happens."

Irwin said, "That's scary—in a powerful, humbling, and awesome way." Together, we savored, stretched out, saturated, and spread this truth. Even though Irwin couldn't trust most others, he accessed his profound trust in his internal system of protectors—his inside family. They embodied his energy and desire to promote positive change and his need to preserve his truth and desire to live at all costs. This energy and mission accompanied him across his whole life.

Irwin is a "lifer," my supervisor's term for those whose trauma continues throughout their life and stay in treatment until our retirement or death—theirs or ours. We provide our lifers co-created and shared moments of trauma healing and transformation as we loyally accompany them through repeated losses, helplessness, and hopelessness. It's a "both/and" experience as we undo their aloneness but cannot undo their pain.

My experience with Irwin reminds me of the book *The Rabbit Listened* (Doerrfeld, 2018), in which little Taylor needed someone to hold space with him, to just be with, listen to, and witness his distress. Rabbit did just that. 'Being with' was the doing—Taylor once safe, seen, and soothed could act together with rabbit to feel better. Even when it seems like trauma treatment has no end point or objectives can't be met, we can remember that we are like Rabbit, providing a deeply reparative experience for a little while by just being with our client. Infusing our playful spirit sweetens the experience as we add positivity, lightness, and even joy. Even if only experienced momentarily, clients feel and are different, which constitutes healing and change.

Bringing It All Together

Throughout this book, we've learned how to invite the spirit of play to treat traumatized clients of all ages to promote positive change that is healing and transformational. To practice integrating playfulness with trauma work, we merged our academically grounded understanding of trauma and its effects with playful approachability. We defined trauma as including the six UNs: Personally feeling UNsafe, UNseen, and UNconnected/alone and subjectively appraising trauma as UNbearable/intolerable, UNwilled/unwanted, and UNresolved. We detailed trauma's effects as three comprehensive levels of disturbance: dysregulated ANS and affect, disintegrated brain functioning, and disconnection from others and Self.

In direct contrast to trauma, we learned how playfulness brings recursive cycles of positivity, ease and flow, curiosity-seeking, and supports our true essence to emerge. While trauma can happen to anyone, engaging playfully can reach anyone—clients of all ages, developmental, cognitive, and physical levels of functioning—because it's wired into our neural circuitry.

We explored what makes play "playful" and defined how play expresses itself differently across development. Since each therapist and client may prefer and engage different types of play, we need sensitivity to best match and integrate our playful style to that of our client to support attuned relational healing. While the innate developmental and therapeutic powers of play were identified as generally supportive of growth and healing, play's superpowers were specifically shown to hold the mechanisms of action that heal and transform trauma and fueled when juxtaposing them with trauma states. Play truly is an ideally suited partner in trauma treatment.

Similar to bottom-up, trauma-oriented therapies, engaging the spirit of play directly and efficiently accesses trauma memories where they live, encoded in the right hemisphere. The spirit of play also speaks the language of trauma memory fragments—sensorimotor, primary process, symbols and metaphors—but challenges them with laughter and joy. Finally, playfully reframing trauma-related symptoms as allies not enemies in treatment changes the healing mindset for therapist and client alike. Engaging the spirit of play to treat trauma is a no-brainer in a thoroughly grounded-in-science sense.

We explored practical ways to create a playful therapy setting that is a safe, sensorimotor-sensitive space, and how to use it to promote exploration and healing. We as therapists learned how to grow our playful spirit and use its positivity to fuel change, boost the healing powers of the healing relationship, and attune on steroids to catalyze earning security with our clients and transform their experience of trauma.

Finally, we synthesized and integrated theory with practice exploring how to be playful with the elements needed to promote change in trauma treatment. We identified the importance of inviting and making space for change to happen through goodbyes, grieving, and playfulness. We learned how to metaprocess to deepen change and promote transformation. The myriad of playful practices and case vignettes interwoven through this book has brought to life how therapists and clients can feel and know they've co-created a healing and transformational experience of trauma. The related and ultimate readiness to complete a course of treatment for now is when a traumatized client both in and outside of therapy can:

1. Effectively tolerate their ANS and affect dysregulation and return from states of danger/life threat and protection back to safety and connection;
2. Hold both/and thinking and embrace the rich multiplicity of their mind with related sensations, emotions, affects, and thoughts;

3. Juxtapose mutually exclusive expectations and wire in new, wise, and positivity-promoting ones;
4. Establish healthy boundaries of closeness and distance to appropriately satisfy and balance their own and others' needs, while supporting their separate identity;
5. Balance relational give-and-receive dynamics physically, emotionally, cognitively, and spiritually/energetically;
6. Earn secure-enough relationships with themselves and others marked by feeling and being safe, seen, and soothed;
7. Develop cooperation, respect, compassion, and care among their parts of mind and with others. Move through internal and external relational challenges with a sense of integrity, clarity, and fluidity;
8. Create a new trauma narrative and related self-beliefs that enable them to pursue their purpose, meaning, and fulfillment intrapersonally and relationally;
9. Develop new, regulated ANS and affective connection to their once-disturbing memories without forgetting the important lessons they hold;
10. Believe they can bring meaningful change to their life, even if momentarily;
11. Re-connect with or touch into hope and faith in themselves, others, and the future;
12. Possibly re-connect or develop connection with a Higher Power (e.g., spirit, God, the Universe) and the sacred;
13. Demonstrate resiliency in the face of adversity;
14. Be and feel playful: take in and savor positivity, joy, freedom to go with the flow, and vitality affects; and
15. Connect with their deepest sense of their truth, essence, and Self.

A Playful Goodbye Lesson from Guido and Giosuè

To end our exploration of inviting the spirit of play to trauma treatment, I'd like to share a poignant example—this time from the movies. In the 1997 comedy-drama *Life Is Beautiful,* or *La Vita è Bella,* Guido Orefice, a Jewish-Italian bookshop owner uses his deeply creative imagination to shield his son, Giosuè, from the horrors of imprisonment in a Nazi concentration camp. To help him survive, Guido explains to Giosuè that the camp is a complicated game where he can win points for successfully performing tasks his father gives him. Guido says he too will play the game and whoever earns 1,000 points first will win a tank. Giosuè is told he will lose points if he cries, complains he wants his mother, says he's hungry and will earn extra points if he hides from the camp guards. By bringing the spirit of play into the horrors of the death camp, Guido not only saves his son's life but also reduces the impact of the trauma.

Guido and Giosuè offer the ultimate example of how we can co-regulate and deeply care for others with a playful spirit while attuned on steroids. Together, we can move through the worst horrors. For some, if not many, of our deeply traumatized clients, the experience of trauma may never be complete, because life circumstances won't allow it. Yet when we accompany these clients on part of their life's journey, our deeply attuned, relationally engaged playful spirit has the power to evoke experiences of:

- Light—even if just sparks and glimmers—to the darkness;
- Calm and ease to dysregulation;
- Flexibility and openness to rigidity and shut down;
- Integration and flow to splits and blocks;
- Ease and unburdening—even if just for a moment—to pain and heaviness;
- Spontaneity and curiosity to the forced and constrained;
- Vitality—even if short-lived—to the deadness;
- Joy and laughter—even if measured—to grief and loss;
- Connection to melt disconnection and aloneness;
- Possibility and hope to shift the impossible and intolerable; and
- Freedom of spirit and life energy.

In some cases, integrating our playful spirit in trauma treatment can be deeply healing, transformative, and support flourishing. When clients have had and know they have had this profound change experience, their life force and transformance strivings are fortified, helping them continue to grow even when they stop treatment.

Thank you for joining me on this playful journey through healing and transforming trauma. I hope you have fun inviting the spirit of play to your practice, and to your life.

Playfully yours,

Monica

References

Doerrfeld, C. (2018). *The rabbit listened*. New York: Penguin.

Rothschild, B. (2021). *Revolutionizing trauma treatment: Stabilization, safety and nervous system balance*. New York: Norton.

Index

Note: *Italic* page numbers refer to figures.